NURSING PERSPECTIVES AND ISSUES

By Gloria M. Grippando, EdD., RN

NURSING PERSPECTIVES AND ISSUES

*Few will have the greatness to bend history itself,
but each of us can work to change a small portion
of events, and in the total of all those acts will
be written the history of this generation.*

— Robert F. Kennedy

NURSING PERSPECTIVES AND ISSUES

Gloria M. Grippando, EdD., RN
Instructor of Nursing, Broward Community College
Fort Lauderdale, Fla.

DELMAR PUBLISHERS
COPYRIGHT ©1977
BY LITTON EDUCATIONAL PUBLISHING, INC.

10 9 8 7 6 5 4 3 2 1

LIBRARY OF CONGRESS CATALOG CARD NUMBER: 76-14090

Printed in the United States of America
Published Simultaneously in Canada by
Delmar Publishers, A Division of
Van Nostrand Reinhold, Ltd.

Consulting Editor — Betty Dean, EdD, RN.

Project Editor — Pamela Culbert, MS, RN.

ADN Series Editor — Angela Emmi, MS, BSNEd, RN.

DELMAR PUBLISHERS • ALBANY, NEW YORK 12205
A DIVISION OF LITTON EDUCATIONAL PUBLISHING, INC.

FOREWORD

Nursing Perspectives and Issues is one of the texts in the Delmar ADN series. However, because each text was designed to meet specific instructional goals common to all, it is felt the texts will be valuable to students in any nursing program. The underlying themes of the series include: (1) the health-illness continuum, (2) developmental stages, and (3) integrated content. Each text is designed to involve the student in a total learning experience. Student objectives are listed for each chapter to guide learning and promote mastery of the content. Activities and discussion topics are suggested. Multiple-choice, matching, and essay-type questions test student achievement. An extensive glossary and bibliography are provided for each chapter for reference and reenforcement of subject content.

To verify the technical content and evaluate student opinions, portions of each title are classroom tested in AD nursing programs. All of the authors, each of whom holds the minimum of a master's degree in nursing, are actively involved in the instruction of ADN students. The editors are former instructors and hold academic degrees in nursing and/or nursing education.

Nursing Perspectives and Issues was written by Gloria M. Grippando. Dr. Grippando has had considerable experience in nursing education. She is particularly interested in the development of the open curriculum. Her background includes teaching and coordinating programs in practical nurse education as well as diploma and associate degree programs for registered nurses. As consultant for the State of Illinois, she was involved in evaluation and research. Her interest in research is well reflected in the analysis of nursing history and current issues.

Dr. Grippando completed postgraduate studies at Marquette University, Northwestern University, Northern Illinois University, and Carthage College before enrolling at Nova University where she received her doctorate. At the time the text was written, she was on the faculty of the College of Lake County, Illinois.

PREFACE

It is generally accepted that in order to fully understand current trends and to plan for the future, one must be familiar with past events and circumstances. *Nursing Perspectives and Issues* examines current and relevant issues facing all nurses today, within the context of the historical development of organized nursing.

While researching course content materials, it became evident that programs in practical, technical, and professional nursing display many degrees of similarity in presenting history and issues in nursing. Rapid, technological advances and changing roles of the nurse necessitate an updated review of ethical responsibilities, moral and legal rights, health team relationships, job opportunities, educational programs in nursing, proposed legislation, laws, and controversies which directly influence the current practice of nursing and will have significant implications for nursing practice in the future. Students in all types of nursing education programs share the same heritage and future in terms of the history of nursing and health care needs. Because of this commonality, it seemed appropriate that a text be developed which may be used in any type of nursing program.

The author's doctoral dissertation, *The Analysis of a Core Course for Community College Nursing Students* (published by ERIC-U.C.L.A. Clearinghouse for Junior Colleges), centered around this text. The purpose of the study was to test the effectiveness of a core course in a nursing history and trends course for RN and PN students. The proposed course utilized *Nursing Perspectives and Issues* as a common text for the two levels of community college nursing students. Student performance was evaluated by testing chapter review items for content validity and the correlation of test scores. A secondary purpose of the study was to evaluate various aspects of the text, such as the objectives, reading level, illustrations, glossary, content, suggested activities, bibliography, review items, and the need for this book. Evaluation of the text by students and faculty of 24 programs in 18 community colleges indicated that the text effectively met the objectives of each chapter and the needs of students and faculty.

The author admits to being one of the nostalgic nurses who finds identity in remembering the accomplishments of the pioneers in nursing; enjoys being an active participant in the turmoils of the present era; and is enthusiastically attuned to the contributions of future nurses in meeting the health care needs of *all* people!

Other Delmar publications for technical and professional nurses are:

Nursing Concepts and Processes — Carolyn Chambers Clark, EdD, RN.

Drug Interactions — Joseph R. DiPalma, M.D.

Basic Readings in Drug Therapy — Joseph R. DiPalma, M.D. and Morton J. Rodman, PhD.

More Readings in Drug Therapy — Morton J. Rodman, PhD. and Joseph R. DiPalma, M.D.

How to Read an ECG — Herbert H. Butler, M.D.

CONTENTS

EVENTS WHICH INFLUENCED THE NURSING PROFESSION

B.C. 4500	Calendars, writing
4000	
3000	Imhotep, Egyptian physician
2500	Egyptian pyramids
2000	First Babylonian Dynasty
1500	Hammurabi
1000	Moses led Exodus; Mosaic Law
	Homer's *Iliad* and *Odyssey*
	Aesculapian medical cult
500	Hippocrates, Buddha, Confucius
0	Birth of Christ
	Phoebe, deaconess nurses, Roman hospitals
100	Galen
300	Official order of deaconesses established
	Constantinople center of government, art
400	First general hospital in Rome
	Fall of Rome
500	Founding of Hôtel Dieu, Paris
600	Benedictine monastery established
	Saints Cosmos and Damian faith healing
800	Rhazes, the Persian physician
	School of Salerno, medical school
900	Monasticism; early English hospitals
	Avicenna wrote *Canon of Medicine*
1000	Feudalism
1100	First Crusade
1300	Founding of St. Bartholomew's Hospital, London
	Plague, St. Catherine of Siena
1400	Guilds of Surgeons, Barber Surgeons
	Leonardo da Vinci
1500	Columbus sailed to New World
	Ambrose Paré
	Reformation
1600	William Harvey, Father of Modern Medicine
1700	Microscope invented
	Industrial Revolution
	American Revolution
	First American Hospitals
1800	Sairey Gamp, Charles Dickens' portrayal of a nurse
	Kaiserswerth School founded
	Florence Nightingale – St. Thomas' Hospital 1900
A.D. 1900	*American Journal of Nursing* established

SECTION 1
INFLUENCES OF THE PAST

chapter 1
PRIMEVAL MEDICINE AND NURSING

STUDENT OBJECTIVES

- Identify the contributions of ancient civilizations to the development of medicine and nursing.

- Explain the development of medicine from witchcraft to the scientific works of Hippocrates.

- Name two symbols currently in use which have their roots in ancient mythology.

Nursing is believed to have originated with the primitive mother who nursed the ill members of her family unit. The term *nurse* stems from the Latin word, *nutrix*, to nourish. It is assumed that men and women were ministering to the needs of their children and the sick from the beginning of civilization. However, very little has been written about nursing as a unique function in ancient times. There are a few brief accounts of men and women involved in activities which can now be identified with modern nursing practice. It is not likely that organized nursing existed before the birth of the Christian church. It is possible, through a study of ancient health care practices, to see the development of medical science and how it indirectly influenced the growth and development of nursing.

Primitive man lived in cave dwellings where small groups congregated together for mutual protection and survival. Knowledge was gained through life experiences and by observations of lower animal forms. The medicinal values of plants, the use of water submersion of afflicted limbs, and the application of heat as therapy, were learned either accidentally or after experimentation.

Individuals who became particularly skilled with these basic remedies were called medicine men. Illness was believed to be caused by evil spirits and the medicine man was called upon to practice black magic to drive out the evil from the afflicted person, figure 1-1. As the cure of disease developed into a ritualistic religious ceremony, medicine men were replaced by priest physicians.

BABYLONIAN MEDICINE

The rules governing medical practice in Babylonia were laid down in the Code of Hammurabi, which is the oldest known book of its kind. Hammurabi, the sixth king of the Babylonian Empire, developed this comprehensive Code of Law around 2100 B.C. It is still preserved today.

Medical practice was limited mainly to the use of magic or *sorcery* (the use of power derived from evil spirits) to drive out the evil spirits associated with ill health. The doctor was paid if the patient recovered and was punished if the patient was not cured or died. Simple surgical procedures and *bloodletting* (removal of blood from the body) were skillfully performed. Abraham, a native of Babylonia, performed circumcisions. Public health regulations were very strict.

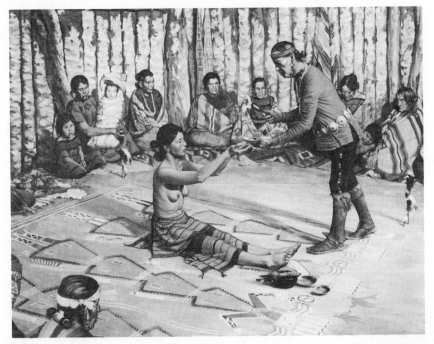

Fig. 1-1 The medicine man performing rituals to cure a sick woman. (Courtesy Parke, Davis and Company, ©1957)

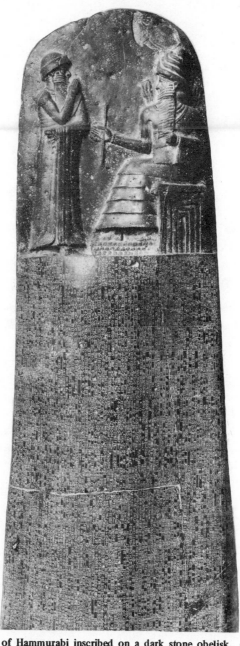

Fig. 1-2 The code of Hammurabi inscribed on a dark stone obelisk. (Photograph from the Mansell Collection, London)

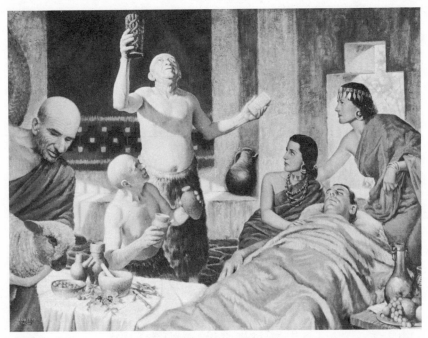

Fig. 1-3   Patient being treated by Babylonian pharmacists. (Courtesy Parke, Davis and Company, ©1951)

It was believed that insects spread disease, and the measures advocated to prevent the spread of disease were the earliest forms of preventive medicine. Babylonians had a practical knowledge of many drugs and herbs including laudanum, an opiate, figure 1-3.

The Babylonian nurse was no doubt a domestic servant or slave and may have been either male or female. There are accounts of *wet nurses* (female servants who breast-fed the infants of the master's household) who often had great affection for their charges.

EGYPTIAN MEDICINE

Both the Babylonians and Egyptians feared evil spirits as a cause of illness. Sorcery and magic were acceptable practices. Health and disease were related to gods who were identified with the sun and stars. Healing was performed by magician-physicians who practiced wizardry and sorcery.

Archeological studies also indicate that the Egyptians practiced medicine thousands of years before Christ. Homer, the Greek poet, referred to the Egyptians as the best doctors of that era. Physicians were skilled in the art of diagno-

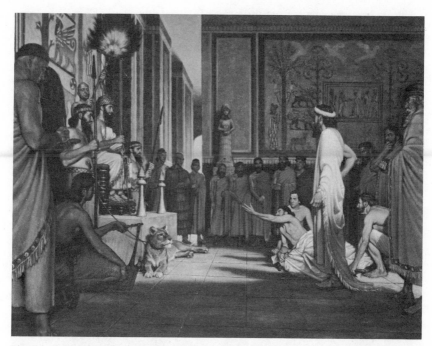

Fig. 1-4 Hammurabi, the Babylonian king, who developed the code which regulated medical practice. (Courtesy Parke, Davis and Company, ©1957)

sis, and prescribed medications in the form of pills and suppositories similar to those in use today. The enema was one of the most frequently used procedures. The treatment of bone fractures was quite sophisticated, as evidenced by mummified remains. Ancient Egyptians had extensive knowledge of anatomy, pharmacy and pathology. Through the mummification ceremony the knowledge of anatomy, antiseptics, dissection and the art of bandaging advanced. Embalming was a major function of the Egyptian physician and the bodies were so well preserved that the mummified bodies still exist today. Many of the mummies have shown evidence that ancient Egyptians suffered from diseases seen today. There is evidence that medical specialties existed and Herodotus, a Greek historian, even described Egypt as being overrun with medical specialists. The pharaohs surrounded themselves with specialists to care for the various parts of the body.

Physicians in ancient Egypt did not practice obstetrics but left this field entirely to midwives. Most births were attended to by friends or attendants serving as nurses. Wet nurses were engaged on contract to breast-feed the infants for six-month periods.

Since Egypt's doctors were priest-physicians, medical practice took place mainly in the temples. The priests recorded their medical lore on rolls of *papyrus,* a delicate substance made from the stems of the papyrus plant. These rolls listed disease classification, description and prescriptions. The most referred to is *Ebers' Papyrus* purchased in 1873 by Dr. Georg Ebers of Germany, figure 1-5. Another papyrus was discovered by Edwin Smith in 1862 which is referred to as the first surgical textbook. Only a few of the books relating to medical practice have been preserved due to the perishable nature of the paper used.

Imhotep, who lived about 3000 B.C., was the greatest physician of ancient Egypt. He did much to improve the care of the sick and was also a great architect and statesman. After his death he was declared a god of medicine and a temple was built for his worship.

HEBREW MEDICINE

Moses, raised as the son of a pharaoh's daughter, practiced preventive medicine in Israel. He advocated food habits, personal hygiene, and appointed public health officials for the detection, prevention and isolation of contagious diseases. Because of his sophisticated education. Moses did not approve of the use of magic in the treatment of disease.

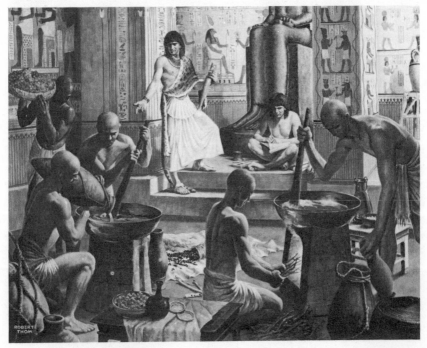

Fig. 1-5 **Days of the Papyrus Ebers.** (Courtesy Parke, Davis and Company, ©1951)

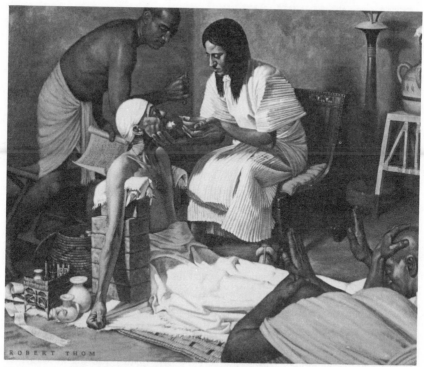

Fig. 1-6 A skilled Egyptian physician. (Courtesy Parke, Davis and Company © 1957)

According to legend, Hebrew medicine began with King Solomon who wrote the *Book of Remedies*. Hebrew physicians, called *rofeh* which means to ease, appeared some 300 years after the death of Moses. They were required to be licensed and usually practiced in the temple. The *Talmud* contains medical concepts and laws which identify the importance placed on personal hygiene. Israelites, as the Egyptians before them, were advocates of cleanliness. They washed hands and utensils, boiled or filtered water, inspected meat carefully for spoilage and even possessed primitive flush-type toilets. Hebrew law forbade spitting and tattooing. Religious ceremonies included purification rites such as bathing and isolation, which were related to hygiene and sanitation.

The ancient Jews believed all men should be entitled to medical care regardless of social status. They provided housing for travelers and possibly even medical care in shelters which were called *xenodochia*.

In the twenty-fourth chapter of Genesis, Rebekah leaves her home to marry Isaac. Deborah, referred to as a nurse, accompanied Rebekah. She was the first nurse to be recorded in history.

AESCULAPIAN MEDICINE IN GREECE

In Greek mythology, Apollo's son, Aesculapius, was the God of Healing. He was usually depicted holding a staff entwined with serpents of wisdom. The emblem, called the caduceus, is today the symbol of the medical profession, figure 1-7.   Aesculapius had two daughters, Hygeia, Goddess of Health, and Panacea, the Restorer of Health, figure 1-8.   The ancient Greeks worshipped Aesculapius and called upon his healing powers in temples erected in his honor. As temples were holy places, where no one was permitted to be born or die, special buildings near the temples were built for worship by the ill and injured. These temples and *sanatoria* (establishments that provide therapy, diet, and exercise programs) were erected in lovely settings, where fresh water, fresh air, sunshine and wholesome food were available.   While enjoying such a setting, cure was sought through complicated rituals.   Music and poetry played a major role in these ceremonies.   Efforts were made to develop the proper mental attitude through the entertainment in theaters, gymnasiums or concert halls.   The poor flocked to the temple where Aesculapius would be satisfied with meager offerings.   The cures were considered miraculous, but what was thought to be a cure was often merely temporary relief brought about by hysteria, as writings show little possibility of physiological changes or permanent cures.   Archeologists have excavated tablets written in the fourth century B.C. entitled "Cures of Apollo and Aesculapius" with some seventy case histories giving accounts of patients, their diseases and cures.

The priests of the Aesculapian temples initially used rituals and magic as well as prayer and sacrifice to cure the ill.   Gradually, these priests began to develop some skill in caring for the infirm worshippers.   In the *Iliad*, Homer inferred that wounds were treated with surgery and drugs.   Surgical instruments and

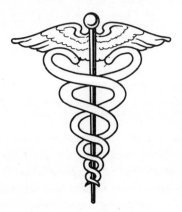

Fig. 1-7 The Caduceus

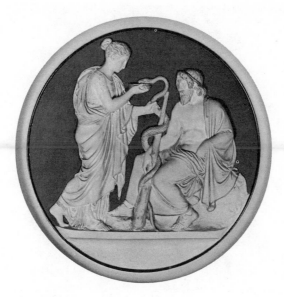

Fig. 1-8 Aesculapius, the God of Healing and his daughter, Hygeia, the Goddess of Health (Courtesy of Josephine A. Dolan)

sutures were not mentioned. Surgery probably consisted of removing foreign bodies from the wounds, application of a topical drug such as powder from a plant, and perhaps some bandaging. Drugs may have been given internally although the epic does not indicate this in early Greece. Knowledge of anatomy centered on large organs, bones and muscles. Eventually, these Aesculapian priests organized themselves as *Asclepiads* and established a crude medical school about the year 800 B.C. With the organization of the Aesculapian medical cult, more scientific medical knowledge developed although religious healing in the temples was prevalent through Greek civilization, figure 1-9, page 10. The priests developed and accumulated empirical knowledge through observation.

According to mythology, Horus, an Egyptian sun god, lost his sight after being attacked by an evil demon. Troth, the God of Health, restored the eye and power of vision. ℞ became the symbol of the eye of Horus and is still written on every prescription today, figure 1-10, page 11.

Hippocrates

In 460 B.C. one of the most remembered Greeks, Hippocrates, was born to one of the Asclepiads, a priest-physician. Brought up in a medical school atmosphere, he apparently gained sufficient knowledge to identify similar symptoms among the ill and subsequently determined these had a common cause. Actually

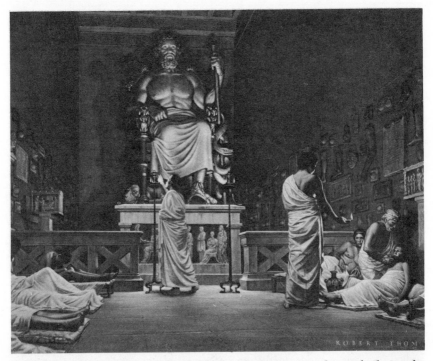

Fig. 1-9 Aesculapian priests care for the sick who have come to seek cures in the temples of Aesculapius. (Courtesy Parke, Davis and Company, © 1957)

very little is known about him personally except that he was a follower of the Aesculapius Cult. He was a well-known physician who taught medicine to students; they, in turn, paid him a tuition fee.

Hippocrates based his work on four major premises. First, he developed the principle that the physician was to aid the natural forces of the body, and that illness was not caused by sin. Secondly, Hippocrates and his followers compiled case histories which became part of the *Corpus Hippocraticum*. For centuries these were considered to be total medical knowledge. The concept of total patient care, as practiced by the twentieth century nurse, was advocated by Hippocrates when he stated that to treat a diseased eye, it was necessary to treat the entire body. Thirdly, through teaching he prepared physicians of outstanding ability who carried on the practice of medicine and surgery, always acclaiming him as their authority. Fourthly, his teaching emphasized empathy and a code of ethics. He required his students to take an oath; today, the Hippocratic Oath is taken by physicians upon completion of their medical education, figure 1-12, page 12. Hippocrates made such significant contributions to the field of medicine that he has been given the title, Father of Scientific Medicine.

ROGER A. SMITH, M.D.   JAMES L. BRYAN, M.D.
                        785 WARREN AVENUE
                      DELMAR, NEW YORK 12054
OFFICE HOURS: TELEPHONE:
BY APPOINTMENT   439-3993

NAME . . . . AGE . . . .

ADDRESS. . . . . DATE . . . .

℞

☐ LABEL

REFIL UT DICT.
1 ☐ 2 ☐ 3 ☐ 4 ☐ TIMES
P.R.N. ☐   NON REP. ☐
REFILLED . . . .

REG. NO. . . . . M.D.

Fig. 1-10 ℞ the symbol for the eye of Horus, is found on all prescription forms.

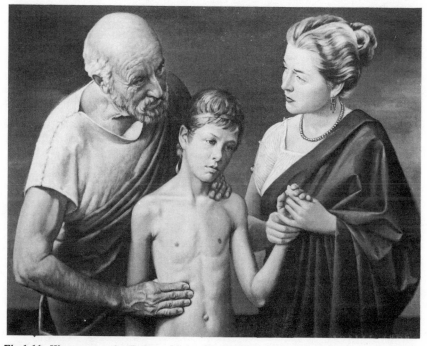

Fig 1-11 **Hippocrates, the Father of Scientific Medicine.** (Courtesy Parke, Davis and Company, © 1958)

I swear by Apollo Physician, by Asclepius, by Health, by Panacea and by all the gods and goddesses, making them my witnesses, that I will carry out, according to my ability and judgement, this oath and this indenture. To hold my teacher in this art equal to my own parents; to make him partner in my livelihood; when he is in need of money to share mine with him; to consider his family as my own brothers, and to teach them this art, if they want to learn it, without fee or indenture; to impart precept, oral instruction, and all other instruction to my own sons, the sons of my teacher, and to indentured pupils who have taken the physician's oath, but to nobody else. I will use treatment to help the sick according to my ability and judgement, but never with a view to injury and wrongdoing. Neither will I administer a poison to anybody when asked to do so, nor will I suggest such a course. Similarly I will not give a woman a pessary to cause abortion. But I will keep pure and holy both my life and my art. I will not use the knife, not even, verily, on sufferers from stone, but I will give place to such as are craftsmen therein. Into whatsoever houses I enter, I will enter to help the sick, and I will abstain from all intentional wrongdoing and harm, especially from abusing the bodies of man or woman, bond or free. And as whatsoever I shall see or hear in the course of my profession as well as outside my profession in my intercourse with men, if it be what should not be published abroad, I will never divulge, holding such things to be holy secrets. Now if I carry out this oath, and break it not, may I gain forever reputation among all men for my life and for my art, but if I transgress it and forswear myself, may the opposite befall me.

Fig. 1-12 The Hippocratic Oath

Early Greek Physicians and Health Care

Most Greek physicians traveled from city to city, selling their services much like craftsmen and artists. Usually the physician and his assistants set up temporary offices in their living quarters. Patients requiring more than outpatient care remained in the physician's home where they were nursed by the assistants and slaves. The wealthy patients called the physician to their private homes.

In time, communities began to realize the advantages of having a physician on a permanent basis. Special taxes were raised and the physician was offered a salary to induce him to remain in the community. The first record of a salaried physician was at the end of the sixth century.

Physicians of the medical schools worked independently of the priest-physicians. The Hippocratic physician was interested in prognosis and treatment. Little emphasis was placed upon diagnosis because of the limited knowledge at that time and the importance placed upon the health of the whole body instead of an afflicted part of the body. Vomiting was induced and enemas were given. Physical fitness through proper diet and gymnastics was stressed. In addition to the bathing and diet regimen, hypnosis was also often used. The physician assisted with difficult or abnormal childbirth although elderly mothers who served as midwives provided most of the obstetrical care. Asepsis was not understood but the early physicians recognized an advantage to treating wounds with boiled clear water or wine. Surgical procedures were performed on outer surfaces of the body such as the eye, nose, mouth and rectum. Fractures and dislocations were exceptionally well treated.

The *Corpus Hippocraticum* written by many authors in the fifth or fourth centuries B.C. reveals the medical knowledge concerning symptomatology, dietetics, pharmacology and surgery. Unfortunately, medical literature was not written before the fifth century B.C. in Greece, probably because the physicians were craftsmen and transmitted knowledge by actual practice and oral instruction.

THE ROMAN EMPIRE

The Greek Hellenistic monarchy ended about 30 B.C., when Roman domination began. About the year 146 B.C., Greece was controlled by Rome. Physicians of the Hippocratic school became slaves of the Romans, and their knowledge of medical practice filtered throughout Rome. Before this time, Rome recognized hygiene and sanitation as the foundation of good health. Quite possibly public health had its beginning here. Of great importance was the building of aqueducts, sewerage systems, and bath houses to promote good health.

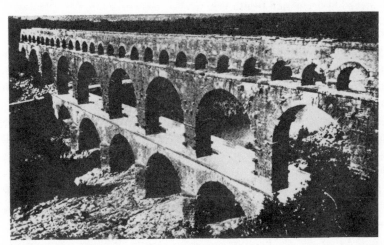

Fig. 1-13 A well-preserved Roman aqueduct. (Reprinted from Ralph H. Major, *A History of Medicine,* Volume I, 1954. Courtesy of Charles C. Thomas, Springfield, Illinois.)

The Romans frequently engaged in war and developed military medicine. First aid was given on the battlefield and a field-ambulance service was provided. The hospital system of Rome was quite successful. Excavations at Pompeii indicate the physician's home may have been used as an infirmary, similar to the present day nursing home. Although the numbers of slaves were vast there was no provision for them when they fell ill. A temple to Aesculapius was erected on an island which became a refuge for the sick poor. The Emperor decreed that if the slaves recovered, they were to be set free.

Roman medicine had a high degree of specialization. Urology, gynecology, and eye, ear, nose and throat specialists prevailed. Roman physicians performed many surgical procedures including plastic surgery; however, their knowledge of drugs was considered to be inadequate. One of the greatest contributions of the Romans was the translation of Greek medical terminology into Latin. Latin terms have been used in medicine ever since.

Roman women, unlike the Greeks, were independent and were involved in many activities and functions outside of the home. Some women cared for the ill members of their households, while others delegated these duties to Greek slaves. Women were allowed to practice medicine. Wet nurses were employed and were expected to be kind, of sound mind, clean, and healthy.

During the third century B.C. Greek physicians began drifting into Rome where Greek medicine was at first opposed but later triumphant. Asclepiades, a Greek physician from Asia Minor, born in 124 B.C., established Greek medicine in Rome. His theory was atomistic; that is, disease was caused by a disturbance of the movement of atoms through the pores of the body. His treatment consisted primarily of diet, baths, and gymnastics. Tracheotomies were frequently performed for upper respiratory distress.

Asclepiades paved the way for another medical sect called the Methodists founded about 50 B.C. The Methodist theory of disease was based on excessive contraction or relaxation of the pores of the body. Treatment was directed toward overcoming excessive contractions and relaxation. One of the most famous gynecologists and obstetricians, Soranus, was a member of the Methodist School and author of many medical books. The Pneumatists, another sect, developed very accurate clinical descriptions of diabetes, tetanus, diphtheria and leprosy.

Celsus was a Roman gentleman who recorded much of the information available on medical practice. Celsus preserved information on surgical use of ligatures, cataract surgery and principles of dermatology. Celsus described fractures and their treatment, and he advocated exercises after the fractures healed, which today are part of rehabilitation therapy.

The greatest physician after Hippocrates was Galen, who was born around 130 A.D. in Asia Minor. After nine years of medical study, he became physician to the gladiators. He gained fame in Rome as a lecturer and medical practitioner.

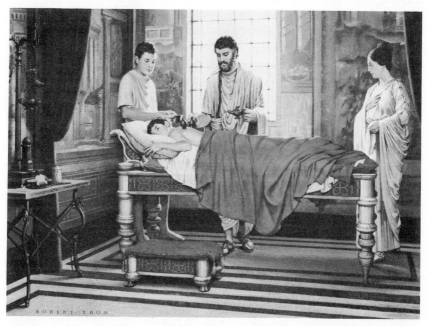

Fig. 1-14 Galen, the remarkable Roman physician. (Courtesy Parke, Davis and Company, ©1958)

He excelled in anatomy and physiology and wrote volumes on scientific medicine. Galen became a good surgeon as a result of the many dissections he performed while studying anatomy and physiology. He firmly believed in physical therapy and in the prevention of disease. Through his volumes of writings, Galen contributed vastly to medical knowledge and is considered by many to be one of the most remarkable of all physicians.

INDIAN MEDICINE

The first civilization in India flourished between 2500 B.C. and 1500 B.C. Excavated remains indicate that there were large cities and a highly developed culture. Elaborate municipal drainage systems existed, evidence that these early Indians had an understanding of the importance of sanitation. Unfortunately the writings left by this civilization cannot be understood because the script has yet to be deciphered. After 1500 B.C. came the Vedic Age, which produced the classical Indian civilization and Hinduism. In the sixth century B.C., Indian life was greatly influenced by the life and teachings of Buddha. Both cultures have made remarkable contributions to medicine.

Hinduism

Hinduism, sometimes referred to as the mother of all religions, greatly influenced the lives of the people of India. Ancient priests preserved the teachings of Hinduism in two collections of sacred books numbering approximately one hundred. These are known as the *Vedas* and the *Upanishads* and are written in Sanskrit language. In the Vedas, man is pictured as free from disease at birth. In the book known as the *Veda of Longevity,* hygiene and prevention of sickness is stressed and smallpox inoculations, materia medica, psychiatry, medical, surgical and pediatric practice are mentioned.

The Hindus practiced a team concept which included the physician, nurse, and patient. Duties, qualifications, and attributes of the team members are identified in the *Charaka-Samhita.* Records indicate that instruments such as the tissue forceps, scissors and catheters were used for surgical procedures, including plastic surgery. Drugs and diet were prescribed in addition to surgical intervention. However, diseases believed to be incurable (such as tuberculosis and diabetes) were not treated because of their poor prognosis.

Buddhism

About 500 B.C., Gautama, who was later known as *Buddha,* which means the *Enlightened One,* was born in India. As a young monk, while meditating, he received enlightenment concerning the meaning of life and aspired to bring contentment to all men. Buddha founded many religious communities which later became a source of help to King Asoka, who reigned at that time. As a follower of Buddhism in 250 B.C., King Asoka founded buildings which today can be compared to hotels and hospitals. Nurses, always male, functioned as does the practical nurse or orderly of today.

By 1 A.D., India had developed a system similar to current licensing practice in that permission of the governing party was required to practice medicine; in this case, the king's permission was necessary. Prevention of disease was of prime importance and hygienic procedures were considered a religious duty. The priest-physician was the medical practitioner and, therefore, religious ceremony and prayer were a prelude to treatment. Women held a high position in India at this time. Although they centered their activities around managing the home, it is assumed that they functioned as nurses when members of the family became ill.

CHINESE MEDICINE

About 500 B.C. Confucius, a famous Chinese philosopher, was born during a politically corrupt and oppressed period. He revived the patriarchal rule, and, based on the foundation of family units, Confucius set out to build an empire ensuring a good life for all. Confucius advocated the *Golden Rule* of treating others as you would like to be treated.

Medical knowledge in early China included dissection techniques, studies of the circulatory system, methods of physical diagnosis, massage, the therapeutic use of baths, and the significance of pulse rates. Emperor Shen Nung originated the *acupuncture technique* (the insertion of needles into the body to cure illness). Surgery was poorly developed, possibly due to the belief that mutilation of the body would remain in evidence in the life after death.

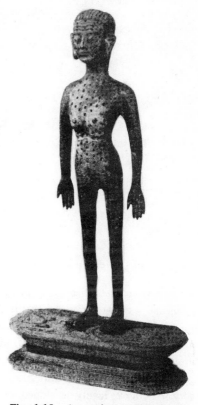

Fig. 1-15   An ancient model showing sites for acupuncture. (Reprinted from Ralph H. Major, *A History of Medicine,* Volume I, 1954. Courtesy of Charles C. Thomas, Springfield, Illinois.)

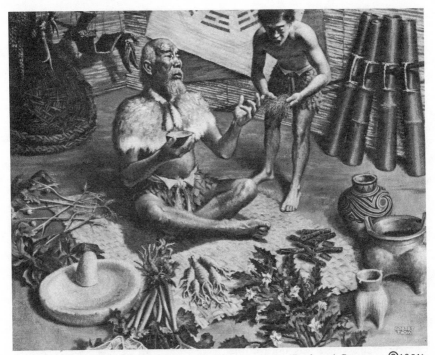

Fig. 1-16 The ancient Chinese pharmacist. (Courtesy Parke, Davis and Company, ©1951)

Physicians were held in high esteem, often at the level of the gods. The Chinese physician based diagnosis on some 200 types of pulses and observation. Very little value was placed upon the patient's medical history. Many drugs used in ancient China are still in use today such as iodine, liver preparations, and opiates.

MEDICINE OF CENTRAL AND SOUTH AMERICA

As was customary in other primitive cultures, medicine men practiced religious and medical duties. Later, priests performed these functions also. Excavations of skulls in Peru provide evidence of *trephine openings* (small circular holes made in the skull with a saw) made on living humans as a surgical procedure, figure 1-17. Archeologists have uncovered evidence that amputations, bone surgery, tumor removal and cauterizations were performed. It is believed that surgery in Peru was highly developed. Ancient pottery depicts the use of prostheses.

The ancient civilizations of Central and South America practiced praiseworthy medicine according to reports of the Spanish conquerors who described their travels to the king of Spain. Medicine of the Aztecs in Mexico was centered around religion. The Aztecs were particularly knowledgeable about narcotics

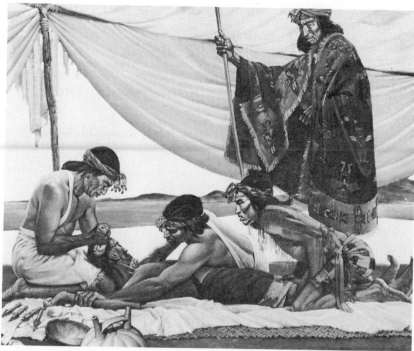

Fig. 1-17 Trephining in ancient Peru. (Courtesy Parke, Davis and Company, © 1957)

and other plants of medicinal value. Surgery was practiced with sutures made out of hair. Fumigation and bloodletting were common procedures. Baths and diet were considered important. It is believed that women were among the medical specialists although no particular reference is made to women as nurses.

SUMMARY

In early civilizations, religious beliefs and myths were the foundations of medical practice. The responsibility for curing and treating the sick and injured was given to the religious leaders. As witch doctors and priests became more adept, their intervention began to be based upon the results of experimentation and observation. With development of empirical knowledge, health care was delegated to priest-physicians and eventually to the secular physician, who was trained in the techniques of his profession. This latter development occurred primarily in the Greek and Roman civilizations. Many civilizations made significant contributions in the development of special procedures, the biological sciences, diagnostic measures, classification of diseases, and recording of observations which transformed medicine from magic into a science.

SUGGESTED ACTIVITIES

- Visit a museum of natural history and examine items, such as primitive surgical instruments, which might be related to ancient medical practice.

- Through a panel discussion in class, present the spiritual and cultural influences of ancient civilizations on the development of medical and nursing professions.

- Plan a bulletin board display to depict scenes of ancient medicine and early nursing care.

- Draw a sketch of the early hospital setting and compare it with modern architecture of medical facilities.

REVIEW

A.   Multiple Choice. Select the best answer.

1. The introduction of thin needles into the skin, which originated in China, is called
    - a. trephination.
    - b. dissection.
    - c. amputation.
    - d. acupuncture.

2. The Babylonian king who wrote a code governing medical practice around 2100 B.C. was
    - a. Imhotep.
    - b. Hammurabi.
    - c. Herodotus.
    - d. Gautama.

3. The Greek god of healing was
    - a. Hippocrates.
    - b. Apollo.
    - c. Panacea.
    - d. Aesculapius.

4. An Egyptian priest who was so outstanding as a physician that he was worshipped as a god was
    - a. Imhotep.
    - b. Moses.
    - c. Horus.
    - d. Hammurabi.

5. The collection of notes and writings of case histories of Greek patients credited to Hippocrates is called
    - a. Ebers' Papyrus.
    - b. Corpus Hippocraticum.
    - c. The Book of Remedies.
    - d. The Vedas.

6. The earliest forms of medical practice were
    - a. acupunctures.
    - b. health codes.
    - c. witchcraft, sorcery and magic.
    - d. mummification.

7. Medical terminology is written in
   a. Greek.
   b. Latin.
   c. symbols.
   d. hieroglyphics.

8. The first mention of a team approach to health care was in
   a. India.
   b. Greece.
   c. Rome.
   d. China.

9. The first nurse in recorded history was
   a. Hygeia.
   b. a midwife.
   c. Panacea.
   d. Deborah.

10. The only civilization which allowed women in medical practice was
    a. Greek.
    b. Roman.
    c. Palestinian.
    d. Egyptian.

B. Match the significant contributions in Column II with the country or civilization listed in Column I.

Column I	Column II
1. Aztec	a. medications in pill form
2. Palestine	b. preventive medicine
3. China	c. the first medical school
4. Greece	d. sewage systems
5. Egypt	e. acupuncture
6. India	f. refined surgical instruments
7. Roman	g. use of narcotics

C. Briefly answer the following questions.

1. What were the four major premises of Hippocrates?

2. Discuss the mummification process of Egypt and its contribution to medical science.

3. Name two symbols which were used in early times and are still in use today.

chapter 2
THE INFLUENCE
OF CHRISTIANITY

STUDENT OBJECTIVES

- Identify the contributions of men and women to nursing which were made possible by the influence of the Christian church.

- Explain how the lack of social services might have contributed to the spread of disease.

- Explain how the progress of medical science was affected by the early Christian church.

At a time when the world was at its wealthiest, Jesus Christ was born in Bethlehem, a town of Palestine. In spite of affluence and riches, this was not a happy era. Pagan ideals which prevailed placed little value on human life. The teaching and works of Christ had a profound effect upon nursing and medicine, figure 2-1. Although His work was confined to Palestine, followers of His teachings spread the philosophy of Christianity throughout the entire world. Men and women committed to both the love of the Church and to the poor and infirm, dedicated their lives to providing nursing care to the ill. Many basic nursing services were rendered with empathy and understanding. Rome began to decline about 325 A.D. and Christianity became the official religion of Rome.

EARLY CHRISTIAN ORDERS OF WOMEN

At the ecumenical congress of the bishops of the Church in 325 A.D., an official order of deaconesses was established. About the sixth century they became orders of sisters, many of which are still in existence today. The deacon-

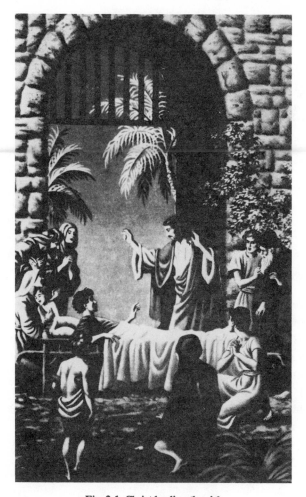

Fig. 2-1 Christ healing the sick

esses of the early Church followed the example of Jesus Christ by showing love of mankind through their works of charity and mercy. They were meek and humble while feeding the hungry, giving drink to the thirsty, providing shelter to the homeless, and caring for the sick and needy. The deaconesses functioned as visiting nurses and social workers and were women of high social status, appointed by the bishops of the Church. By becoming deaconesses, women who were widows or virgins were able to find a respectable place in society by performing duties considered meaningful. One of the most acclaimed deaconesses was Phoebe who lived about 55 A.D., figure 2-2, page 24. She is remembered as the first visiting nurse and the first deaconess. Phoebe was

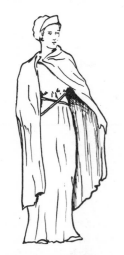

Fig. 2-2   Phoebe, the first visiting nurse

introduced to the Christian world by St. Paul and her duties were to minister to the sick. Christian men functioned as deacons performing the same nursing functions as the women although each ministered to members of their own sex.

EARLY CHRISTIAN HOSPITALS

Although the deaconesses visited the sick and administered to them in their homes, a need existed for hospital-type institutions. Often, the bishops provided a place of shelter and refuge by opening their own homes to the sick and weary. Even though these early hospitals provided shelter, food and nursing care, little or no medical care was available. Hygienic conditions were poor. Ill mothers were often forced to bring their well children with them and expose them to the illnesses of others. Social services were not provided nor were doctors available in these early Christian hospitals.

Around 330 A.D. a large hospital was founded by Emperor Constantine the Great, who was influential in calling together the ecumenical congress for the First Council of Nicea in 325 A.D. It was decreed by the Council that each attending bishop would build a hospital in every city where a cathedral had been erected; its purpose was to meet the needs of the Christians and promote the propagation of the faith.

St. Basil of Athens built the largest hospital in Asia Minor about 370 A.D. It was a huge complex of buildings housing lepers, children, the aged, and possibly others in separate dwellings. Known as the Basilias, it resembled the large hospital of today.

EARLY NURSING LEADERS

Christians made pilgrimages to the Holy Land seeking miraculous cures. Many of them required food and lodging before reaching their destination and found refuge shelters provided along the way. This inn-type abode was known as a *hospice.* In the middle of the fourth century some women of Roman nobility converted their spacious homes into hospices or hospitals. Marcella, a Roman matron of great wealth, who had been widowed at an early age, turned to Christianity for solace. Marcella was interested in the care of the sick and works of charity. She made her home into a convent and devoted her life to the many women who followed her. Because of her devoted leadership she became known as the Mother of Nuns.

The first general hospital established in Rome about 380 A.D. was built by one of Rome's most beautiful and prestigious women, Fabiola. Fabiola was dissatisfied with her two unsuccessful attempts at marriage and turned to Christianity. In atonement for her past, she dedicated her life to the care of the sick.

Paula, considered the most learned woman of this period, entered Marcella's convent and became a close friend of Fabiola. She and one of her daughters established many hospices for the pilgrims enroute to Palestine. They erected several hospitals and tended to the basic nursing needs of the patients.

EARLY CHRISTIAN MEDICINE

The physicians of the Christian church practiced faith healing and overlooked the value of the administration of drugs and other elements of scientific medicine. All people were treated equally regardless of race or social status. The concept of brotherly love prevailed. Faith in Christ as the supreme healer, and hope for cure from illness through the intercession of saints, formed the nucleus of Christian medicine.

One of the Apostles of Christ known as St. Luke, the beloved physician, describes in detail many accounts of medical cures wrought by Christ and His disciples. Terminology used by St. Luke in his Gospel indicates his knowledge of Hippocratic medicine. From his writings it can be concluded that St. Luke possessed the attributes of a fine physician. The parable of the Good Samaritan, as recorded in the Gospel of St. Luke, clearly indicates knowledge of the administration of first aid treatment

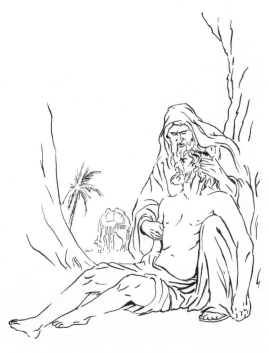

Fig. 2-3 The parable of the Good Samaritan demonstrates concern for fellowmen and the use of first aid.

as well as the value of pouring wine, with its alcohol content, over wounds to prevent infection.

After Constantinople became the capital of the Byzantine Empire about 476 A.D., the church fathers carried on the medical traditions of the Greeks before them. Faith healing prevailed and numerous accounts of healing, attributed to intercession by saints, have been recorded. According to legend, Saints Cosmas and Damian, who were brothers, had a church in Rome erected to them; accounts of faith healing have been depicted in famous paintings of the Renaissance Period. At the time of their martyrdom, 683 A.D., another martyr named Sebastian was being invoked to cure the plague victims in Rome.

Many other saints suffered varied tortures and were martyred by nonChristians for their faith. Christians associated afflicted parts of their bodies to specific saints who suffered similarly in their death tortures. Hence, they became the patron saint of headaches, backaches, intestinal disorders, and nursing mothers to name a few. Many modern day Christians continue to invoke medical cures from the saints.

MONASTIC MEDICINE AND NURSING

The Roman Empire ended in 476 A.D. and Europe was divided into many kingdoms. Christians retreated into convents and monasteries. Several religious

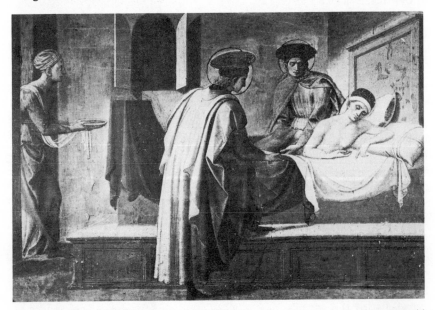

Fig. 2-4 Miracle of Saints Cosmas and Damian. (Reprinted by permission of Photographie Giraudon, Paris)

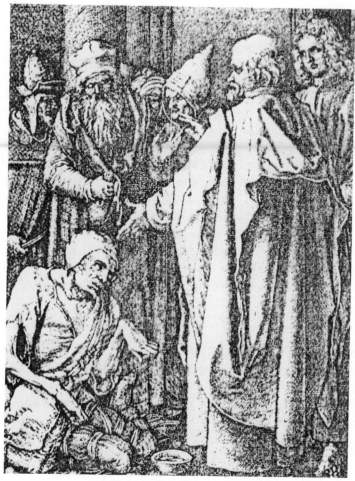

Fig. 2-5 St. Peter heals the lame.
Copy of the engraving by Albrecht Dürer. (Courtesy of Cornell
University Press)

orders included care of the sick among their duties. Prior to the coming of
Christianity to the world, men were paganistic and life had little or no real meaning. Christianity brought a reverence for life and was responsible for saving
many people from total destruction.

Medicine as practiced by monks had little scientific basis. Theory and scientific data related to anatomy, physiology and pharmacology were no longer the
major focus. More emphasis was placed on the comfort and care of the sick, and
the recitation of prayers for saintly intervention. Nursing duties were performed
by monks and nuns. Some of the monks attempted to provide visiting nurse

services to the ill in the towns but the Church was fearful that their spiritual obligations might be neglected. The nursing duties were therefore confined to infirmaries and clinic settings within the monastery walls.

Benedict founded a monastic colony about 529 A.D. between Rome and Naples from whence came the Benedictine Rule still followed today. One of the functions of the monks was to copy the manuscripts of past physicians. Physicians of this era preferred to study these writings and base their practice on past knowledge instead of making new scientific discoveries or developing new techniques in the treatment of the ill. A major function of the Benedictine monks was growing herbs, which were rich in medicinal value.

Although the Church essentially opposed the writings of Galen and Hippocrates, the basic concepts of Roman and Greek medicine were preserved in the monastic libraries. Aside from St. Benedict, Cassiodorus was very influential in preserving medical works. After serving as a Roman statesman, he founded a monastery and donated his vast collection of Hippocratic books and classical writings to it. Cassiodorus was the first to advocate the use of reference to medical illustrations to clarify writings difficult to understand.

SUMMARY

In some ways, early Christians followed the practices of the Aesculapians. Temples of Aesculapius were transformed into churches of Christ. Medical practice was based on a faith healing concept. The Christian faith offered new hope and meaning to a human race tired of paganism. Medical practice was concerned with prayer and faith rather than the existing scientific theories of medicinal knowledge. Christianity, however, gave women who were not married a role to fulfill that was dignified and meaningful. These women were the roots of organized nursing.

SUGGESTED ACTIVITIES

- Locate passages in the New Testament which relate various accounts of faith healing. Make a list of the kinds of afflictions mentioned.

- Start a notebook in which the contributions of men to nursing will be entered, beginning with this unit. Make entries as you progress through the remaining units.

- Make a list of attributes desirable in a nurse practicing today. On a separate sheet of paper list the attributes of the early Christians who cared for the sick. Compare the two lists and note similarities and dissimilarities.

REVIEW

A.   Multiple Choice. Select the best answer.

1.   The first to advocate the use of illustrations to clarify difficult medical concepts was
     a. Hippocrates.   c. St. Luke
     b. Cassiodorus.   d. St. Cosmas.

2.   The terminology used by St. Luke in his Gospel indicates that he was a follower of
     a. Hippocrates.   c. St. Benedict.
     b. monastic medicine.   d. Aesculapius.

3.   The first visiting nurse in recorded history was
     a. Marcella.   c. Phoebe.
     b. Fabiola.   d. an Augustinian nun.

4.   The first organized group that provided nursing services was
     a. an order of sisters.   c. the newly converted Christians.
     b. an order of monks.   d. an order of deaconesses.

5.   A large hospital built in Asia Minor about 370 A.D. was called
     a. St. Basil.   c. The Temple of Aesculapius.
     b. a hospice.   d. Basilias.

6.   A Roman woman who has been named the "Mother of Nuns" for her devotion to the women in her convent was
     a. Marcella.   c. Phoebe.
     b. Fabiola.   d. Paula.

7.   The first hospital was established in Rome about 380 A.D. by
     a. St. Paul.   c. St. Luke.
     b. Fabiola.   d. St. Damian.

8.   When saints are invoked to cure the ill, it is called
     a. Byzantine medicine.   c. faith healing.
     b. a miracle.   d. a petition.

9.   One of the earliest accounts of first aid and emergency care is found in
     a. the biblical parable of the Good Samaritan.
     b. the texts of Cassiodorus.
     c. the writings of Galen.
     d. Greek mythology.

10. The new interest in caring for the sick and poor was a result of
    a. the establishment of religious orders.
    b. Greek teachings.
    c. Benedictine rule.
    d. the philosophy of Christianity.

B. Briefly answer the following questions.

1. Explain what role social service might have played in the lives of the patients in early Christian hospitals.

2. What effect did Christianity initially have on the development of scientific medical practice?

chapter 3
MEDIEVAL
HEALTH CARE

STUDENT OBJECTIVES

- Identify contributions made by groups and individuals to the organization of nursing.

- Explain the social conditions of the Middle Ages which led to the organization of health care services.

- Describe the nursing activities of the Middle Ages.

The great Roman Empire collapsed in chaos after being devastated by invaders. The Middle Ages, or Medieval Period (500-1450 A.D.) which followed, was characterized by the growth and domination of the Christian church. The focus of the Church was the civilization and conversion of the barbarian invaders and the pagan world. The Crusaders, religious orders of priests, brothers, and knights, traveled throughout Europe and the Near East, with the mission of regaining the Holy Lands for the faithful. When the zealous Crusaders returned to their homelands, they brought with them new ideas, products and treasures from the pagan world. In the eleventh century, towns and cities began to flourish, reflecting the growing volume of commercial trade which the Crusades had facilitated. Industries were developed to provide goods for trade in the world market. Universities were established for the purpose of collecting and recording knowledge and to systematically explain the phenomena observed in the universe. Monasteries and the papacy provided the impetus and leadership for the restructuring of the Western World. The roots of Western civilization and organized nursing are to be found in this Medieval Period.

MEDIEVAL NURSING

During the Crusades the military orders discovered that their Moslem enemies cared for the sick in organized facilities, so the Crusaders built similar hospitals near the battlefronts. The members took turns fighting and nursing the wounded. Later, monasteries and regular religious orders were established to carry out the work of Christ. In addition to their religious duties, the members of these orders devoted their lives to helping the heathen, poor, orphaned, and ill. Secular orders developed when it became obvious that some members of religious orders did not like nursing or did not have time to devote to nursing. Lay persons organized groups who would be responsible for nursing services only.

Military Orders

Historically, the three primary military orders were the Knights of St. John, the Teutonic Knights, and the Knights of St. Lazarus. Of these, the Knights of St. John were the most outstanding. Under the leadership of Brother Peter Gerard, a group of monks nursing in two Christian hospitals, which had been established in Jerusalem in 1050, founded an order and dedicated it to St. John, the Almoner. The "Hospitalers," as the Knights of St. John were called, were extremely successful and the order grew in size and influence. Being a military order, the hierarchy of authority was clear; obedience and devotion were maintained with rigid discipline. These characteristics were an integral part of organized nursing for hundreds of years and it is only recently that this approach has

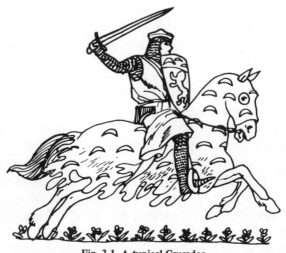

Fig. 3-1 A typical Crusader

been modified to allow individual participation in decision making. The Knights of St. John still have a viable organization in England today. Because of its involvement in the organization of the International Red Cross, the insignia of the order was adopted for use by the Red Cross.

The German counterpart of the Knights of St. John were called the Teutonic Knights. The order was established in the early twelfth century, in a German hospital in Jerusalem. The organizational structure followed that of the Order of St. John, which probably initially exerted some control over its new German affiliate. The Teutonic Knights were involved in the wars of the Holy Land and in 1190 A.D. they established a tent hospital for their wounded. Eventually, the order cut the ties with the Order of St. John and moved headquarters to Germany. Only men could be full members of the order, but women were granted sisterhood and held secondary positions. Both men and women performed nursing duties until the order changed its role after the Crusades and the sisters took over the nursing responsibilities.

The Knights of St. Lazarus was organized solely for the purpose of nursing the lepers in the conquered city of Jerusalem. When leprosy began to abate, the order was taken over by the Knights of St. John.

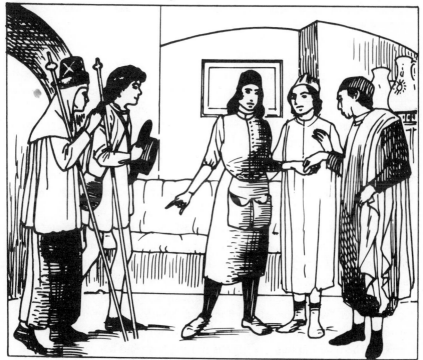

Fig. 3-2 Weary travelers seek shelter in a medieval hospice.

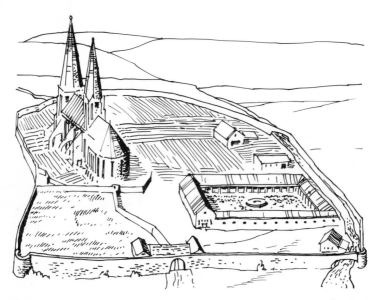

Fig. 3-3   The medieval monastery was a self-sufficient village and farm behind walls, and dominated by the large church or cathedral.

Religious Orders

Christian men and women established religious communities, each having its own unique vows, rituals, and purpose. The trend of the Middle Ages was to seek the security, peace, and protection found within monastery walls. Christians who once tended to the needs of the ill in their homes joined groups of priests, brothers, and sisters who established hospices within monasteries. The hospice provided lodging for travelers, the poor and the sick—all under the same roof. Eventually it became obvious that the sick should be separated from others in the hospice. Using the Persian and Arab hospitals as models, hospitals were built and staffed by members of the religious or regular orders.

In the Twelfth century, St. Francis of Assisi and St. Clare, his disciple, founded two orders that have grown vastly over the centuries and are actively functioning today in many parts of the world. St. Francis cared for the lepers and the poor. He attracted many followers who became known as the First Order of St. Francis. Clare became one if his disciples. She went to live in a Benedictine convent, where she attracted many followers of her own. She formed a nursing group, the Second Order of St. Francis, which today is called the "Poor Clares." The order no longer performs nursing functions but cares for the poor and aged.

Secular Orders

Persons who were dedicated to particular orders, but did not want to take the binding vows of regular orders and live in a monastic community, established tertiary orders for lay people. The secular orders attracted people with real desire to nurse and, therefore, they were very successful and effective. Many of these orders are still in existence.

St. Francis founded the Third Order of St. Francis which consisted of lay persons who desired to follow him but did not want to live the secluded life of the regular order. Lay members did not take the vows of poverty and chastity; neither did they have to denounce the world as the members of the regular order were required to do. This group made many contributions to nursing and served the sick and poor in their own communities. During the Middle Ages they also did some hospital nursing.

The Beguines were organized in Liegi, Flanders about 1170 A.D. and spread to France, Germany, and into the Netherlands. Their leader was a priest named Lambert le Begue. Originally, four or five women lived together and tended to the sick in a community, as a means of supporting themselves. Although not bound by rigid rules and regulations, they mutually agreed upon a code of conduct and uniformity of dress. By the fourteenth century, they numbered almost 200,000 and expanded their duties to hospital staff nursing.

Another influential order still in existence today is the Oblate Order which began in the twelfth century. Founded in Italy, its main function was to staff the hospitals of Florence. Members were given specific training for the nursing duties they were expected to assume.

One of the most outstanding nursing leaders and hospital nurses of this period was St. Catherine of Siena (1347-1380) who as a young child pledged her life to religion and was inclined toward nursing. Catherine wanted to join the second Order of St. Dominic (which was a cloistered order), but could not because she was too young. Therefore, she became active in the tertiary order of St. Dominic (which was composed of lay persons who nursed). Under its auspices she gained fame as a nurse in the hospital at La Scala, during the epidemic of the plague.

Medieval Nursing Practice

Nursing in the regular and secular orders was very organized. It is easy to see the roots of traditional nursing in these early orders. The young new members of the order were probationers and wore regular clothes on duty. When they advanced, they were able to wear the uniform, a white robe. Upon successful

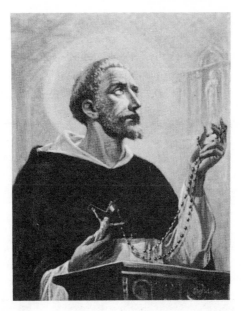

Fig. 3-4 Saint Dominic. (Courtesy St. Dominic's Mission Society and Fr. Joseph D. Nash, O.P.)

completion of the novitiate period, they received the hood. All nurses were responsible to the director of nursing, then called a maîtresse. Unselfish, obedient and total devotion was expected of all members of the order. Because the orders were sponsored by the Church at a time when the Church was the ultimate power, the vitality and strength of the orders grew. Nursing became an acceptable pursuit for women and, thus, many talented, intelligent, and wealthy women entered the orders. Medicine, as an occupation, on the other hand, did not win favor with the Church. In fact, the Church probably thwarted the growth of medical science. Because of this, medicine was not able to exert authority or control over nursing.

The Church dictated nursing practice to a great extent. The human body was basically thought to be unclean, so the Sisters of God were prevented from doing those things which were of "unclean" character; perineal care, enemas, and douches were not acceptable procedures. On the other hand, meeting the spiritual needs of the patient was the priority of the nurse. Nurses fed and bathed the patients, changed and washed the bed linen, administered medications, dressed wounds, and did the general cleaning. Some hospitals had salaried doctors but most had the services of a visiting physician. Medical practice was rudimentary and equipment was primitive. The nurses were really the main providers of health care which was mostly custodial and *palliative* (reducing the severity of the symptoms) rather than treatment of the disease.

THE MEDIEVAL HOSPITAL

The Crusaders observed the Arabs and Persians and brought back many Moslem ideas concerning hospital construction and organization. The military nursing orders followed the Moslem concepts and erected hospitals resembling their architectural design. The hospital was not only functional but a place of artistic beauty. Gothic windows of stained glass; carved, vaulted ceilings; and magnificent paneling created an atmosphere of peace and celestial beauty. Beds were separated by intricately-carved removable partitions, and curtains of beautiful fabric. Ceilings and walls were often decorated by magnificent paintings and sculptures, figure 3-5.

The early hospital was called a *Hôtel Dieu.* The Hôtel Dieu in Paris was founded in 650 A.D. In the twelfth century the Augustinian nuns took charge of the hospital and kept meticulous records which provided most of the information about hospitals and nursing in the Middle Ages. Although the hospital was

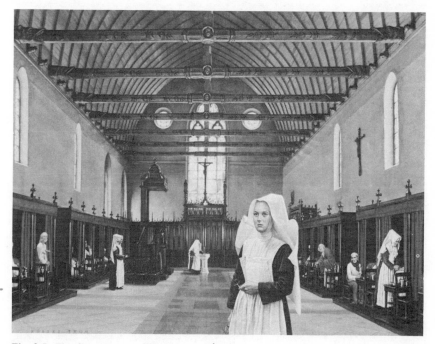

Fig. 3-5 The Great Room of the Poor at Hôtel Dieu in Paris. (Courtesy Parke, Davis and Company, © 1958)

beautiful, it is obvious that modern nursing would be restricted in such a facility. The high windows provided poor light and inadequate ventilation. Heating and plumbing were nonexistent and the fixed position of patient beds would make patient care difficult. In some medieval hospitals, two and three patients occupied one bed, which reflected the lack of appreciation of the communicability of disease and asepsis.

MEDIEVAL MEDICINE

Arab and Persian medicine was at its prime between 850 and 1050 A.D. The Arabs had developed the numeral system, mathematics, and algebra. Great hospitals were built and physicians who staffed the hospitals were educated in academies. Medicine, as a body of knowledge, began to expand. Rhazes, a Persian, (860-932) was an excellent physician of his time, figure 3-6. He studied communicable disease, and was able to explain the difference between measles and smallpox. Avicenna (980-1037) wrote a medical text, the *Canon of Medicine,* which was used in medical schools for six centuries. The text covered pharmacology and symptomatology. Avicenna advocated the separation of the duties

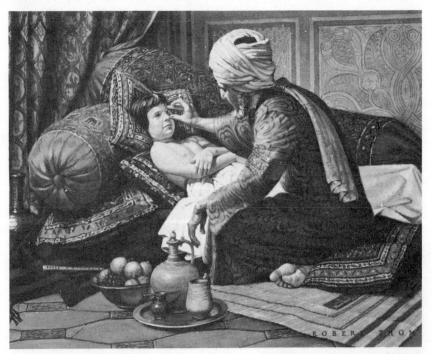

Fig. 3-6 Rhazes, the Father of Pediatrics. (Courtesy Parke, Davis and Company, © 1958)

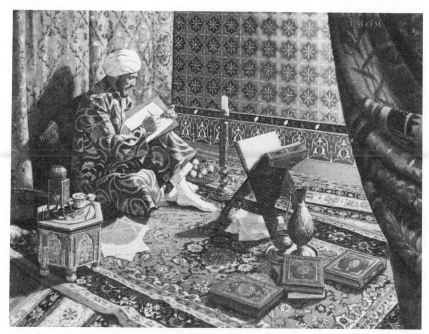

Fig. 3-7 Avicenna, the Prince of Physicians. (Courtesy, Parke, Davis and Company, ©1953)

of the pharmacist and physician which brought about the first apothecary shops. Albucasis, also a Persian physician, introduced cauterization in the treatment of fifty diseases. Surgery was limited to tonsillectomies and care of wounds. Persia, now Iran, honored Avicenna in 1954 as the *Prince of Physicians* and Rhazes in 1964 as the *Father of Pediatrics,* by placing their portraits on postage stamps.

In Europe, medicine was stagnated by the restrictions of the Church. Dissection of the human body was prohibited and so anatomy ceased to be studied. The genitals were considered unclean, which made the study of urine questionable. The barber-surgeon, who rid the body of ill humours by bloodletting, fell into ill repute because of his distasteful work.

In 848 A.D. the School of Salerno, a medical school, was established. Although the school was affiliated with the Benedictine Abbey at Monte Cassino, the Church did not have complete authority or control over the school. Men and women served on the experienced faculty. One of the early female physicians was St. Hildegarde (1099-1179), a German Benedictine abbess. In addition to her practice of medicine, she taught courses in the care of the sick to prepare young titled women to function as nurses. The school produced many books on the subjects of therapeutics, prescriptions, obstetrics, gynecology, epilepsy, and oral disease. The school developed a well-planned curriculum and required an examination be taken before the faculty, prior to practicing medicine. The school taught philosophy, law, and theology, in addition to medicine and thereby resembled the university system today. Clinical surgery was taught for many years and Roger Frugardi's *Roger's Surgery,* the first medieval textbook on surgery, dominated surgical practice for a hundred years. Included in the text were surgical treatment of nasal polyps, hemorrhoids, fractures of the jaw, intestinal anastomosis, bladder stones, and skull fractures. Inspired by Hippocrates, the doctors centered their attention on the patient and diet.

EPIDEMICS OF THE MIDDLE AGES

People flocked to the cities in the late Middle Ages but the city was not ready for the mass crowds, and confusion and contagion reigned. Garbage was thrown in the ditches and along the streets where cattle and pigs roamed. Body wastes were disposed of through the windows. Fresh water was scarce and uncleanliness of both body and home existed. Public bathing in sweat houses was an attempt to bring about a degree of cleanliness, but they proved to be sources of infection and its spread, as well as moral degradation. The practice was restricted when the plagues of the fourteenth century developed.

Leprosy was mentioned in the Code of Hammurabi and was believed to have been carried from Egypt by the Israelites. It was discussed by Moses, Confucius in China, and Charaka in India. Greek and Roman physicians encountered leprosy and it became widespread until it reached epidemic stages in the thirteenth century. Lepers were not isolated but were permitted to live freely following specific rules and regulations, such as identifying themselves with black cloaks, large black hats and carrying a stick and rattle. The rattle was to warn others of their approach and the stick was to handle merchandise. The weakened condition of the lepers caused many to fall victims of the bubonic plague which was generally fatal to them. Thus leprosy declined in numbers of victims and few cases were reported after the sixteenth century.

Bubonic plague, known as the *Black Death* first appeared in China in the fourteenth century. There were numerous speculations as to the cause of the disease. Some blamed it on astrology; others blamed the Jews and many of them were persecuted. Physicians began to isolate the victims and the first quarantine of ships began in Venice in 1377. This is standard procedure in most ports even today as a preventive measure. The plague had great impact on the economic and moral status of the world. Medically, physicians were unable to cope with the devastating effects of the disease. Priests of the Church perished as victims of the disease; therefore, many persons lost belief in the super-

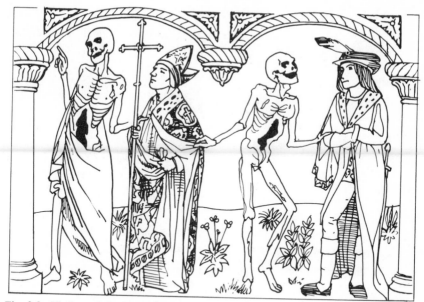

Fig. 3-8 Victims of the Black Death return to destroy a bishop and nobleman, symbols of the church and wealth.

natural and a decline in morality ensued. Some have proclaimed the Black Death a prelude to the Reformation Period.

SUMMARY

The Crusades had a profound influence on the development and formal organization of nursing. The Crusaders themselves organized nursing out of necessity. Under the leadership of the Church, religious and lay groups organized to perform nursing tasks by meeting the spiritual and physical needs of the ill. The Crusaders spread the knowledge they acquired in their travels and all of Europe benefited by the improvement of hospitals.

SUGGESTED ACTIVITIES

- Contact a local hospital operated by a religious order and report to the class on the origin of the order and the contributions it has made to nursing at the present time.

- Compile a list of all the men and women who made contributions to nursing during the Middle Ages. Identify the century, the geographic location, and the nature of their contributions.

- Write a paper conceptualizing a typical day on a nursing unit in a medieval hospital. List specific nursing procedures and the conditions under which they might have been performed.

REVIEW

A.   Multiple Choice. Select the best answer.

1. A woman who devoted her life to nursing and is remembered for her work in hospitals caring for victims of the plague was
   a. St. Hildegarde.   c. St. Catherine of Siena.
   b. St. Clare   d. St. Louise de Marillac.

2. Monks and nuns who cared for the sick and wounded and also went to battle were called
   a. Hospitalers.   c. a Christian nursing order.
   b. Kinghts of St. John.   d. all of these.

3. Secular nursing orders which are still in operation today are
   a. The Oblates and The Second Order of St. Francis.
   b. The Knights of St. John and St. Lazarus.
   c. a and b.
   d. neither a nor b.

4. An epidemic which raged across Europe in the late Middle Ages was
   a. bubonic plague.   c. typhoid.
   b. leprosy.   d. smallpox.

5. The concept of the modern hospital was developed by
   a. the Crusaders.   c. monks and nuns.
   b. the Moslems.   d. the Greeks.

6. Nurses in the Medieval Period probably
   a. changed bed linens   c. passed medication
   b. bathed patients   d. did none of these.

7. The most significant advances in medicine during the Middle Ages were brought about by
   a. the Crusaders.
   b. the interest of the Church in medicine.
   c. the establishment of a medical school in Salerno.
   d. the development of hospitals.

8. The orders made up of lay persons who were not bound to religious vows were called
   a. military orders.   c. regular orders.
   b. religious orders.   d. secular orders.

9. Women in the Middle Ages were not likely to be found
   a. on the faculty of a medical school.
   b. as full members of the Teutonic Knights.
   c. in uniform while performing nursing duties.
   d. working in hotels.

10. The Church prohibited
    a. human dissection and autopsy.
    b. giving perineal care by nurses.
    c. administering enemas by women.
    d. all of the above.

B. Briefly answer the following questions.

1. Cite an example of how the nursing orders may have been restricted by their close association with the Church.

2. Give three reasons why nursing services were organized.

chapter 4
THE DARK AGES
AND NEW IDEAS

STUDENT OBJECTIVES

- Name the leaders of reform and state the contributions each has made to society.

- State reasons for the detrimental effect the Reformation had upon nursing.

- Identify the positive influence the renewed interest in the arts and sciences had upon medical advancement in the Renaissance period.

During the Middle Ages (500-1450 A.D.) nursing services were provided by organizations within the Church. Motivated by charity, women from prominent families compassionately rendered nursing care. Little progress was made in medical treatment even though universities began to develop in an effort to preserve and expand knowledge. Toward the end of the period papal government began to deteriorate. Europe was ravaged by plagues, famines, and wars which decimated the population and led to economic crises. The time was ripe for change.

THE RENAISSANCE

By the beginning of the fifteenth century, the chaos of the Middle Ages subsided with man's quest for new knowledge and beauty. The civilization of ancient Greece and Rome was reborn; thus the period is called the *Renaissance*. Interest was focused on classical literature, humanism, and expressions of beauty.

Artists became very interested in the human body. Cadavers were dissected and body structures studied, so that the artist might more accurately reproduce

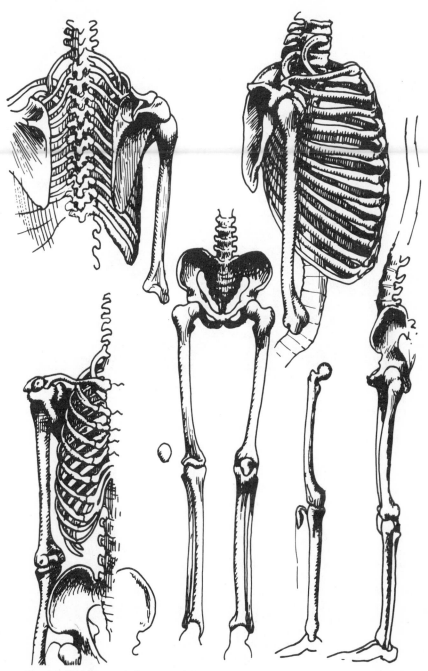

Fig. 4-1 Sketches made from actual dissection. (Adapted from a da Vinci drawing.)

nature.   Leonardo da Vinci (1452-1519), in addition to being one of the greatest artists of the Renaissance, had a keen interest in the realm of medicine.   He is believed to have dissected over thirty bodies in the Santo Spirito mortuary in Rome.   Working by candlelight, he made anatomical sketches in great detail, figure 4-1, page 45.   He was the first to study fetal membranes, cerebral nerves,

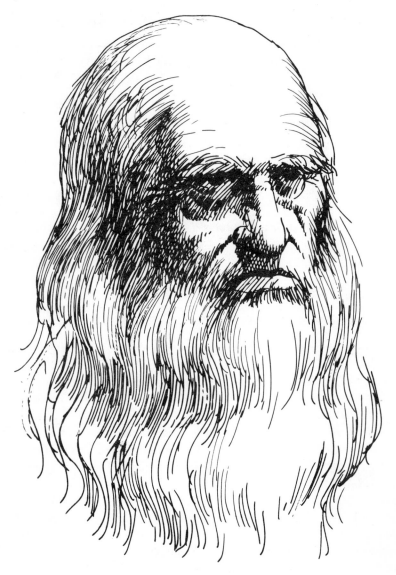

Fig. 4-2 Leonardo da Vinci

the eye, muscular function, and the human brain. Artists such as da Vinci were influential in the development of anatomy, and their knowledge led to the development of physiology as a science.

Medical Conditions

Medicine was facing two new conditions heretofore relatively unknown or unrecognized. These were gunshot wounds and syphilis. Gunshot wounds developed after the thirteenth century invention of firearms, including the cannon. Treatment of wounds required surgery and new procedures were developed to treat amputations, wounds, and infections resulting from untreated gunshot wounds. Cauterization of wounds became a common practice. Syphilis raged through all of Europe and Asia and was believed by some to have originated in America around 1494. At first, it was often mistaken for leprosy. There were conflicting views regarding the origin of syphilis but the fact remains that an epidemic raged throughout Europe in the late fifteenth century.

Mental illness was believed to be caused by witchcraft and demons. Witches were believed to be insane and were burned at the stake. Those who were not put to death were chained in dungeon cells or chased away from the villages. Few medical institutions housed the insane. One of the first was Bethlehem Hospital in London, England. Tourists found it amusing and entertaining to tour the hospital and observe the patients.

Medical Practitioners

In Paris in the fifteenth century, there were three types of practitioners who made up the medical profession. Physicians who were graduates of a school of medicine but did not perform surgery comprised one group. Another group called surgeons, treated wounds, did cauterizations, and applied plasters and ointments, but did not do surgery. The third group, barber surgeons, practiced bloodletting, tooth extraction, did crude surgery, and even gave enemas in addition to doing their barbering. The red and white striped barber pole, symbol of the barber shop today, originated with the bloodletting function of the barber. The blood-soaked bandages were hung out to dry and flapped in the wind, winding around the pole to which they were attached. Doctors relied on urinalysis, bloodletting and the four *humours* in the diagnosis of disease. The humours referred to four fluids or semifluids present in the body. They were: aqueous, crystalline, ocular, and vitreous humours.

In order to support himself economically, the doctor confined his practice mainly to the upper class. The academically trained physician spoke Latin

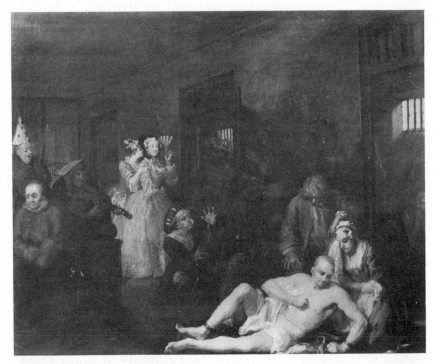

Fig. 4-3 **Bethlehem Hospital in London which housed the insane was more often called Bedlam.** (Courtesy Sir John Sloane's Museum, London)

fluently and dressed in long robes made of furs and costly materials. His position was one of high esteem and he preferred to give directions rather than perform surgery himself. Unqualified medical practitioners took over the care of the poor.

Surgery in England was initially subordinate to medicine. In 1369, army surgeons formed the society known as The Military Guild of Surgeons. Their members had an apprenticeship of six years and then had to pass an examination given by the masters of the guild. If they failed, they spent another six years as an apprentice and if they failed the exam a second time they could not practice surgery.

The Guild of Barber Surgeons was formed in 1300 and incorporated in 1462. Apprentices of this guild were given lectures, observed dissections and were later licensed to practice. An Act of Parliament in 1540 united the two guilds and declared barbers could not function as surgeons and vice versa. The official licensing bodies in England were the universities, the bishops, the Royal College of Physicians, the Guild of Military Surgeons, and the Company of Barber Surgeons.

THE REFORMATION

The Reformation which began in Germany in 1517 was a religious movement brought about by Protestant revolt against the deteriorating patriarchal rule of the Roman Catholic church. The rebellion against the pope and the patriarchal rule of the Church was led by Martin Luther (1483-1546) of Germany. Luther had been an Augustinian monk who opposed some fundamental doctrines and practices of the Church. Luther proposed some ninety-five debatable items which provoked religious dissension. This led to the formation of the Protestants, a group which was to be comprised of many religious denominations. Followers of Martin Luther were called Lutherans and the Lutheran church today still embraces his doctrine.

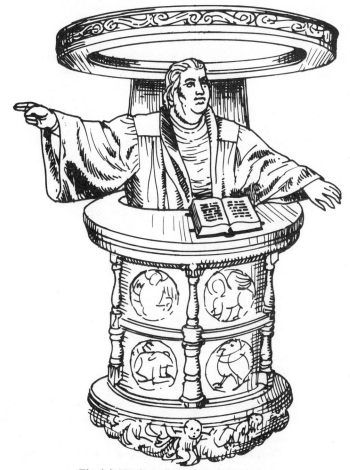

Fig. 4-4 Martin Luther, Leader of the Reformation

The Role of Women

The Reformation brought about a tremendous change in the role of women in society. Prior to this time women were revered by the Church. Women of prominent families were encouraged to be involved in charitable activities outside the home. Nuns who nursed and taught were recruited from the finest families in Europe. Women had many opportunities to contribute to society. The Reformation brought about religious freedom but not freedom for women. Women became subordinate to men and were expected to remain in the family home caring for offspring. No respectable woman worked outside the home. There were no job opportunities for women, except for destitute women who found positions as servants in domestic service.

Nursing in Protestant Countries

The Reformation had a disastrous effect upon nursing. Hospitals operated by Roman Catholic religious orders were closed or controlled by the Protestants. Hospital personnel fled to other parts of the world to avoid persecution, leaving deserted buildings behind. Monasteries in England were also closed. The abrupt demise of religious orders created a tremendous shortage of people to care for the sick. In order to fill the nursing ranks, women were recruited from all sources. Generally, these women were the wayward who were assigned to nursing duties in lieu of serving jail sentences. Sairey Gamp and Betsy Prig in the book, *Martin Chuzzlewit,* written by Charles Dickens in 1844 represent the nursing image of what is called the dark period of nursing, figure 4-5. These private duty nurses were neglectful of their duties, drank alcohol while on duty, used profanity freely, and were often cruel to the patient. Sairey Gamp was, in reality, not a fictitious character of the book but an actual nurse the author's friend had hired for a member of his family. Today, an individual who lacks the desirable attributes of a nurse and does not adhere to an ethical code of conduct is often referred to as a "Sairey Gamp."

Nursing in Catholic Countries

The Catholic countries escaped this dark age to some extent. The surviving religious orders continued to care for the sick and indigent. In France, a priest and a social reformer, St. Vincent de Paul, developed the concept of vocational education, believing the poverty situation might be alleviated if the poor were taught a skilled trade. For those persons who were unable to work, he organized a charitable organization to provide necessary subsistence. St. Vincent de Paul

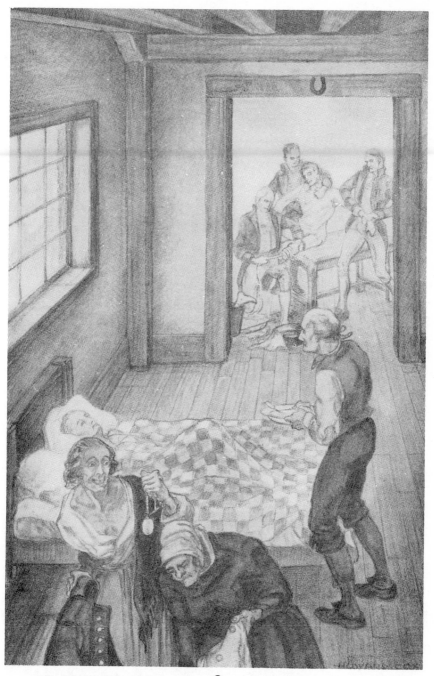

Fig. 4-5 The dark period of nursing. (©1935 Physician's Record Co., Chicago)

organized a society of women to assist him in his community work. They gave nursing care to the patients in the Hotel Dieu Hospital in Paris which was operated by the Augustinian nuns. Mlle. Louise La Gras assisted him by organizing the religious order known as the Daughters of Charity. These Sisters were not confined to the convent but were allowed to go out into the community and meet the needs of individuals where the problems existed. This Order of St. Vincent de Paul, which took over the nursing care in many European countries and later Canada and North America, was the beginning of organized charity.

NEW IDEAS IN MEDICINE

The Renaissance and Reformation were responsible for stimulating new thinking, which led to the birth of the scientific method of inquiry. Modern

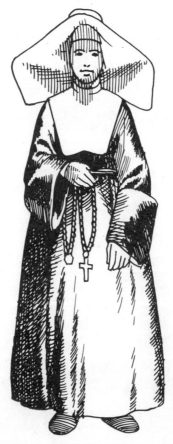

Fig. 4-6 A nursing sister of St. Vincent de Paul

science was developed in the seventeenth century and this had a profound influence on the development of medicine; it also paved the way for the Industrial Revolution.

An early outstanding physician was Ambroise Paré (1510-1590), a surgeon, who practiced at the Hôtel Dieu in Paris. Paré made great strides in the treatment of fractures, dislocations, and obstetrical techniques. He introduced the use of *ligatures* (threads or filaments) to tie off blood vessels during surgery, and he wrote many surgical textbooks.

Seventeenth Century Developments in Medicine

William Harvey (1578-1657) practiced medicine in London in the early part of the seventeenth century on the staff of St. Bartholomew's Hospital. Although Hippocrates used the term, *circulation of the blood,* and many others made reference to it, William Harvey was the first to actually unlock the door of mystery concerning the circulatory system. Harvey's most valuable contribution, however, was the establishment of physiological experimentation, which has earned him acclaim as the *Father of Modern Medicine.*

The development of the clinical method was the contribution of Thomas Sydenham (1624-1689). He advocated subjecting old theories to new scientific observation. Independent research led him to describe chorea and gout, common ailments of the time.

Anton van Leeuwenhoek (1632-1723) first used the microscope. He described bacteria and protozoa, which had never before been seen. Unfortunately, the significance of microscopic study was not realized for many years.

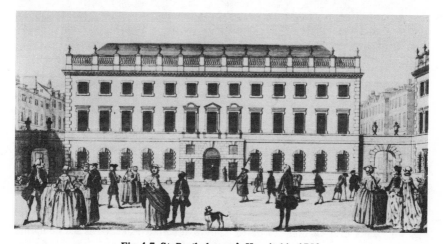

Fig. 4-7 St. Bartholomew's Hospital in 1752

During the seventeenth century, autopsy was found to be useful in determining the cause of death and the effect of disease on the body. The autopsy offered the physician the opportunity to study gross anatomy and to practice surgical technique. Pathology became a science.

Significant Medical Discoveries of the Eighteenth Century

In the eighteenth century smallpox was prevalent and took many lives. Edward Jenner (1749-1823) developed the first immunization after the discovery that cowpox virus prevented smallpox. This success sparked new interest in the prevention of communicable disease.

William Withering (1741-1799) discovered that tea brewed with foxglove, a garden plant, cured dropsy or heart failure. The ingredient that brought about the improvement was digitalis.

James Lind was the first to discover that scurvy, which killed many pilgrims en route to America, was caused by the lack of vitamin C. He introduced citrus fruits as a means of preventing the disease, figure 4-8. This earned English sailors the nickname, "limeys."

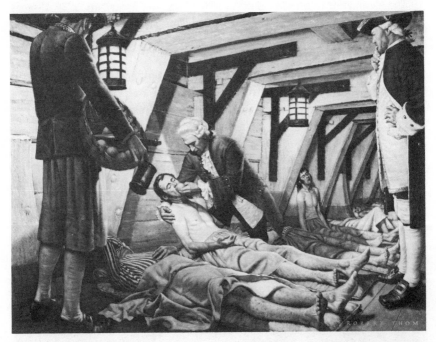

Fig. 4-8   James Lind discovers a cure for scurvy.   (Courtesy Parke, Davis and Company, © 1959)

The art of *percussion* (tapping of the chest and abdomen) was first used and perfected by physicians during the eighteenth century. Prior to this time, the art was unique to innkeepers who tapped wine kegs to determine the remaining volume.

As a physician and director of two hospitals in Paris, Phillipe Pinel (1755-1826) saw the need to stop the inhumane treatment of the mentally ill. Due to the lack of understanding of psychiatry, mental disorders were believed to be caused by demons. Patients were put into chains and treated cruelly. Pinel advocated acceptance of the mentally ill as human beings in need of medical assistance, nursing care and social services, figure 4-9.

SOCIAL REFORM AND NURSING

In the eighteenth century there was a growing awareness of the need to improve social conditions. Interest in reform grew steadily throughout the eighteenth and nineteenth centuries, and the movement brought about many changes which influenced health care and nursing.

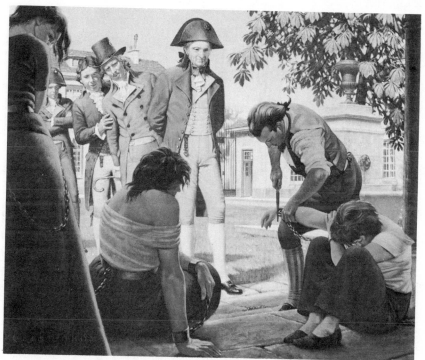

Fig. 4-9 **Pinel unchains the insane.** (Courtesy Parke, Davis and Company, ©1960)

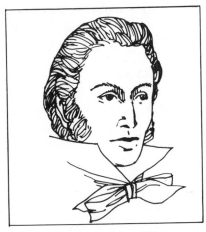

Rene Laennec (1781-1826)
Laennec described the pathology of tuberculosis.

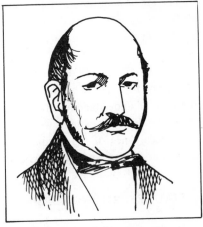

Ignatz Semmelweis (1818-1865)
Semmelweis proved that puerperal sepsis could be prevented if those caring for the patient washed their hands.

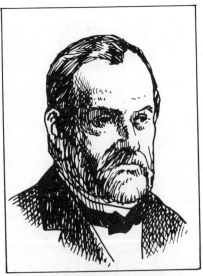

Louis Pasteur (1822-1895)
Pasteur has been credited with the discovery of anaerobic bacteria and the process of pasteurization.

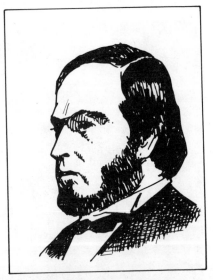

Lord Joseph Lister (1827-1912)
Lister capitalized on the work of Pasteur and developed aseptic technique.

Fig. 4-10 Nineteenth century advances in medicine

John Howard

One of the most dedicated, hardworking leaders of reform, John Howard (1726-1790) was a fighter for the cause of public health. He found fault with the physicians who did not recognize the plague as a contagious disease. John Howard exposed the deplorable treatment of prisoners herded together into cells with no light or sanitation and insufficient diet. Although a native of London, he studied hospital, quarantine, and prison systems of more than a half dozen countries. He promoted vast prison reform and conditions were vastly improved because of his work and dedication.

Theodor Fliedner

Theodor Fliedner as a young minister in Kaiserswerth, Germany, decided to travel to Holland and England in an effort to study means of combating the problems of poverty among his flock. He observed the work of those actively

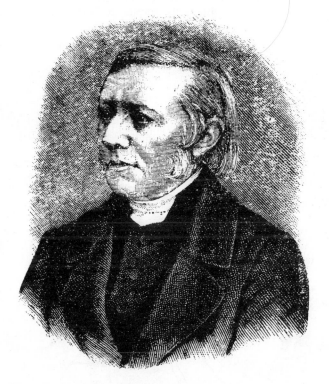

Fig. 4-11 Pastor Theodor Fliedner dedicated his life to prison reform and hospital administration.

engaged in reform and he began to formulate plans that involved his first wife, Fredericke. He was highly motivated by the prison reform work of Elizabeth Fry. He was also aware of the deplorable conditions of nursing services and recognized a need for nursing education. In 1836 he opened a hospital in Kaiserswerth and Gertrude Reichardt entered as the first deaconess. Theodor and Fredericke Fliedner were unusually capable administrators and organized the hospital as it grew into a systematic division of services. By 1864, the number of deaconesses rose to 1,600 who served not only the sick, but wayward girls and the orphaned. The Kaiserswerth Institute School of Nursing exists even today. Pastor Fliedner and four deaconesses traveled to North America in 1849 and established a hospital in Pittsburgh, Pennsylvania under the direction of Pastor William Passavant.

Elizabeth Fry

Elizabeth Fry (1780-1845) was a Quaker philanthropist who carried on the work of John Howard. After visiting the hospital at Kaiserswerth and observing the functions of the deaconesses, she became motivated to do similar nursing care for the poor in London, England. Although the group of women she

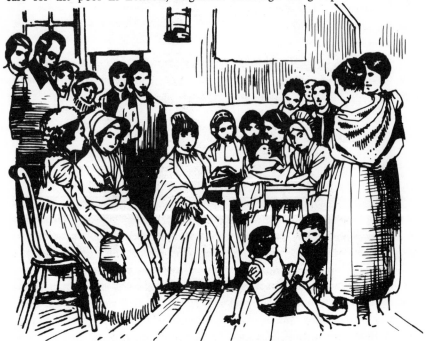

Fig. 4-12 Elizabeth Fry visits with prisoners.

organized to perform nursing services were initially called the Protestant Sisters of Charity, they were not affiliated with any church. They were later known as the Institute of Nursing Sisters.

Mother Mary Catherine McAuley

Born in Dublin into a family of wealth, Mary McAuley grew up in a circle consisting of many physicians and pharmacists. Mother McAuley is the founder of the Sisters of Mercy. The original purpose was to aid destitute girls; as the order grew in numbers, it spread to many parts of the world and became actively involved in nursing. This Roman Catholic order nursed the victims of a cholera epidemic in

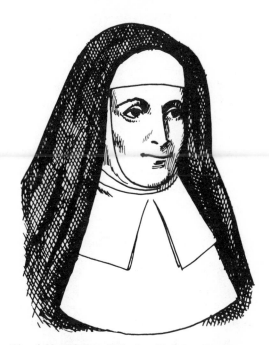

Fig. 4-13 Mother Catherine McAuley, founder of the Sisters of Mercy

1832 and the ill in Dublin hospitals. Today these nuns care for the ill in all parts of the world including North America where the Order operates several hospitals.

EARLY LEADERS IN AMERICAN MEDICINE

Migrants left Europe for America and brought to the new country serious health problems. Infectious diseases such as scarlet fever, diphtheria, influenza, and yellow fever produced epidemics in the crowded, dirty cities. There was not enough housing or food to accommodate the growing population. There were few medical supplies and fewer doctors. To study medicine required a return to Europe, which few could afford. In 1765, America's first medical school was established in Philadelphia, which is now the University of Pennsylvania. However, by the time of the American Revolution, there was still a tremendous shortage of doctors, nurses, and medical supplies. Medical treatment was unsophisticated and nursing was provided by women who cared for their sick relatives in their own homes. The first hospital built in America, in 1737, was Charity Hospital of New Orleans. Pennsylvania General Hospital (1751), New

York Hospital (1781), Massachusetts General Hospital (1821), and Bellevue Hospital in New York (1848) were early hospitals and are great medical centers today.

The men whose contributions are noted in this text are not by any means the only outstanding people identified with medical progress during this period. They are few among many notable scientists, educators, and physicians who brought about significant advances in medicine.

Benjamin Rush

Benjamin Rush (1746-1813) held a faculty position in chemistry at the College of Philadelphia school of medicine. He was also one of the signers of the Declaration of Independence and the most famous physician of the Revolu-

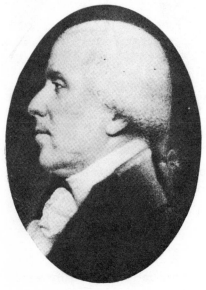

tionary period. He wrote extensively and his works had great impact on medical practice. He wrote the first American text on psychiatry and because of this book, based on his humane treatment of the mentally ill, he has been remembered as the first American psychiatrist. He has also been linked with the beginning of chiropractic medicine.

Rush was a highly controversial figure and many of his theories found opposition. He based his views on the belief that there was one cause and one cure for all disease and advocated bleeding and purging techniques. Criticism of Rush stems from his lack of scientific approach and indifference to statistics and laboratory research. He

Fig. 4-14   Benjamin Rush, the first American psychiatrist

had a humanistic approach and was mainly concerned with psychosomatic relationships. Although limited by his narrow approach to medicine, he remains a noteworthy contributor to twentieth century medical thinking.

William Morton

Dr. Morton (1819-1868) was a graduate of the Harvard Medical School and a practicing dentist. He used local applications of ether when filling teeth. He experimented with dogs in ether inhalation and felt so confident about its anaesthesizing properties that he sought permission to administer ether prior to the surgical removal of a tumor from the jaw of a patient of Dr. John C. Warren, Jr., Professor of Surgery at Harvard Medical School. Although this was the initial introduction of the use of ether, much controversy existed as to who was the first American to introduce ether as a surgical anesthetic. The discovery of anesthesia made possible the great advances in surgical technique during the nineteenth and twentieth centuries.

The Mayo Story

Located in Southern Minnesota surrounded by dairy farms, lies Rochester, Minnesota and the Mayo Clinic. The Mayo legacy began with Dr. William Worrall Mayo, born and educated in England and Scotland. At the age of 26, he arrived in New York and began his career as a chemist at Bellevue Hospital. Completing studies begun in Europe, he received a medical degree from Indiana Medical College in 1850. In that period of American medicine, men were trained as practitioners of frontier medicine.

In 1854, tired of practice with little remuneration and an annual bout with malaria, the impulsive Dr. Mayo left for Minnesota. He tried to earn a living in a variety of ways and finally, in 1865, he established a medical office in

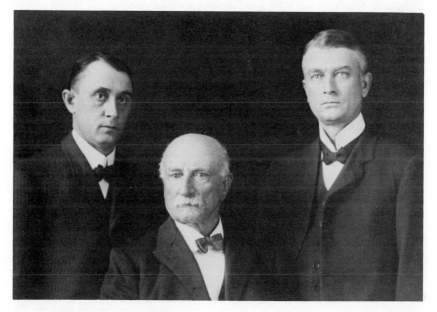

Fig. 4-15 The Mayo doctors: Dr. William W. Mayo (center), and sons Dr. Charles H. Mayo (left) and Dr. William J. Mayo (right)

Rochester. In 1869, he returned to Bellevue Hospital to study surgical techniques and gynecological surgery, which became his specialty when he returned to Rochester.

Dr. William Worrall Mayo had two sons who credited their parents and especially their father for their success. William James Mayo (1861-1939) graduated from the University of Michigan Medical School in 1883 and Charles Horace Mayo (1865-1939) graduated from Chicago Medical College in 1888. Although engaged in general practice, surgery was the chief love of the Mayos, who spent every free moment dissecting eyes from sheep obtained from the slaughterhouse.

The volume of patients who flocked to the famous Drs. Mayo for surgery were generally cared for by local women who performed basic nursing duties because Rochester had no hospital. The tornado of August 21, 1883 hit Rochester and left many wounded who required not only surgery but postoperative nursing care. The motherhouse of the Sisters of St. Francis was turned into an impromptu hospital and, although the order was a teaching order, the sisters served as nurses. In 1889, the sisters opened St. Mary's Hospital, figure 4-16.

The clinic grew due to the steady flow of patients from many geographic locations and doctors in search of newer concepts of medical and surgical techniques. The International Surgeons' Club, later known as the Surgeons' Club, was organized on June 7, 1906 and included visiting physicians among its members. From this club developed the Mayo postgraduate school of surgery.

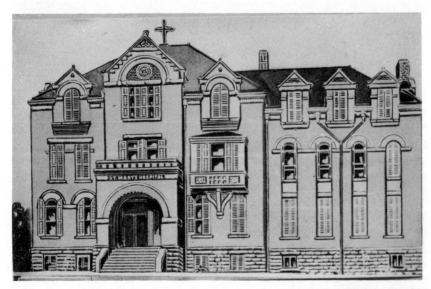

Fig. 4-16 St. Mary's Hospital, Rochester, Minnesota as it appeared when it opened in 1889

The growing numbers of patients was paralleled by an increase in personnel. The number of diagnosticians and clinical staff members grew and expanded to include all areas of medical specialization. Teaching and education became a vital

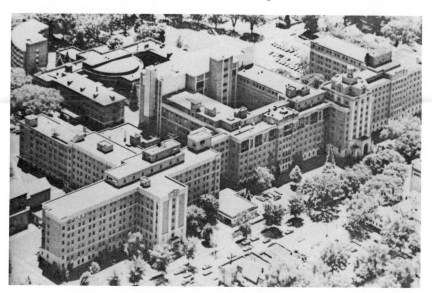

Fig. 4-17 St. Mary's Hospital in 1975

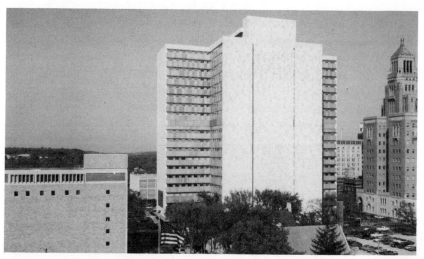

Fig. 4-18 The Mayo Clinic. Buildings pictured, left to right: the Harwick Building; the Mayo Building (main diagnostic and outpatient treatment center); and the Plummer Building (which houses many patient care services, medical education and medical research departments)

force on the Mayo scene. On February 8, 1915, the Mayo Foundation for Medical Education and Research was formed and an affiliation between the University of Minnesota and the Mayo Clinic was contracted. Today, the Mayo Clinic is internationally renowned and a visitor to Rochester cannot help but be impressed by the spirit of the city, the magical aura of the clinic, and the empathy and prevailing spirit of brotherhood.

EQUAL RIGHTS FOR WOMEN

The Code of Hammurabi stated that women were the exclusive property of men. Throughout the ages this creed has been challenged by women. The Reformation served to reinforce the ancient norms, but the Industrial Revolution brought about changes which stimulated women to seriously take action which would once and for all abolish the myth of male supremacy. This movement, which continues today, was necessary before nursing could develop into the profession it is today.

The Industrial Revolution has been defined as a change in the economy; it was characterized by the introduction and use of powered machinery. However, this change in the late eighteenth century was more complex. The revolution was facilitated by many developments. Exploration of a new continent brought wealth to Europe. New thought led to improved agricultural methods and larger harvests. Fewer farmers were needed on the feudal estates so families moved to cities and developed businesses and crafts. Private enterprise developed and the individual was no longer a victim of the restrictive feudal social state. As basic needs were more easily met, the individual had more time to devote to thought, education, religion, politics, and leisure. Scientific discoveries were made which, in turn, made practical application possible. With the development of machinery, a new age was born.

The theme of individual rights was apparent throughout the eighteenth and nineteenth centuries. Women became aware of many injustices and the abrogation of the rights they did have. In an effort to change the status of women, American women demanded the right to vote. English women later began suffrage efforts. After nearly seventy-five years of frustration and resistance, in 1920 the Constitution was amended allowing women to vote. With the vote, women found new power. They could introduce, support, defeat and influence local and federal legislation. Unfortunately, even today much of this power goes unused.

The freedom of women is growing. Women want equal legal status with men and, even more, women are demanding psychological acceptance of this equality at every level of society. The education of women is now accepted. More women are leaving the home and returning to work. More women are returning to school in search of technical and professional education.

The development of nursing has paralleled and reflects this movement. Men and women are seeking a career in nursing at the associate and baccalaureate levels. More women and men are making nursing a career rather than a short-term job. Nurses are demanding legal independence from and acceptance by the physician. Nurses are demanding salaries and benefits commensurate with other professional groups. Nurses are learning to use their power to their advantage; like all women, nurses are developing a new image and status.

SUMMARY

The Reformation was a religious movement against the Church, resulting in the formation of Protestant religions. It had a devastating effect on nursing because of the closing of monasteries, where the religious orders cared for the sick. This period is known as the dark period of nursing. During the Renaissance there was a movement toward the revival of the arts and sciences in Europe. Nursing did not advance scientifically or technically for at least three centuries. Medical knowledge, on the other hand, experienced a renaissance or rebirth. Using the scientific method, scientists and physicians developed the sciences and techniques which are the foundations of modern medicine.

SUGGESTED ACTIVITIES

- Investigate the historical account of medicine and nursing as it began in a geographic location of interest to you. Compare its contributions to the health field with other areas.

- Make a comparison of the desirable characteristics of today's nurse with the characteristics of the nurse in the dark period of nursing.

- Visit the campus art department or a nearby school of art in search of Renaissance art. Study the artist's conceptualization of physical and mental distress.

REVIEW

A.   Multiple Choice. Select the best answer.

    1.   The Father of Modern Medicine was
       a. Hippocrates.   c. William Harvey.
       b. Leonardo da Vinci.   d. Philippe Pinel.

2. The Reformation, which was a rebellion against the patriarchal rule of the Church, was led by
    a. Martin Luther.
    b. Theodor Fliedner.
    c. Fredericke Fliedner.
    d. St. Vincent de Paul.

3. The new disease which raged throughout Europe in the fifteenth century was
    a. leprosy.
    b. syphilis.
    c. plague.
    d. tuberculosis.

4. Detailed study of anatomy by artists and sculptors in the fifteenth century led to a new science called
    a. pathology.
    b. biology.
    c. neurology.
    d. physiology.

5. A Quaker philanthropist who studied at Kaiserswerth and later organized a group of women who provided nursing services in London, England was
    a. Florence Nightingale.
    b. Betsy Prig.
    c. Elizabeth Fry.
    d. Mother McAuley.

6. Progress in surgical technique was made possible by the discovery of
    a. anesthesia.
    b. dissection.
    c. anatomy.
    d. bloodletting.

7. One of the first hospitals to provide facilities for the mentally ill was
    a. St. Bartholomew's Hospital.
    b. Hôtel Dieu.
    c. Kaiserswerth.
    d. Bedlam.

8. One of the most detrimental effects of the Reformation on nursing was
    a. the closing of the monasteries.
    b. the belief that women belonged in the home.
    c. the closing of hospitals run by religious orders.
    d. the shortage of doctors.

9. At the time of the American Revolution, the ill and injured were cared for
    a. by women in their own homes.
    b. by religious orders.
    c. in large city hospitals.
    d. in doctor's offices.

10. The social and economic changes which greatly influenced the development of nursing were a product of
    a. the Reformation.
    b. the Crusades.
    c. the Industrial Revolution.
    d. the Renaissance.

B.   Briefly answer the following questions.

1.   Describe the typical nurse in the seventeenth century.

2.   Explain the value of human dissection in the study of medicine.

SECTION 2
THE BIRTH OF ORGANIZED NURSING

chapter 5
THE NIGHTINGALE
CONCEPT

STUDENT OBJECTIVES

- List the accomplishments of Florence Nightingale in the areas of nursing, public health and social services.

- Explain the Nightingale concept of nursing.

- Compare present day basic nursing education to the curriculum offered in The Nightingale School for Nurses in 1860.

In the early nineteenth century, the Industrial Revolution was well under way. Medical science was developing rapidly and medical practitioners were frustrated in their efforts to provide adequate health care to the growing population because hospital facilities, and the personnel that staffed them, were grossly inadequate. Efforts had been made to prepare skilled nurses, but training programs were scarce and unsophisticated. Nursing needed someone to organize nursing education and service. Florence Nightingale perceived this need. Through her leadership, determination and influence, organized nursing was born.

EARLY LIFE

Born May 12, 1820 in Florence, Italy to British parents on a trip abroad, Florence Nightingale was named for the city of her birth. Her family experienced the best in life as a result of vast inheritances received from relatives. Their religious affiliation was Unitarian. Florence's grandfather was a member of Parliament and her father was an intellectual with a thirst for knowledge; an attribute Florence was to inherit. In the tradition of the wealthy of the Victorian era, she was reared by governesses in the comfort of the family's several lavishly furnished homes. She received the best education available and traveled throughout Europe with her family so that she might have a broad outlook and be introduced to the elite of European society. Having inherited the brilliant mind of her father, she easily mastered many subjects including several languages which were to be very helpful to her in later years.

As a young girl, Florence was sometimes overemotional and supersensitive. She had a very creative mind and a marvelous sense of humor, which together occasionally led her to gross exaggeration. Florence was very sympathetic and tenderhearted, and even as a child she loved to care for injured animals or visit the sick and poor of the neighborhood. As she matured, Florence became a serious young lady, characterized by a systematic mind, sound judgment, and firm purpose. She was also quite attractive and had many suitors. It was expected that Florence would find a suitable, wealthy gentleman, marry and raise a family.

However, Florence did not find it easy to conform to the expectations of her family and the norms of a Victorian society. She found little satisfaction in gracious living and extensive travel. She was bored having only art, music and embroidery to fill her time. Most significantly, she rebelled against the widely accepted idea that women of position did not seek careers. Florence believed she experienced a calling from God and was drawn toward nursing, education, and social reform. The more her family tried to dissuade her from such fields, the firmer her purpose became. Having the advantages of a wealthy family, influential friends, and social prestige, in addition to her own determination and persistence, Florence was well equipped to pursue those goals she set for herself.

FORMATIVE YEARS

By the time Miss Nightingale reached the age of adulthood, she had definitely made up her mind to become a nurse. Her parents were unwilling to permit her to enter nursing and had difficulty understanding her motivation. A woman with her social background could not join the ranks of the "Sairey Gamps." At the age of 24, she was given encouragement by Dr. Ward Howe, a philanthropist from the United States and friend of the Nightingale family. She was also encouraged by one of the first female physicians in America, Dr. Elizabeth Blackwell, a close friend and confidante.

Since there were no schools of nursing, Miss Nightingale visited hospitals in an attempt to observe nursing as it was practiced by untrained individuals. She not only visited hospitals in England but traveled abroad to tour hospitals and orphanages in France, Egypt, and Greece. A trip to Kaiserswerth, Germany in

1850 was the most significant. Although the training program offered was inadequate in many respects, Miss Nightingale was pleased with the Institution of Protestant Deaconesses under the direction of Pastor Theodor Fliedner and his wife. In 1851, at the age of 31, she became a student nurse and spent three

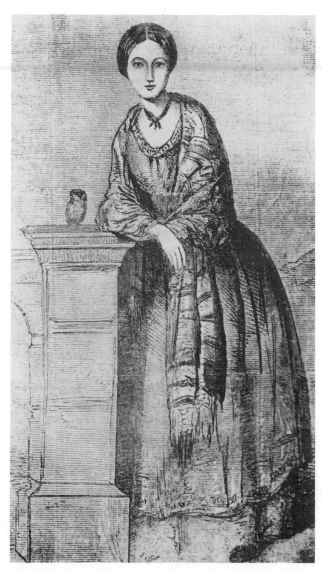

Fig. 5-1 Florence Nightingale was an attractive young girl and it was expected that she would marry and raise a family.

months in training. Although bred as a lady and accustomed to being waited upon, she never shirked the hard duties assigned to her at Fliedner's School. After completing the training program at Kaiserswerth, she went to Paris to work with the Sisters of Charity and to observe surgery performed by famous and skilled French physicians.

Although Miss Nightingale was delighted to have the training in Germany and France, she was very much aware that the programs were inadequate to prepare the kind of nurse she envisioned. It was these experiences which motivated her to later devote much of her time to the upgrading of nursing education.

As a graduate nurse her first position was superintendent of the Establishment for Gentlewomen During Illness, where she cared for homeless women and governesses. In addition to providing nursing care, she became concerned about their social needs. Through her friend, Sir Sidney Herbert, she was able to find homes for many after discharge from the hospital. In some cases, positions were arranged for the governesses in England and America.

THE CRIMEAN WAR

In 1853, war broke out in the Crimea. England and France were assisting Turkey against Russia. Nursing care was provided for the French and Russian soldiers by the different orders of nursing sisters from the two countries. However, the British soldier was nearly neglected as there were no organized services to care for the wounded and sick. A newspaperman, W. H. Russell of the *Times,* gave an account of the disgraceful conditions which existed and the English people were horrified. This expose forced the English government to take action. Sir Sidney Herbert, the Secretary of War, immediately thought of Florence Nightingale and wrote to her asking her to consider going to the battlefield. Miss Nightingale in the meantime, having read the *Times* account of the conditions in the Crimea, decided that going to the Crimean theater would give her an opportunity to utilize her knowledge and experience. She wrote to Sir Herbert offering her services in the organization of nursing services for the wounded. Their letters are believed to have crossed in the mail.

Miss Nightingale found thirty-eight women, some of whom were untrained as nurses but were committed to providing nursing care to the sick and wounded soldiers. Initially there were ten Roman Catholic sisters, fourteen Anglican nuns, and fourteen nurses with practical hospital nursing experience. The number later grew to 125 nurses and untrained volunteers.

On October 21, 1854, the British nurses set out for Scutari. The conditions they encountered were extremely frustrating and utterly chaotic. The resident medical officers resented women being assigned to the front lines and antici-

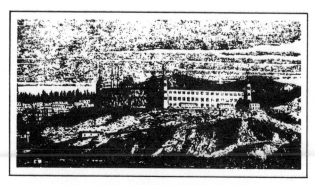

Fig. 5-2 The barrack hospital at Scutari

pated problems would be caused by their presence. The women were assigned to barrack hospital in Scutari, which was built to accommodate 1700 patients; yet, three times that number of patients were crowded together on the wards. Soldiers were lying on beds of unclean straw, in dirty uniforms saturated with old, dried blood. Dirt was everywhere, cholera was prevalent and amputations were frequently performed without anesthesia. Sanitation was poor and toilet facilities were deplorable. Rats and mice scurried across the ward floor while lice and bedbugs added to the discomfort of the patients. Food was not nutritious and hardly even edible. The men often ate with their fingers as eating utensils were nonexistent. The nurses found no soap, towels, basins or clean linen to bathe the patients.

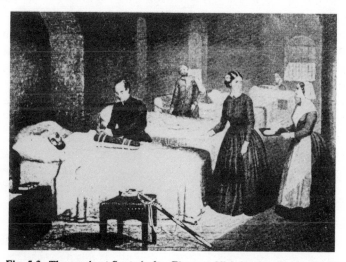

Fig. 5-3 The wards at Scutari after Florence Nightingale arrived and took over the hospital

Ignoring the scorn of the medical staff, who were not in agreement with women being assigned to the warfront, Miss Nightingale and her nurses went about the tasks at hand. Patiently, the nurses tended the ill and wounded soldiers and did what they could to improve the deplorable conditions. It did not take the doctors and officers long to realize that Miss Nightingale was a valuable asset. Not only could she organize nursing care, but she also had money and many influential friends. Finally, with the full support of the medical staff, Miss Nightingale and her staff began to make changes. From the age of thirty-two, she had received an annual allowance of $2,500 from her father, and in characteristic philanthropic style, Florence Nightingale used the allowance to purchase the badly needed supplies. She ordered hundreds of scrub brushes and the nurses set about cleaning. She set up diet kitchens and provided hot, balanced meals. She had screens built and placed between beds to provide a measure of privacy and to shield patients from watching amputations and other crude surgery. Miss Nightingale also realized the needs of convalescing soldiers. She established a canteen, reading room, diversional activities, allotment deduction plan for families of soldiers, and had volunteers write letters for those soldiers who could not write home.

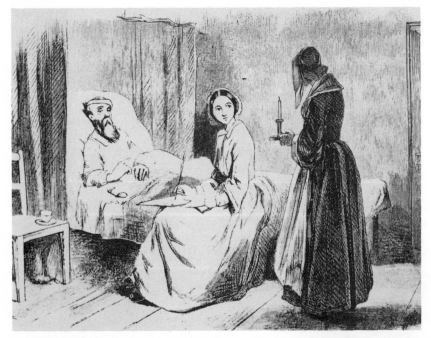

Fig. 5-4 This scene shows Florence Nightingale making her evening rounds. One of her nurses is writing a letter for a dying soldier.

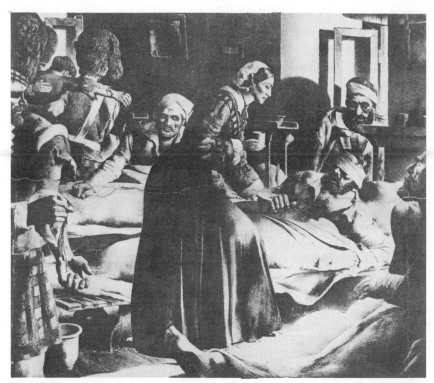

Fig. 5-5 Florence Nightingale in the Crimea. (Courtesy Parke, Davis and Company, ©1953)

When the nurses arrived in Scutari, the death rate was 50 to 60 percent. Within six months, that rate was reduced to 2 percent. Miss Nightingale found initially that no care at all was provided during the night, and many men died that could have been saved if some kind of supervision had been provided. Thus, every night she made rounds with her lamp. This activity which she performed religiously, endeared her to the wounded and ill, and immortalized her as The Lady With the Lamp, figure 5-6, page 78.

POSTWAR ACHIEVEMENTS

While in the Crimea, Miss Nightingale contracted Crimean fever, which was possibly typhus or typhoid fever. The illness sapped her physical strength and left her a semi-invalid for the rest of her life. However, Miss Nightingale's determination and mental vitality was quite intact. She returned to England in 1856 with plans to do something about improving the training of nurses. Her own training experiences and the observations she made of poorly trained nurses in the Crimea, convinced her that an organized program was badly needed.

Miss Nightingale's work in the Crimea had not gone unnoticed in England. Queen Victoria bestowed upon her the badge of honor that carried the Cross of St. George, England's royal emblem. The English queen and the Sultan of Turkey gave Miss Nightingale lavish jewels in gratitude for her unselfish service. Because of the vast statistical reports she had prepared based upon original research projects she had undertaken, Miss Nightingale was made a Fellow of the Royal Statistical Society. Grateful soldiers, their families, and private citizens contributed about $220,000 to a fund, later named the "Nightingale Fund," which was to be used in the establishment of a training school for nurses. The school was established in 1860 at St. Thomas Hospital in London.

While in the Crimea, Miss Nightingale had become interested in the off-duty life of the British soldier. She had implemented numerous reforms which provided services for the families of soldiers living in the camp: entertainment which was more wholesome than that locally available, better food, clothing, and housing. After her return to England, her attention turned to the British soldiers assigned to India, where the death rate due to disease was phenomenal. She began to study the situation and soon discovered that the lack of sanitation was undoubtedly contributing to the high death rate of soldiers. Through her leadership, a sewage disposal system was installed, more suitable clothing for the warm environment was provided, and better food was made available for the soldiers. The death rate dropped from 69 percent to 5 percent.

The Nightingale School for Nurses

Miss Nightingale advocated nursing as both an art and a science. She strongly believed that the focus of a training

SANTA FILOMENA

Whene'er a noble deed is wrought,
Whene'er is spoken a noble thought,
    Our hearts, in glad surprise,
    To higher levels rise.

The tidal wave of deeper souls
Into our inmost being rolls,
    And lifts us unawares
    Out of all meaner cares.

Honor to those whose words or deeds
Thus help us in our daily needs,
    And by their overflow
    Raise us from what is low!

Thus thought I, as by night I read
Of the great army of the dead,
    The trenches cold and damp,
    The starved and frozen camp,—

The wounded from the battle-plain,
In dreary hospitals of pain,
    The cheerless corridors,
    The cold and stony floors.

Lo! in that house of misery
A lady with a lamp I see
    Pass through the glimmering gloom,
    And flit from room to room.

And slow, as in a dream of bliss,
The speechless sufferer turns to kiss
    Her shadow, as it falls
    Upon the darkening walls.

As if a door in heaven should be
Opened and then closed suddenly,
    The vision came and went,
    The light shone and was spent.

Fig. 5-6   Henry Wadsworth Longfellow wrote this poem about "Santa Filomena," which means Saint Nightingale.

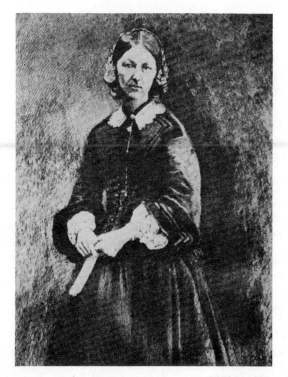

Fig. 5-7 Florence Nightingale about 1856, taken by order of the Queen shortly after her return from the Crimea

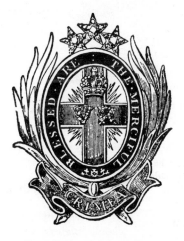

Fig. 5-8 The Nightingale Jewel

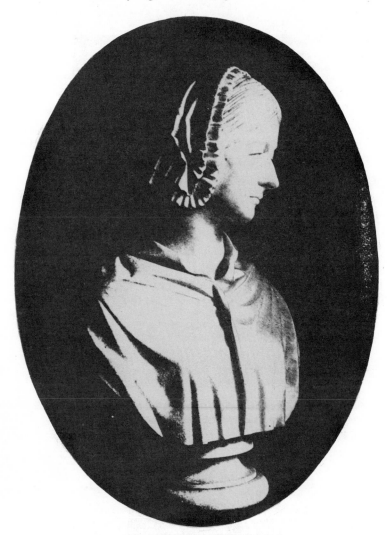

Fig. 5-9 This bust was presented to Miss Nightingale after the Crimean War, by the soldiers she had nursed. The bust is the work of Sir John Steele.

school should be nursing education rather than nursing service. She felt the curriculum should be flexible and should stress compassion and empathy for the patient. She insisted that the patient was to be treated as a whole person and not as a disease entity. She also realized that clinical practice and theory must be correlated to ensure quality education. Miss Nightingale's philosophy of educating nurses in an endowed school, independent of nursing service in the hospital, is widely accepted by nursing educators today.

With monies from the "Nightingale Fund," a building was purchased to house the nursing students. Under Miss Nightingale's supervision a matron was appointed for the school and St. Thomas Hospital was selected for the clinical experience. The purpose of the school was to train women to work as hospital nurses and district nurses for the sick poor. This trained nurse was a forerunner of the public health nurse. It was expected that these educated nurses would ultimately establish nursing education programs in England and abroad. Admission criteria were developed and all applicants were thoroughly screened according to these criteria. The highly selective nature of the admission process is reflected in the numbers of applicants and students. Annually, 15 to 30 students were selected from 1,000 to 2,000 applicants. Expenses were paid by the Nightingale Fund for those students who could not afford the cost of the program.

Fifteen probationers constituted the first class when the school opened in 1860, under the direction of the matron, Mrs. Wardroper. The program was one year in length. Students were given thirty-six hours of theoretical study, consisting of twelve hours of Anatomy and Surgical Nursing, twelve hours of Physiology and Medical Nursing, twelve hours of Chemistry, Food and Sanitation and

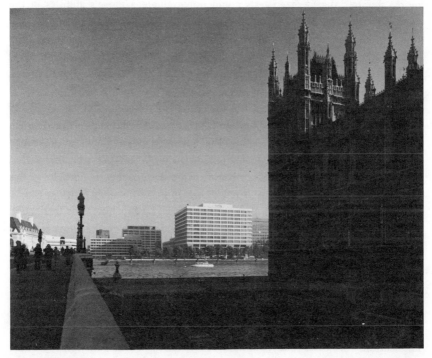

Fig. 5-10 St. Thomas Hospital in London as seen from Westminster Bridge by the Houses of Parliament

lectures on ethics and professionalism. Case studies were required. Evaluation and testing was done by the school matron. In 1875, a clinical instructor was hired to take the students on rounds with doctors to observe symptoms, treatment and response to treatment. The instructor acted as a role model in demonstrating nursing procedures and other aspects of nursing care. All faculty members were paid by the Nightingale Fund and closely supervised by Miss Nightingale herself. Miss Nightingale gave an annual address to her students, counseled them frequently, and wrote letters of encouragement.

As Miss Nightingale observed the nursing students, she began to see the need to promote efficiency and to conserve the nurse's time and energy. The changes she brought about hardly seem innovative today, but in the nineteenth century hospital they were very exciting. Dumbwaiters were constructed to carry the diet trays to the upper floors; hot water was piped to each patient ward; and a call-bell system was installed.

Graduates of the school were not licensed as they are today. In fact, Miss Nightingale did not approve of licensing examinations because she felt there were no outside groups capable of testing the knowledge of nurses. Furthermore, she felt that written tests could not evaluate a nurse's abilities in the "arts" of nursing or clinical practice. She did encourage her students to continue their education after graduation and stressed that learning must not stop upon graduation. Graduates of the Nightingale School were later head nurses in Scotland, Germany, Norway, Sweden, Canada, the United States, South Africa, India and Australia.

Being a semi-invalid most of her life, Miss Nightingale spent her days and nights doing research and writing books and articles. She kept a diary, which was customary in her day, and kept in touch with friends and colleagues through volumes of correspondence. Because Miss Nightingale was such a prolific writer, it is impossible to review all of her books, pamphlets, papers, and articles in this short chapter. Therefore, only a few of her more well-known writings can be mentioned. Miss Nightingale's first publication was a brochure, *The Institution of Kaiserswerth on the Rhine for the Practical Training of Deaconesses under the Direction of the Rev. Pastor Fliedner, Embracing the Support and Care of a Hospital, Infant and Industrial Schools, and a Female Penitentiary,* which interestingly was printed by the inmates of the London Ragged Colonial Training School in 1851. At her own expense, Miss Nightingale printed *Notes on the British Army,* which discussed the improvement of sanitation in the camps of peacetime soldiers, a topic on which she was well versed. An article which has implications for nurses today, *Subsidiary Notes as to the Introduction of Female Nursing into Military Hospitals in Peace and War,* brought about substantial changes in attitudes concerning the usefulness of nurses. *Notes on Nursing:*

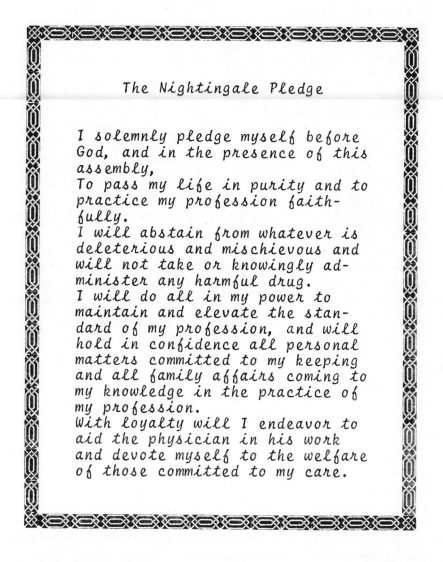

The Nightingale Pledge

I solemnly pledge myself before God, and in the presence of this assembly,
To pass my life in purity and to practice my profession faithfully.
I will abstain from whatever is deleterious and mischievous and will not take or knowingly administer any harmful drug.
I will do all in my power to maintain and elevate the standard of my profession, and will hold in confidence all personal matters committed to my keeping and all family affairs coming to my knowledge in the practice of my profession.
With loyalty will I endeavor to aid the physician in his work and devote myself to the welfare of those committed to my care.

Fig. 5-11 The Nightingale Pledge was formulated in 1893 by a committee of which Mrs. Lystra E. Gretter, R.N., was the chairman. It was first administered to the 1893 graduating class of the Farrand Training School, now the Harper Hospital, Detroit, Mich.

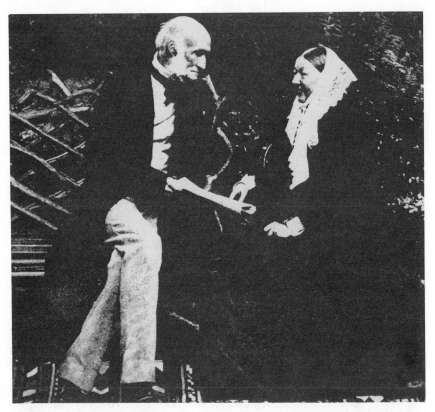

Fig. 5-12 Miss Nightingale chats with a friend on the lawn of Claydon House, 1889.

What It Is, and What It Is Not, was a best selling textbook which she wrote for her students and was translated into several languages.

Florence Nightingale died in her sleep on August 13, 1910 at the age of ninety. It was her wish to be buried in the family grave in Willow, Hampshire, and although it was proposed that she be interred in Westminster Abbey, her wishes were fulfilled.

SUMMARY

Although Florence Nightingale made valuable contributions to health reform in prisons, workhouses, and in the military, she is best remembered for her work in hospital organization and nursing education. During her lifetime she was the leading authority on all matters regarding nursing and acted as a consultant throughout the world. Miss Nightingale envisioned nursing as it exists today. She is credited with giving to nursing, concepts based on sound educational principles and a high regard for professional ethics.

SUGGESTED ACTIVITIES

- Make a poster or decorate a bulletin board which depicts the contributions Florence Nightingale made to society.

- Make a list of attributes and characteristics other than those mentioned in the text, which Florence Nightingale might have considered desirable for nurses in her era.

- Obtain a copy of the philosophy of the nursing program in which you are enrolled and compare it with the philosophy of the Nightingale School.

REVIEW

A. Multiple Choice. Select the best answer.

1. Florence Nightingale received her basic training in nursing
   a. from her governess.
   b. at the Institution of Protestant Deaconesses.
   c. from the Sisters of Charity.
   d. during the war.

2. The first nursing position held by Miss Nightingale was
   a. hospital nurse in Paris.
   b. night nurse in the army barracks.
   c. instructor of practical nurses.
   d. Superintendent of the Establishment of Gentlewomen During Illness.

3. A title given Miss Nightingale by Longfellow, based upon her nightly rounds in Scutari, was
   a. Angel of Mercy.   c. The Organization Woman.
   b. The Lady With the Lamp.   d. none of these.

4. Miss Nightingale was a semi-invalid most of her life after being stricken, probably with
   a. smallpox.   c. yellow fever.
   b. diphtheria.   d. typhoid fever.

5. The first formal nursing education had its beginning
   a. at St. Thomas Hospital.
   b. at The Nightingale School for Nurses.
   c. at The Fliedner's Institute.
   d. a and b above.

6. After the war, Florence Nightingale devoted many years of her life in improving health and environmental conditions for British soldiers in
   a. England.   c. The Crimea.
   b. Scutari.   d. India.

7. The purpose of the Nightingale School was
   a. to train hospital nurses.
   b. to prepare nursing leaders and educators.
   c. to train public health nurses.
   d. all of the above.

8. Miss Nightingale's success in Scutari can best be seen in
   a. the great admiration for her by patients, doctors and officers.
   b. the improvement in nursing care.
   c. the drastic reduction in the mortality rate.
   d. the many honors bestowed upon her.

9. Miss Nightingale's famous nursing text was called
   a. *On Trained Nursing.*
   b. *Notes on Nursing: What It Is and What It Is Not.*
   c. *A Summary on the Ethical Practice of Trained Nurses.*
   d. none of the above.

10. Miss Nightingale made great contributions in the areas of
    a. public health.   c. education.
    b. nursing.   d. all of these.

B. Briefly answer the following questions.

1. (a) How did Florence Nightingale's social status, contacts with influential persons, and family finances help in her pursuit of a nursing career?

   (b) What are some evidences that Florence Nightingale upgraded the nursing profession?

2. State reasons why Miss Nightingale opposed registration (certification, licensure) for nurses.

chapter 6
THE VANGUARDS OF NURSING IN AMERICA

STUDENT OBJECTIVES

- Identify some of the early nursing leaders in the United States.
- Describe the disaster relief activities of the American Red Cross.
- Identify the major contributions made by American leaders in nursing.

In the early nineteenth century, the status of nursing in the United States was not unlike that in England prior to the influence of Florence Nightingale. Large city hospitals were in existence and nurses were haphazardly trained in the hospital. There were few trained nurses and no formal training programs. The Civil War, much like the Crimean War in the case of England, brought the need for skilled nurses to the attention of government agencies, and brought about the first major reforms in nursing in this country. In the latter half of the century, the growing sense of social responsibility for health, the improved status of women in society, and the influence of the Nightingale concept, all contributed to the development of nursing education and improved nursing practice. The United States produced many women who greatly influenced nursing during the same period that Florence Nightingale made her reforms, and later. Unfortunately, because of necessary limitations, only a few of these leaders can be mentioned in this text.

DOROTHEA LYNDE DIX (1802-1887)

Born in Maine to a poverty-stricken family, Dorothea Dix experienced an unhappy childhood. At the age of twelve, she left home to live in Boston with a grandmother who was later to leave Dorothea financially self-sufficient. At the age of fourteen, encouraged by her grandmother, Miss Dix embarked on a teaching career. She studied to be a teacher and taught wealthy girls in her grandmother's home, and poor children in a room over the stable.

By the time Dorothea Dix reached the age of twenty-one, her health began to fail as a result of the driving force which governed her work habits. She developed tuberculosis and spent over a year resting in the home of William Rathbone in England. Returning to Boston in 1837, she was asked to teach a Sunday school class in an institution where conditions were inhumane. It was this initiation to the plight of the mentally ill, confined to cages and often beaten, chained, and naked in a cold and filthy environment, that aroused the sense of social justice within her. She traveled all over America convincing state legislators to pass bills providing more humane treatment for the mentally ill. Through tireless efforts over a twenty-year period, Dorothea Dix brought about government control of state mental hospitals. As a result, commitment to a mental institution was based on diagnosis by the physician; treatment and care was carefully supervised; and the use of restraints became limited.

When the Civil War broke out in 1861, Miss Dix became a volunteer nurse and was appointed the Superintendent of Women Nurses for All Military Hospitals. This was the first United States Army Nurse Corps. She was never educated as a nurse but, nonetheless, was an exceptionally capable administrator and organizer. She was not afraid to reprimand physicians or nurses for neglect of duty. Like Florence Nightingale, Miss Dix did not seek public acclaim and never accepted remuneration for her efforts.

CLARA BARTON (1821-1912)

Born in North Oxford, Massachusetts on Christmas Day, Clara Barton was destined for great accomplishments in life, figure 6-1. Although she was shy, her determination and independence won her many friends and followers. At a time when career women were looked upon with skepticism, Miss Barton made great strides. She was a teacher during a period when teaching positions for women were limited. She worked in the offices of the federal government in Washington and paved the way for women in the volunteer service during the Civil War.

Clara Barton was granted permission to take the volunteer services to the field hospitals. For these efforts, she was affectionately referred to as *The Angel of the Battlefield*. She is remembered for the impartiality expressed in the nursing care she rendered to both whites and blacks, Northerners and Southerners. The armies were in need of medical supplies, proper clothing, food and bedding. She delivered supplies to the medical officers, cooked for the soldiers, and nursed the wounded. Miss Barton, however, recognized the need for more than the necessities of life and rendered services to meet the emotional and spiritual needs of the men. After the war had ended, she assumed responsibility for locating missing soldiers and marking the graves of soldiers in a national cemetery on the Andersonville grounds.

In 1869, Clara Barton visited friends in Geneva, Switzerland who introduced her to the Red Cross idea and the book, *A Memory of Solferino,* written by

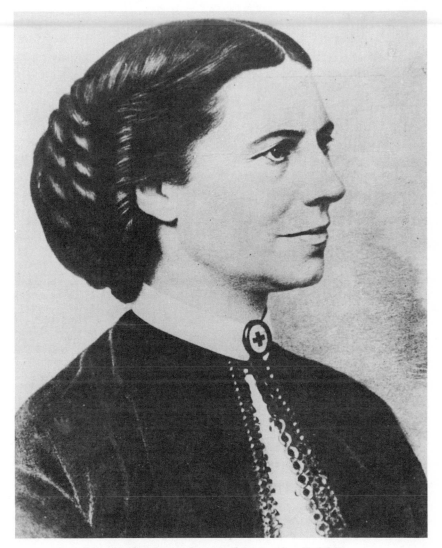

Fig. 6-1 Clara Barton, founder of the American Red Cross

Jean Henri Dunant, figure 6-2. In this book, printed in 1862, Henri Dunant described the deplorable war conditions from which the Red Cross idea evolved. He conceived of a neutral organization, devoted to nursing the wounded of war. In 1881, Clara Barton formed the American Association of the Red Cross, and served as its first president. Disaster relief has been one of the chief tasks of the Red Cross and the organization today is recognized for its invaluable services to the victims of floods, fire, earthquakes, epidemics, and war, to name just a few.

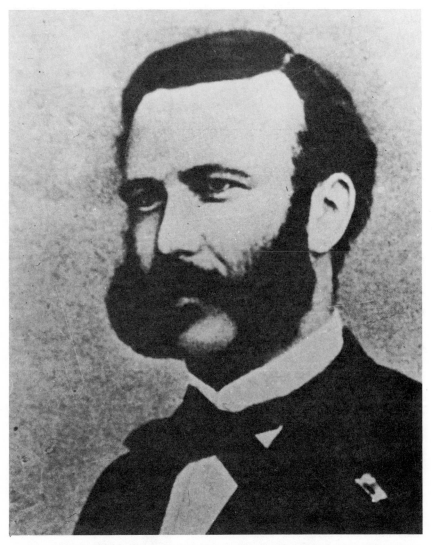

Fig. 6-2 Jean Henri Dunant formulated a plan for the relief of war victims.

Disaster services include first aid stations for patient care, assistance to families in finding and identifying their dead, supplementation of nursing services in hospitals, and assistance in immunization programs. The Red Cross Blood Program provides blood without charge to hospitals and physicians for victims of disasters. Food, clothing and shelter are provided to individuals and families who have lost their homes.

The Red Cross also offers three home nursing courses: Home Nursing, Mother and Baby Care, and Mother's Aide. There are also programs in blood bank nursing and training programs for volunteer nurses' aides. The Red Cross works in cooperation with all community, national and international health organizations.

Miss Barton built a home in Glen Echo, Maryland in 1897, constructed in part from lumber salvaged from the emergency shelters built during the 1889 Johnstown flood. The house also served as the national headquarters of the American Red Cross until 1904. The home was deeded to the National Park Service and is open to the public.

LINDA RICHARDS (1841-1930)

After graduation from the New England Hospital for Women and Children, Linda Richards became the first trained nurse in America. She completed the one-year program in Boston in 1873. Immediately upon graduating, she accept-

ed a position as night superintendent at Bellevue Hospital in New York. In an attempt to make an accurate, detailed report to the nursing director each morning, she made notes on each patient. Physicians also found this system of value to them and from this, the system of medical records evolved. In 1874 Miss Richards became superintendent of the nursing school of the Massachusetts General Hospital, where she assumed teaching duties in addition to providing direct patient care. Today this school is called the Massachusetts General Hospital School of Nursing.

Linda Richards went to England to study nursing methods and became acquainted with Miss Nightingale. Upon

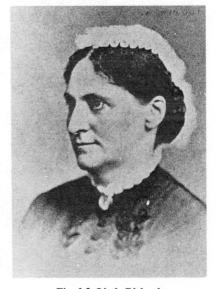

Fig. 6-3 Linda Richards

her return to the United States, she served as a consultant in organizing nursing service in hospitals throughout the country. In 1885 Miss Richards again left her homeland and went to Japan to set up the first nurse training program in Kyoto. The school opened in 1887 with Miss Richards acting as both director and lecturer. Textbooks were translated into Japanses and the classes were conducted with the aid of an interpreter. She remained in this position for four years. The latter years of her career were devoted to the establishment of nursing schools in hospitals for the mentally ill.

The National League for Nursing presents the Linda Richards Award to a nurse actively engaged in nursing who has made a significant contribution to nursing. Criteria in the selection of the recipient of the award are that the contribution be unique, of a pioneer nature, and be deserving of national recognition. Nominations are submitted by the NLN members, constituent leagues, nursing school faculties and agency members. The award is presented in a special ceremony during the National League for Nursing biennial convention.

ISABEL HAMPTON ROBB (1860-1910)

One of the most outstanding graduates of the Bellevue Hospital Training School, Isabel Hampton did not enter nursing until the age of twenty-six. Having been a school teacher in Canada, she brought educational theory to her role as the superintendent of the Illinois Training School. She implemented a graded system of theory and practice. Students received clinical experience on the wards of Cook County Hospital in Chicago and Miss Hampton arranged for private duty experience by means of affiliation. She was a firm believer in a three-year training program and worked tirelessly to institute an eight-hour day for nurses rather than the usual twelve-hour day. She also advocated rest periods and study hours. Miss Hampton was among the first nurses to recognize the importance of licensure as a protection for the patient.

Miss Hampton married Dr. Hunter Robb in 1894, which dismayed some of the active feminists who were her colleagues; however, Mrs. Robb demonstrated that it was possible to have

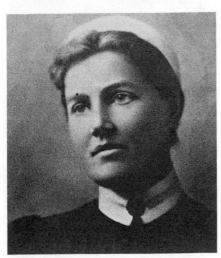

Fig. 6-4 Isabel Hampton Robb

both a career and a marriage. She wrote nursing textbooks, became involved in the formation of the first national nurses organization, Nurses Associated Alumnae of the United States and Canada, and was one of the founders of the *American Journal of Nursing.*

LAVINIA L. DOCK (1858-1956)

One of the early graduates of the Bellevue Hospital Training School, Miss Dock was night superintendent at Bellevue Hospital. Later, she became assistant to Isabel Hampton Robb at Johns Hopkins and the Illinois Training School. Miss Dock made a study of professional organization bylaws and was instrumental in using her knowledge in the establishment of an organization of nursing school superintendents in 1894. This Society of Superintendents became the National League of Nursing Education, which is today The National League for Nursing. Miss Dock is best known for her *History of Nursing* which has become the classic text on nursing history.

MARY ELIZA MAHONEY (1845-1926)

Miss Mahoney graduated from the New England Hospital for Women and Children in 1879 as the first black professional nurse in America. In 1909, she

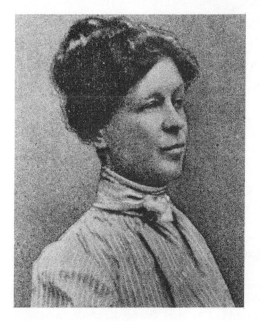

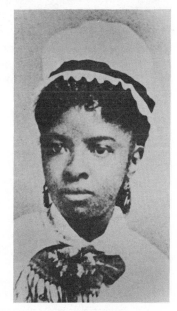

Fig. 6-5 Lavinia L. Dock.   Fig. 6-6 Mary Mahoney.

gave the welcoming address before the gathering of the National Association of Colored Graduate Nurses. She devoted her life to giving quality nursing care to private duty patients. She worked for the acceptance of the blacks in the nursing profession. After her death in 1926, the National Association of Colored Graduate Nurses established an award to be presented to an outstanding black nurse. The first award was presented in 1936. Today, the American Nurse's Association

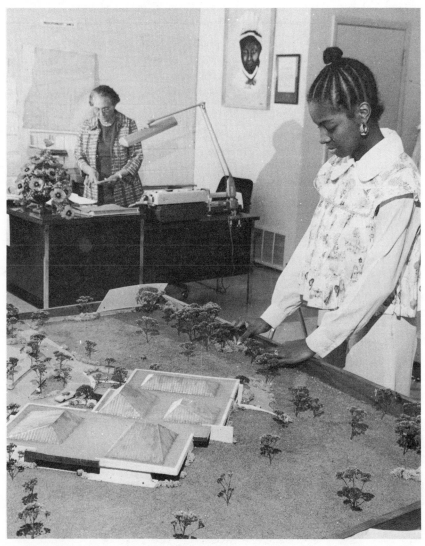

Fig. 6-7 Prospective student observing model of the Mary Mahoney Health Center facility. Portrait of Mary Mahoney hangs on right wall

presents the Mary Mahoney award biennially to persons instrumental in promoting equal opportunities in nursing to minority persons. The Community Health Project, Inc., a nonprofit corporation funded by the Department of Health, Education and Welfare (DHEW) has established a center in her memory; it is located in Oklahoma and provides health care services to isolated communities.

LILLIAN D. WALD (1867-1940)

In 1893, Lillian Wald founded the Henry Street Settlement in New York City. The goal of this endeavor was to provide free nursing care to the sick poor on the lower east side of the city. This was the beginning of public health nursing in the United States.

Miss Wald's chief concern was that nursing school graduates be capable of providing quality nursing services in the home. She became interested in the need for nursing and social services among the poor, soon after she graduated from the New York Hospital School of Nursing. Her contributions to the development of public health nursing include lecturing at the Department of Nursing Education of Columbia University and serving as the first president of the National Organization for Public Health Nursing in 1912. The accomplishments of the Henry Street Settlement are recorded in two books authored by Miss Wald, *House on Henry Street* and *Windows on Henry Street.*

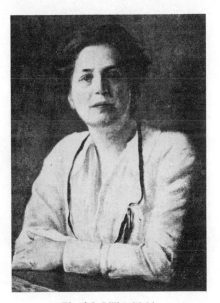

Fig. 6-8 Lillian Wald

MARY ADELAIDE NUTTING (1858-1947)

As a graduate of the first class of the Johns Hopkins School of Nursing, Miss Nutting continued the work of Isabel Hampton Robb. She raised the standards of nursing education and developed the department of nursing at Teachers College, Columbia University. She was given the title *First Professor of Nursing* and in 1944, the National League of Nursing Education awarded her the first medal for leadership. Members of the National League for Nursing submit, to an awards committee, nominations of individuals or groups whose achievements have made a significant contribution to nursing service or nursing education. During the biennial convention of the NLN, the Mary Adelaide Nutting award is presented in a special ceremony.

Miss Nutting was successful in establishing the eight-hour day for student nurses (something that Isabel Hampton Robb had advocated previously but did not accomplish). She established the three-year program with a probationary period prior to clinical experience. Many original concepts of nursing education were conceived by Miss Nutting. She coauthored a four-volume *History of Nursing* with Lavinia Dock and she was one of the persons responsible for the formation of the International Council of Nurses.

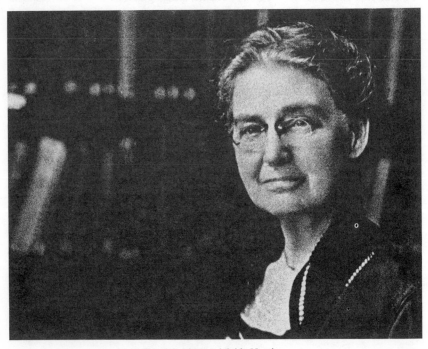

Fig. 6-9 Mary Adelaide Nutting

ANNIE W. GOODRICH (1876-1955)

Annie W. Goodrich was born into a family of professional persons and enjoyed an early life of extensive travel and social contacts; these were later to be an asset to her career. At the age of twenty-four, she entered the two-year nursing program at the New York Hospital Training School for Nurses. As Inspector for Training Schools in New York in 1910, she proved her ability as an outstanding leader, capable of making vital decisions to promote nursing to a professional status. She adhered strongly to high standards. Annie W. Goodrich assessed the ideas of Lillian D. Wald and Mary Adelaide Nutting and implemented them. Miss Goodrich and Miss Nutting were both strong-willed and determined and, although they were sometimes opposite in their views, they supported each other in nursing education endeavors.

Other accomplishments included serving as the president of the International Council of Nurses from 1912 to 1915, the American Federation of Nurses, the American Nurses' Association and the Association of Collegiate Schools of Nursing. She was Director of the Visiting Nurse Service of the Henry Street Settlement and Dean of Nursing at Yale University. She was Yale University's first female dean.

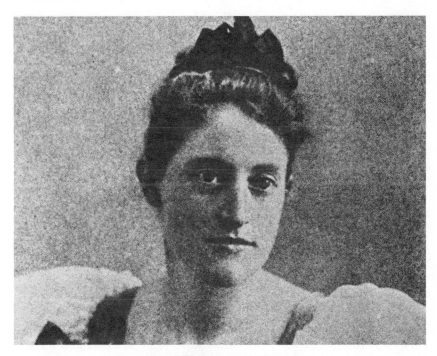

Fig. 6-10 Annie W. Goodrich

When World War I was declared it became apparent that more nurses were needed. Miss Goodrich laid plans for an Army School of Nursing. This earned her the Distinguished Service Medal in 1923. She was also involved in the development of the Vassar Training Camp, which was a twelve-week course for college women. Those who finished this course could then complete their nursing education in a two-year nursing program at selected general hospitals.

CLARA MAASS (1876-1901)

In 1895, 19-year-old Clara Maass graduated from the Nursing School at Newark German Hospital, and three years later became head nurse there. During the Spanish American War, she volunteered to become a contract nurse with the U.S. Army and served in Florida, Georgia, Cuba and the Philippines. After her discharge, she volunteered again in response to Major William C. Gorgas' call for nurses in Havana, where experiments were being carried out to prove the stegomyia mosquito was the yellow fever culprit. Miss Maass volunteered as a test subject and allowed herself to be bitten by a mosquito on June 4, 1901. She contracted a mild case of yellow fever, recovered, and because she doubted the slight fever gave her immunization, volunteered again and was bitten on August 14. She died ten days later at the age of 25. Miss Maass was the only American and the only woman to die during the experiments, which proved the stegomyia mosquito to be the yellow fever carrier and permitted conquest of the disease. In 1976, a commemorative stamp was issued by the U.S. Postal Service. It was the first stamp issued by the United States to honor an individual nurse.

A special medal commemorating Miss Maass' 100th birth anniversary was struck by the Franklin Mint as a part of its Special Commemorative Issues series for collectors. All proceeds, beyond expenses, are to be used for nursing scholarships.*

CONTEMPORARY LEADERSHIP IN NURSING

In 1973, the American Nurses' Association established a national Academy of Nursing. The Academy has as its central purpose, the exploration of broad issues and problems which affect nursing and health care. Thirty-six charter fellows were elected by the Board of Directors of the ANA and additional fellows are elected annually by members of the Academy. A nurse must demonstrate

*Medals are available for shipment by contacting Howard B. Hurley, Clara Maass Medal, Box 1248, Oradell, N.J. 07649. The Bronze medal is $6.50; the sterling silver is $19.50. Check or money order payable to RN Magazine should be sent to Mr. Hurley.

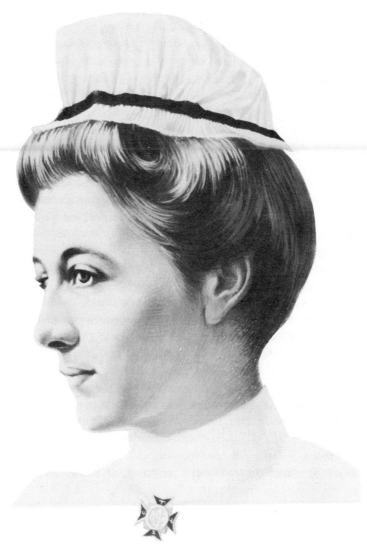

Fig. 6-11 Clara Maass gave her life to conquer yellow fever. (Courtesy RN Magazine, Oradell, N.J.)

outstanding contributions to nursing in order to be considered for a fellowship and thus the Academy gives formal recognition for excellence in nursing.

It would be impossible to name in this text all nurses who have made significant contributions to nursing. Therefore, only a few will be mentioned, and they will represent educators, administrators, researchers, and practitioners in the major divisions of practice.

One of the twentieth century's most creative and dynamic nurses was **Lydia Hall**. Ms. Hall had a particular interest in the way health care was delivered and what effect it had on patients and their families. After considerable experience and observation, she noted that when the patient began to recover and had to adjust to a medical regimen and residual weaknesses or disabilities, he was usually deprived of the attention of the nurse. Instead, because he was feeling much better, an auxiliary health worker was responsible for his care. Ms. Hall, however, felt that the nurse could be most helpful when the patient started to become involved in his recovery. She was so convinced of her hypothesis that she was able to influence the authorities of Montefiore Hospital and Medical Center in New York City to construct and open a health care facility which would be run by nurses. In 1963 Loeb Center for Nursing and Rehabilitation opened for business. The primary purpose of the facility was to demonstrate that nursing care provided by registered nurses only, to patients in the recovery phase of illness, reduces the period of hospitalization and prepares the patient to cope with his unique health problems at home. Ms. Hall's hypothesis was valid.

The Loeb Center facilitates and rewards excellence in clinical nursing and was one of the first innovations in clinical practice which allowed the nurse to function to the fullest potential. Ms. Hall, who died in 1969, is remembered for her unique perceptions of and approaches to clinical nursing.

The work of **Luther Christman** is centered around the improvement of nursing practice. His reputation was first established through his clinical practice. He has since been involved as an administrator, educator, and researcher in trying to develop a base for practice: organizational designs to facilitate the expression of clinical practice and educational programs to develop nursing as an applied science. The goal—to sharpen clinical practice. Dr. Christian has served as a consultant to many programs and has served on numerous professional and multidisciplinary committees in the United States and internationally. He has published in a wide variety of journals and books. Dr. Christman has received many honors for his work and is a Fellow of the American Academy of Nursing and of the Institute of Medicine of Chicago.

Research in nursing has been the significant contribution of **Dr. Faye Abdellah**. Dr. Abdellah served on the faculties of Yale University School of Nursing and Teachers College, Columbia University, where she was also a research fellow. She was chief of the Nursing Education Bureau, Division of Nursing Resources, United States Public Health Service, Department of Health, Education and Welfare, from 1949 to 1959. She has served as a nursing research consultant to the federal government and has written *Patient-Centered Approaches to Nursing* and *Better Patient Care Throgh Nursing Research.* Dr. Abdellah is one of the thirty-six charter fellows of the Academy of Nursing. She continues to provide leadership by directing and coordinating national health services research.

Dr. Hildegard Peplau has long been involved in graduate education in psychiatric nursing and has been responsible for redefining and upgrading psychiatric nursing practice. Dr. Peplau's innovations have established her as an authority on psychiatric nursing and her contributions to nursing have earned her a fellowship in the American Academy of Nursing. Dr. Peplau is the author of numerous professional texts and articles.

Dr. Mildred Montag was responsible for the establishment of nursing education programs in the community college setting. In 1952, her doctoral dissertation, *Education of Nursing Technicians,* led to the development of the Cooperative Research Project in Junior and Community College Education for Nursing, which she directed. Dr. Montag held many positions in nursing education and she has written many books and articles on nursing education and practices. She has received honorary degrees and she was a recipient of the NLN, Linda Richards Achievement Award, among many others.

Dr. Ruth Matheney was a pioneer in the establishment of associate degree programs in New York City and state university systems. She was a professor at City College of New York School of Nursing at the time of her death in 1973. Dr. Matheney was a leader in curriculum design and did considerable research on associate degree and baccalaureate nursing education.

Dr. Laurie M. Gunter, an educator, has long been interested in the unique problems of the elderly. Frustrated by the fact that preparation in geriatric nursing was not offered in most schools of nursing, Dr. Gunter became actively involved in the development of geriatric nursing practice and education on a national scale. As head of the ANA interim certification board for the division on geriatric nursing, Dr. Gunter has been responsible for bringing about recognition of excellence in geriatric nursing practice. She has also been instrumental in the development of graduate education in geriatrics. A recipient of numerous grants, Dr. Gunter has authored numerous professional papers and articles.

A graduate of the Frontier Nursing Service School of Midwifery and a certified nurse-midwife, **Reva Rubin** has had considerable experience in maternal-child health nursing and is one of the profession's foremost authorities on maternity nursing. She was among the first to introduce natural childbirth and the concept of *rooming-in* (the mother and newborn share a room). She also developed the first graduate and doctoral programs in maternity nursing. Ms. Rubin is recognized as one who seeks new knowledge, applies that knowledge and disseminates it, not only in the United States but on a worldwide scale. She serves as a consultant on maternal-child health nursing practice and education to many colleges and universities. She is much sought after as a speaker and is the author of many texts and articles.

The activities of the major professional nursing organizations have increasingly reflected the concerns and interests of the nursing community, the allied health professions, and the public. This responsiveness to the needs of nurses has given nursing organizations new growth and vitality. The profession in turn has benefited tremendously from the efforts of the professional organizations. Because of these organizations, nursing is now recognized and respected as one of the most vital and significant health professions. The nursing organizations can attribute this success to their members and leaders. Executive directors of professional organizations have provided leadership necessary to develop viable organizations and to promote the interests of the profession.

In 1970, when **Dr. Eileen Jacobi** assumed the position of executive director of the American Nurses' Association, the organization was in precarious condition. Recognizing potential and challenge, Dr. Jacobi set about to improve the ANA. Under her direction, the focus of ANA activities became assurance of quality. One of the most significant developments in the seventies was the establishment and implementation of standards for nursing practice. Dr. Jacobi stressed that when nurses recognize the need to be responsive and accountable to the public, the profession inevitably moves forward. Innovations in continuing education, improvements in the economic security of nurses, and the certification of practitioners, have been brought about through Eileen Jacobi's efforts.

As executive director of the New York State Nurses' Association, **Dr. Veronica M. Driscoll** identified the issues and provided the organization with the necessary leadership to bring about significant changes. Dr. Driscoll was the engineer behind the Nurse Practice Act passed in 1972, which was the first legal definition of nursing recognizing it as an independent practice. She also developed one of the early and most effective economic and general welfare programs on a state level. Through the process of collective bargaining, salaries, benefits, and working conditions of nurses employed in New York are being substantially improved and many practice issues are being resolved. Dr. Driscoll served as chairperson of the ANA Commission on Economic and General Welfare. She has written numerous professional articles and has served on many national committees.

Anne Zimmerman has spent most of her professional career in administrative positions of professional nursing organizations. She has been on the staff of the ANA, and the Montana, California, and Illinois Nurses Associations. She has received numerous awards and honors for her contributions to nursing. Most significant was the 1968 ANA honorary membership recognition for twenty-five years devoted to promoting and defending the right of nurses to organize and bargain collectively with employers through the professional organization. She served as the first chairperson of the ANA Commission on Economic and General Welfare. Ms. Zimmerman also served as the ANA representative to the Medical Workers Union Moscow Conference and as the U.S. representative to the World Health Organization-International Labor Organization. In June 1976, Anne Zimmerman was elected president of the American Nurses' Association.

Dr. Martha Rogers, former head of the New York University nursing division, has received numerous awards for her leadership and innovations in nursing. She has done considerable research and held a number of positions in the field of public health nursing as well. In 1976, as part of the bicentennial celebration of New York University alumni, a portrait of Dr. Rogers was unveiled; it now hangs in the nursing division offices.

Virginia Henderson deserves mention because she made great improvements in nursing library resources. Ms. Henderson served as director of the Yale project which developed *Nursing Studies Index*. She also founded the Interagency Council on Library Resources for Nursing. Through her influence the National Library of Medicine has expanded its scope to include nursing literature. She has worked very hard to obtain library resources and facilities for nursing by demonstrating that nursing is not unlike the other health science professions in terms of its need for resources.

Another leader, specifically in public health nursing, was **Pearl McIver.** Ms. McIver died in 1976. A story told about this perceptive, humane nurse centers around her student days. Assigned to night duty on pediatrics, during the 1918 flu epidemic, she ignored the restrictions placed on nursing care and proceeded to pick up the frightened, critically-ill children and rocked them to sleep one by one. This was done after her tour of duty was over. As a graduate, Ms. McIver served with the U.S. Public Health Service for twenty-four years. She was also a past president of the American Nurses' Association and vice-president of the American Public Health Association. She held other positions and received many honors during her lifetime. Among these was the highest international Red Cross nursing honor, the Florence Nightingale Medal.

In April of 1976, **Anna Fillmore,** the first general director and secretary of the National League for Nursing died at the age of 72. She was an outstanding leader in the field of community health services. She was instrumental in establishing the League as a national organization with membership open to professional and lay people who were interested in the improvement of nursing education and service. In her honor, the NLN established the Anna M. Fillmore Award which will be presented to a nurse "who is demonstrating, or has shown, unusual leadership in developing and administering community health services on a local, state or national level."

Ann Magnussen was an internationally recognized nursing leader. After serving in various capacities for the Red Cross, Ms. Magnussen retired as the national director of the American Red Cross Nursing and Health Programs in 1964. During her career she was chairman of the Nursing Advisory Committee of the League of Red Cross Societies in Geneva, Switzerland. She was the first vice-president of the American Nurses' Association board of directors. She, too, was a recipient of the Florence Nightingale Medal. Ann Magnussen died in 1976.

Again, the author emphasizes that it is impossible to list those many individuals who have contributed to the advancement of nursing: Lucile Notter, Jessie Scott, Lucile Petry Leone, Ruth Freeman, Mabel K. Staupers, Lucille Knopf, Carrie Lenburg, Jo Eleanor Elliott, Agnes Gelinas and countless others. Leaders are emerging daily to join the many who have made nursing the dynamic, vital profession it is today.

SUMMARY

The progress in organized nursing in the past one hundred years can be attributed to the dedicated efforts of many nurses. Many individual nurses have made significant contributions and the limits of space prevent recognition of all the devoted pioneers and innovators in nursing. The newly established Hall of Fame contains the names of some pioneers. The American Academy of Nursing provides for formal recognition of nurses who have demonstrated excellence and leadership in nursing, although that is not a central purpose of the Academy. Exploration of broad issues and problems which affect health care and nursing is the goal of its prestigious members.

SUGGESTED ACTIVITIES

- Interview a representative of the American Red Cross and obtain information on the functions of the local chapter in the school district. Inquire as to how the office is prepared to meet emergencies such as sudden war, tornadoes, earthquakes, floods, or epidemics.

- Select a nursing pioneer from those named for the Hall of Fame. Prepare a report and document your findings with bibliography references.

- Contact local hospitals, the district and state nursing associations and inquire about historical memorabilia which might be preserved. Ask

Dorothea Lynde Dix	Civil War superintendent of Army Nurses, pioneer in reforming care of the mentally ill.
Lavinia Lloyd Dock	Author of *Materia Medica for Nurses,* one of the first nursing textbooks; co-author of *History of Nursing;* first secretary of the International Council of Nurses; political activist.
Martha M. Franklin	Active campaigner for racial equality in nursing. Organizer and first president of the National Association of Colored Graduate Nurses.
Annie Warburton Goodrich	Crusader, educator, and diplomat, active in nursing affairs at local, state, national, and international level.
Stella Goostray	President of the National League of Nursing Education, secretary of the National League of Nursing Education for eleven years, director of nursing services and school at Boston Children's Hospital.
Clara Louise Maass	Dedicated nurse who gave her life for scientific research on the cause of yellow fever.
Mary Eliza Mahoney	America's first black professional nurse. Biennial ANA award and health center facility for health aid to isolated communities named for her.
Mary Adelaide Nutting	Noted educator who was instrumental in the development of university education for nurses. Co-author of *History of Nursing.* First nurse to be named a university professor at Columbia University. Principal of the nursing school at Johns Hopkins.
Sophia F. Palmer	First editor of the *American Journal of Nursing.* First president of the New York State Board of Nurse Examiners.
Linda Judson Richards	America's first trained nurse. Pioneer in industrial and psychiatric nursing.
Isabel Hampton Robb	A prime force in creation of the Nurses' Associated Alumnae of the United States and Canada (later the ANA).
Margaret H. Sanger	Founder of the birth control movement in America.
Isabel Maitland Stewart	Author of classic texts on nursing curricula and leader in nursing research.
Adah Belle Samuel Thoms	Crusader for equal rights for blacks in nursing in the American Red Cross and U.S. Army. President of NACGN.
Lillian D. Wald	Founded the forerunner to the Henry Street Settlement (later the Visiting Nurse Service of New York City), champion of improved child labor, pure food, and immigration laws; worker for city parks, recreation centers, better housing, education for the mentally retarded, and national health insurance.

Fig. 6-12 The first nurses named to Nursing's Hall of Fame

permission to examine the items pertinent to this era in nursing history and report findings to the class.

- Research two contemporary leaders in nursing and prepare a paper on their background, philosophy and accomplishments. Document your report.

- Arrange to visit the former home of Clara Barton in Glen Echo, Maryland near Washington, D.C. The home has been turned over to the National Park Service and is open to the public.

- Plan a visit to view the Nursing Archive Collection, Boston University.

REVIEW

A.   Multiple Choice. Select the best answer.

1. The early major reforms in England and the United States were brought about by
    a. establishment of large city hospitals.   c. the onset of war.
    b. Florence Nightingale.   d. the government.

2. Nursing practice and education were improved at the end of the nineteenth century because of
    a. a growing sense of social responsibility for health.
    b. the changing status of women.
    c. the influence of Florence Nightingale.
    d. all of the above.

3. An early reform in the care of the mentally ill was
    a. the establishment of endowed mental hospitals.
    b. administrative control of mental hospitals by doctors.
    c. diagnosis of mental illness by a physician before commitment was made.
    d. the use of restraints to control psychotic patients.

4. The first system of organized medical records was started
    a. at Bellevue Hospital.   c. by army officers.
    b. by Nightingale nurses.   d. none of these.

5. The Linda Richards Award is given to a nurse actively engaged in nursing who has made a significant contribution to nursing, by the
    a. ANA, annually.
    b. NLN, at its biennial convention.
    c. Bellevue Hospital School of Nursing Alumnae.
    d. Public Health Service.

6. The Society of Superintendents organized in 1894 later became
   a. the Council of Directors of Nursing.
   b. the American Nurses' Association.
   c. the National League for Nursing.
   d. the Illinois State Nurses Association.

7. The Mary Mahoney award is given to persons who have promoted equal opportunity in nursing for members of minority groups by the
   a. ANA, biennially.
   b. NLN, annually.
   c. National Association of Colored Graduate Nurses.
   d. NAACP.

8. The twelve-week summer nursing program established during World War I was
   a. developed by Isabel Robb.
   b. to prepare nurses for college teaching.
   c. the Cadet Corps.
   d. the Vassar Training Camp.

B. Match the statement in Column II with the appropriate nursing leader in Column I.

Column I	Column II
1. Annie Goodrich	a. An early leader in public health nursing.
2. Mary Eliza Mahoney	
3. Lillian Wald	b. Called the First Professor of Nursing.
4. Clara Barton	c. One of the first nurses to advocate licensure for consumer protection.
5. Mary Adelaide Nutting	
6. Isabel Hampton Robb	d. Brought about reforms in the care of the mentally ill.
7. Linda Richards	
8. Dorothea Dix	e. Founder of the American Red Cross.
	f. Yale University's first female dean.
	g. The Community Health Project, Inc. funded by HEW, was established in her memory.
	h. The first trained nurse in the United States.

C. Briefly answer the following questions.

1. Compare Florence Nightingale with Dorothea Dix in respect to family background, career education, goals and influence on government.
2. List several activities of the American Red Cross today.

chapter 7
THE EVOLUTION OF NURSING EDUCATION

STUDENT OBJECTIVES

- Recognize the influence of the early European schools of nursing on the development of nursing schools in the United States.
- Identify events and studies which brought about upgrading of nursing education.
- List changes which can be considered as improvements in nursing education.

The evolution of nursing education was influenced by the conditions and changes in society over the past 130 years. The development of science, medicine, humanitarian reform, the hospital industry, the feminist movement, and war, all brought about conditions that helped to carve the patterns of nursing education. In order to better serve society, nurses progressed from a very simple apprenticeship training to a highly organized, theoretical, and technical education.

EUROPEAN SCHOOLS OF NURSING

Early nurses did not receive formal training specifically designed to prepare them to care for the sick. Most often, women learned the art of nursing by working under the direction of experienced *nurses* or physicians. The school at Kaiserswerth was one of the first programs which was established to train women to care for the sick and poor. Theodor Fliedner, a Lutheran pastor and his wife, Fredericke Munster, operated the school which was first not to require religious vows and permitted students to leave at will. Students were taught simple nursing procedures, ethics, and religious doctrine. Upon completion of the brief training program, the graduate was qualified to perform nursing duties in homes, prisons, and hospitals and teach nursing.

The La Source program was founded in 1859 to prepare lay women to care for the sick in their homes. Countess Agenor de Gasparin founded the Normal Evangelical School of Independent Nurses for the Sick. The theory consisted of an hour class, held daily for five months, for a total of 120 hours. The students studied anatomy, physiology, hygiene, pathology, and nursing procedures. The length of each course was one month and each topic was studied in depth and completed before another subject was begun. Clinical lab experience occurred in private homes or clinics. At the completion of the program, the student was given an oral examination. The students wore no uniforms and were not called nurses.

The program later developed into a three-year program. The first nine months were considered a probationary period. After passing a comprehensive examination, the students became regular students and completed the three-year program. Clinical experience was received in a number of hospitals throughout Switzerland. The students qualified for a diploma in public health nursing after graduation, since the final four months were devoted to that specialty. In 1966, the government subsidized the school with an agreement that a minimum of 250 nurses would serve the country in times of emergency or war.

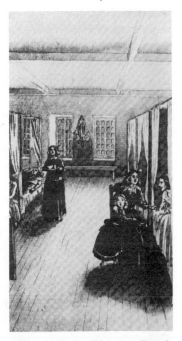

Florence Nightingale was the first to envision nursing education as a preparation for nursing practice. She advocated the establishment of nursing education in an endowed school, where the chief purpose was education rather than service. She also felt students should be taught and supervised by competent personnel. One of her goals for the Nightingale School was to produce educated, trained nurses who would be qualified to establish other training schools. She wanted nurses to be taught by nurses. Miss Nightingale firmly believed that nursing was a profession based on fundamental principles, and that it was distinct from the medical profession. She wanted nurses to be trained in a program of

Fig. 7-1 Jeanne Mance, a French nurse who established nursing services and education at the Hôtel Dieu in Montreal

systematic instruction, which included both theory and nursing skills. She felt nurses should provide quality services which were directly related to the needs of society. She believed that educators of nurses were responsible for the quality of nursing practice.

Miss Nightingale thought it necessary that nursing students live in a disciplined and closely supervised environment; therefore, the students were boarded in a nurses' home and carefully supervised by a housemother. Furthermore, she felt all graduate nurses should live in a nurses' home so that the school could continue to influence the lives and practice of its graduates. Miss Nightingale was very much concerned about the character and morality of nurses; both had to be beyond reproach.

EARLY NURSING EDUCATION IN THE UNITED STATES

During the first part of the nineteenth century the only organized preparation of nurses was in Catholic sisterhoods. Training was an apprenticeship and restricted to members of the order. The Nurse Society of Philadelphia, under the direction of Dr. Joseph Warrington, organized a school of nursing in 1839 which was patterned after the work of Elizabeth Fry in England. Basic lectures and demonstrations were offered, with a *Certificate of Approbation* granted if the student proved proficient. In 1861, the Women's Hospital of Philadelphia offered a six-month course designed to appeal to a higher class of young women. The courses included medical and surgical nursing, materia medica, and dietetics. A diploma was awarded upon completion of the program.

The first organized training schools were developed in the United States after the Civil War. They were established in large city and charitable hospitals. Hospitals were increasing in size and quantity and trained nurses were in short supply. The American Medical Association established a committee to study the shortage of trained nurses. In 1869, the committee made the recommendation that every large hospital should establish a school of nursing. In 1873 three nursing schools were opened. These first schools were sponsored by hospitals but were independent of the hospitals. There were many close ties between early leaders in the United States and Florence Nightingale, which explains why the new schools opened in this country were so similar to the Nightingale concept. Unfortunately, many of the independent schools soon found their funding inadequate and were forced to become a part of the hospital to which they were connected. This gradually led to the exploitation of students by hospitals who had found a new source of free labor. Formal education became secondary to nursing service in the hospital, a trend which did little to improve the quality of nursing practice.

Students were recruited from the ranks of wealthy, single, educated, and well-bred young women. Generally, schools sought mature young ladies who were college educated and between twenty-five and thirty-five years of age. The feminist movement in the United States was gaining momentum. Many young women were career-minded and looking for opportunities to leave home. Nursing was considered a humanitarian endeavor. Therefore, it was quite proper for a single woman to choose nursing as a career.

In the early schools instruction was all too frequently associated with practice rather than principles. In fact, formal instruction was quite limited for several reasons. First, there were very few educated nurses who were qualified to teach, and secondly, no one was quite sure what nurses should be taught. In 1894, Mary Agnes Snively, Superintendent of Nurses at Toronto General Hospital, presented a paper entitled, *A Uniform Curriculum for Training Schools,* at the first meeting of the Canadian Society of Superintendents of Training Schools for Nurses. However, most curriculums evolved from the experiences of the head nurses who determined the theory and practice essential to prepare a nurse. Hours of duty were long and students had one afternoon off every two weeks. The nurses often slept in rooms between patient rooms, as students were expected to tend to patients during the night. Student nurses lived in a hospital dormitory or nurses' home. Obedience was expected and discipline was severe, figure 7-2, page 112.

At first, America's nurses wore no uniforms. The early nurses saw no need for uniformity of dress and some even presented opposing views on the subject. Bellevue Hospital's nursing leaders agreed that it would be more sanitary and economical for the nurses to dress in regulated attire. The first cap appeared in 1875. It was not a fashion fetish but rather was intended to cover long hair that frequently was unclean due to the difficulty encountered in a shampoo-and-set procedure when plumbing and shampoo soap was very limited or nonexistent. Women often wore their hair long and straight, at waist level. The cap afforded the opportunity to push the hair up under the cap, out of view.

A tall, stately, and well-dressed young Bellevue student was asked by the school authorities to go home for two days and return with a proposed uniform. Euphemia Van Rensselaer became the first student nurse to wear a uniform. It was a blue and white striped cotton dress with a white apron, collar and cuffs, and a white cap. The length of the uniform in that period was two inches above the floor. Many variations of the uniform and cap were developed by nursing schools. Each school adopted an original cap, in which every nurse possessed deep pride. The well-groomed nurse wore a crisp white uniform after graduation and displayed her school pin and cap, symbols of major accomplishments.

In addition to caring for your 50 patients, each nurse will follow these regulations:

1. *Daily sweep and mop the floors of your ward, dust the patients' furniture and window sills.*

2. *Maintain an even temperature in your ward by bringing in a scuttle of coal for the day's business.*

3. *Light is important to observe the patient's condition; therefore, each day fill kerosene lamps, clean chimneys, and trim wicks. Wash windows once a week.*

4. *The nurse notes are important in aiding the physician's work. Make your pens carefully; you may whittle to your own individual taste.*

5. *Each nurse on day duty will report every day at 7 am and leave at 8 pm, except on the Sabbath on which day you will be off from 12 noon to 2 pm.*

6. *Graduate nurses in good standing with the director of nurses will be given an evening off each week for courting purposes, or two evenings each week if you go regularly to church.*

7. *Each nurse should lay aside from each pay day a goodly sum of her earnings for her benefits during her declining years, so that she will not become a burden. For example, if you earn $30.00 a month you should set aside $15.00.*

8. *Any nurse who smokes, uses liquor in any form, gets her hair done at a beauty shop, or frequents dancehalls, will give the director of nurses good reason to suspect her worth, intentions and integrity.*

9. *The nurse who performs her labors, serves her patients and doctors faithfully and is without fault for a period of 5 years, will be given an increase by the hospital administrator of 5¢ a day, providing there are no hospital debts that are outstanding.*

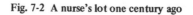

Fig. 7-2 A nurse's lot one century ago

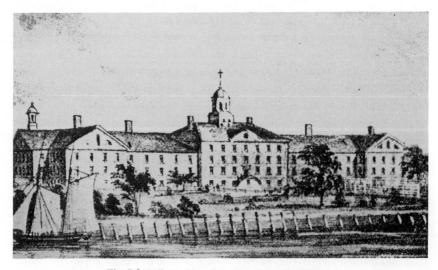

Fig. 7-3 Bellevue Hospital as it appeared in 1848

Three schools, Bellevue Hospital Training School in New York, Massachusetts Hospital Training School in Boston, and the Connecticut Training School in New Haven appeared in America during 1873. These schools greatly influenced the development of nursing education.

Bellevue Hospital School of Nursing

With the war behind them, women involved in the reform movement turned their interests and efforts toward the improvement of hospitals by improving nursing care within the existing institutions. One such group was the New York State Charities Aid Association, of which the Bellevue Hospital Visiting Committee was an integral part. Chairman of the committee was Louisa Lee Schuyler. The committee was influential in soliciting funds to aid the movement. Dr. Gill Wylie, a Bellevue intern, was sent to England to study the nursing schools established under Florence Nightingale. Although the Nightingale system was followed in New York, it was called the Bellevue System. The first director of the school was Sister Helen Bowden who trained in England.

The training program was one year in length, but students were required to remain a second year in service. Duties in the second year included private duty nursing in the patient's home, and head nursing. Nursing students received lodging, board and wages for their service. There was no formal class work. Students gained knowledge through practical experience on the hospital wards, figure 7-4. The head nurses on each ward were the instructors. In 1876, the school published the first nursing manual.

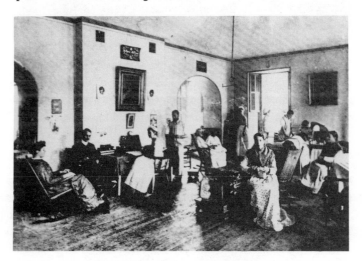

Fig. 7-4 Ward scene of the early days

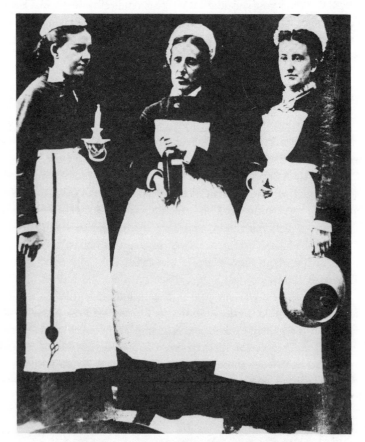

Fig. 7-5 Three of Bellevue's early head nurses

The Bellevue Hospital school continues to be one of the leading schools of nursing. In 1967, it became a part of Hunter College of the City University of New York. The school has produced many nursing leaders; among the early alumnae were Jane A. Delano, Isabel Hampton (Robb), and Lavinia L. Dock.

The New England Hospital for Women and Children

Dr. Marie Zakrzewska, an obstetrician, attempted to establish a training school for nurses at the New England Hospital for Women and Children in Boston, Massachusetts in 1861. Not until 1872, when Dr. Susan Dimock took charge, was the program very successful. Trained in Europe, Dr. Dimock was an advocate of the Kaiserswerth training school methods. The one-year program offered both lectures and practical experience. Both women doctors supervised the training of the nursing students. Probably the most famous of their alumnae was Linda Richards, America's first trained nurse.

Massachusetts General Hospital

The training school of the Massachusetts General Hospital in Boston was opened on November 1, 1873, with a class of six students. Because this was the first school to attempt a formalized instructional program, it is recognized as one of the pioneering schools in nursing education. However, the superintendent of the school, Mrs. Billings, was not a trained nurse. She had been a chief nurse in an army hospital during the Civil War and had worked for several months at Bellevue with Sister Helen. One of the early superintendents of the Massachusetts General Hospital school of nursing was Linda Richards. Miss Richards totally reorganized the school and implemented the Nightingale or Bellevue system.

The Connecticut Training School

At the request of the medical staff of New Haven Hospital, the Connecticut Training School was established in 1873. A graduate of Women's Hospital in Philadelphia, Miss Bayard, was the first superintendent. The school was totally independent of the hospital; this may have brought about its great success. The school quickly grew in size and its graduates became superintendents in other schools of nursing. Doctors and nurses collaborated to write a comprehensive nursing textbook, *The New Haven Manual of Nursing,* which was published in 1879. The text was used by nearly all the nursing schools being organized throughout the United States. The school was one of the first to obtain university affiliation and an endowment. Today it is the Yale University School of Nursing.

THE DEVELOPMENT OF NURSING EDUCATION

The early schools soon proved their value to the hospitals, and it was obvious that there existed a vital need to expand nursing schools. In 1879, there were eleven training schools in the United States. In 1885, the reported number rose to thirty-four. Twenty-four of these schools provided a two-year program. Programs offered by the others were one year or one and one-half years in duration. By 1893, Isabel Hampton Robb addressed the International Congress of Charities in Chicago and reported on the forty-seven educational programs in nursing in America. This rapid expansion continued because of the growing

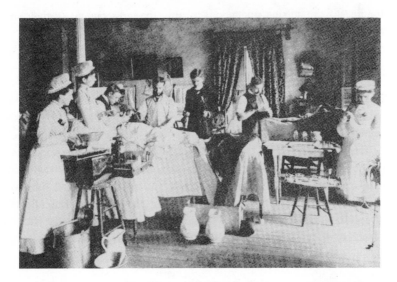

Fig. 7-6 An early operating room

demand for trained nurses. The rapid growth of scientific medicine necessitated more hospitals and thus more nurses. Also, as a consequence of the development of science and the practical application of scientific principles, nurses needed more knowledge and skills. More time was necessary to adequately prepare a nurse.

Early Trends

In 1894, the American Society of Superintendents of Training Schools for Nurses was organized. This group was concerned with the improvement of nursing curricula and standards of admission. In 1912, the association changed its name to the National League of Nursing Education. In 1917, a *Standard Curriculum for Schools of Nursing* was published, which outlined the curriculum for a three-year course. In 1927, *A Curriculum for Schools of Nursing,* a revision of the 1917 edition, advocated including courses in public health, prevention of disease, and sociology. It also discussed the need to upgrade nursing education by providing technical education, rather than apprentice training. The *Curriculum Guide for Schools of Nursing,* which was the third edition, was published in 1937. It established guidelines for curriculum planning and discussed the need for clinical instruction to augment the theoretical courses. It also referred to professional education and collegiate programs for nurses.

Educators did make sincere efforts to develop educationally sound programs. Many times nursing programs were planned beautifully on paper but were not actually implemented as planned. Faculty were often poorly prepared and schools were limited by many intervening variables, such as the state boards of nurse examiners, and service needs of the hospital, and the experiences available in the hospital and community.

Early nursing leaders were motivated to upgrade nursing education and practice. They felt that in order to improve the quality of both education and practice, entrance requirements should be more stringent. Such thinking led to the development of college preparatory courses and the affiliation of nursing schools with the university system. These ambitious leaders felt nurses needed to know *why* things were done, in addition to *how*. Collegiate nursing education was thought to be the remedy to upgrade nursing knowledge, education, and practice. This concept was the source of much controversy. Many people felt that nurses did not need a college education and that nursing was a technical occupation, requiring technical training.

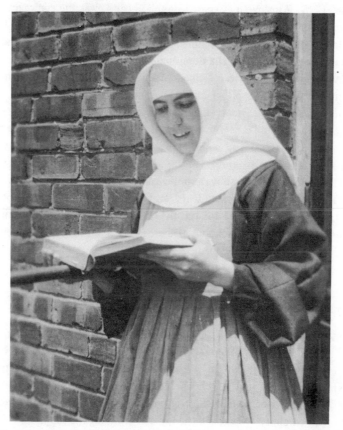

Fig. 7-7 Student nurse in 1921. Order of the Poor Handmaids of Jesus Christ

In 1907, the American Hospital Association decided there were three classifications of nurses: (1) administrators and educators, (2) bedside nurses, and (3) the attendant or subsidiary nurse. The AHA believed all three groups needed special training, but that the nurses in the first two classifications should be examined and licensed by the state. Members of the third group were to be supervised by administrative and bedside nurses.

The Winslow-Goldmark Report

When World War I broke out, more nurses were needed. The schools of nursing waived their admission criteria in order to recruit as many students as possible. After the war, there were as many different educational standards as there were nursing programs. The Rockefeller Foundation became interested in health care and decided to fund the Committee For the Study of Nursing Education. Dr. C. A. Winslow, an expert in public health, was the chairman of this committee, but his secretary, Josephine Goldmark, was responsible for the study. In its 1923 report, the committee made a number of recommendations which had great influence on the development of nursing education. First, the study revealed that there was a tremendous need for health workers who were trained in public health. The committee recommended that public health nurses be prepared in a twenty-eight month basic program, followed by eight months of study in public health. The twenty-eight month program was recommended for all nurses. The committee further recommended that auxiliary workers be trained to assume duties which did not require the expertise of the graduate nurse. The study also revealed that there were few qualified nursing instructors and that students in training programs were not being educated, but were being used to staff the hospital wards. Thus, the committee recommended that nursing schools affiliate with a college or university and that the schools should be funded. It was felt that the affiliation would raise entrance requirements and lead to a better prepared faculty.

The Committee on the Grading of Schools of Nursing

In 1925 another committee was developed to continue the study done by Winslow and Goldmark. Representatives of the National League of Nursing Education, the American Nurses' Association, the National Organization for Public Health Nursing, the American Medical Association and the American Hospital Association comprised the Committee on the Grading of Schools of Nursing. The committee was given the tasks of studying the supply and demand for nurses, analyzing nursing practice and education, and the grading of nursing schools. The study took over seven years. The findings of the committee indicated that nursing education was inadequate to prepare nurses who could meet the expectations and needs of the consumers of nursing services. The actual grading of nursing schools was never done by this committee. However, the study led to reform in nursing education. Admission requirements were raised, requiring a high school education. Most nursing programs were at least three years in length and the nursing educators were better prepared to provide quality instruction. Nursing students were receiving better formal instruction and were not expected to meet the needs of the hospital.

Accreditation

The National League of Nursing Education (NLNE) was a forerunner of the National League for Nursing (NLN), which was established in 1951. Because the Committee on the Grading of Nursing Schools was not able to complete its task, the National League of Nursing Education assumed the responsibility for grading nursing schools. The committee on accreditation developed standards for the evaluation of nursing schools. In 1941, the first list of accredited schools was published. Accreditation by the National League for Nursing indicates that the school has met the standards of excellence, as defined by that agency, in response to the changing needs of society.

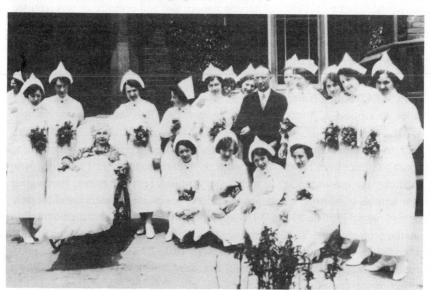

Fig. 7-8 Graduates of a nurse training program in the 1920s

Federal Funding

Florence Nightingale had stated that nursing schools should be responsible to the public for the quality of the work of their graduates. In turn, she felt that nursing education was a responsibility of the public and that public funds should support schools of nursing. Such funding did not begin in the United States until 1943. The second World War, like all wars, brought the need for nurses into public awareness. The Bolton Act, which became law on July 1, 1943, stated that any accredited nursing school could apply for federal funding if the three-year training program was reduced to thirty months. The program was administered by the United States Public Health Service, Division of Nursing Education, which was headed by Lucile Petry. The standards of nursing education were greatly improved across the country, because in order to obtain federal monies, schools had to meet the requirements developed by the National League of Nursing Education. The Bolton Act also required that the nursing schools must admit all qualified applicants regardless of race or religion. In order to accommodate the enormous influx of nursing students, the Lanham Act was passed, which provided funds for dormitories, libraries, classrooms, and other physical facilities needed for nursing education.

The Nurse Training Act of 1943 provided for the establishment of the Cadet Nurse Corps, postgraduate education, and refresher courses. Again, standards were established by the official nursing associations and compliance was required for federal grants. Students enrolled mainly in the thirty-month diploma programs and provided service to local hospitals, releasing graduate nurses for military service. Students received lodging, meals, uniforms, and a monthly stipend for services rendered.

In 1964, another Nurse Training Act was passed, which provided federal assistance to schools of nursing and nursing students. This federal money brought about a traineeship program for graduate nurses, construction grants, and assistance to diploma schools. Fortunately, these federal appropriations for nursing education have been renewed and when possible, expanded. In 1971, the Nurse Training Act was expanded to include student aid, research grants, funding for new schools of nursing, capitation (a uniform per capita payment), and preparation of nurse specialists. In 1975 appropriations were made for construction grants, project grants, institutional support, financial distress, nurse practitioner preparation, traineeships, and student loans. In 1976 and 1977, federal appropriations through the Nurse Training Act were generally reduced. This was a reflection of the cutbacks in federal spending due to the economic decline throughout the country.

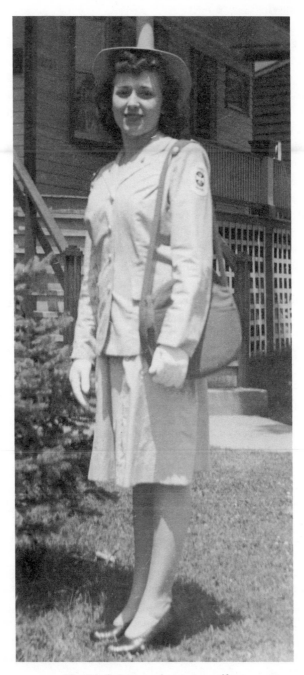

Fig. 7-9 Cadet nurse in summer uniform

The Brown Report

In 1944, a postwar planning group, the National Nursing Planning Committee, was established to develop professional objectives and to determine the areas which required study and research. It was found that a comprehensive study of nursing education was necessary. In 1947, Dr. Esther Lucile Brown undertook a study of the schools of nursing. The study was funded by a grant from the Carnegie Foundation. This study, published in 1948, is known as the *Brown Report* or *Nursing for the Future.* The findings of the study had a profound impact on nursing education in the decade of the fifties. The study recommended that all existing schools of nursing in the country form affiliations with universities. The schools of nursing should have their own budgets. It was recommended that *professional nurses* (graduates of professional schools) should be educated at the baccalaureate level and that two-year college courses be developed to prepare nurses to relieve the nursing shortage. The schools of nursing were encouraged to seek national classification and accreditation. The study also discussed the changing role and growing responsibilities of the nurse in relation to other health professionals. Regional planning for nursing education and service was recommended in order to adequately meet the needs of the community in the future.

SUMMARY

Florence Nightingale was the first to realize that nurses needed special preparation in a supervised, educational setting. Her reforms greatly influenced the development of the early nursing schools in the United States. The growth and development of nursing education in this country is rooted in the growth of hospitals, scientific and medical advances, the role of women in the society and perhaps most significantly, in the nurses themselves. Over the past century, nurses would not tolerate inferior, haphazard, and dangerous nursing practice and education. They also were not satisfied with mediocrity. Nurses have sought to improve care because they are proud of their nursing profession and feel the health care consumer deserves quality nursing. The efforts to upgrade nursing education have met with great obstacles. However, nursing education has made great strides in spite of the opposition, primarily from members of the medical profession and hospital administrators. Progress has been slow but consistent, and it will continue because nurses themselves are demanding more and better education.

SUGGESTED ACTIVITIES

- List in Column I, the admission requirements of the early training schools and in Column II, list the admission criteria of the school in which you are now enrolled. In a third column, cite the similarities and differences.

- Research the history of the uniform and cap of your school, going back to the original uniform worn by the first graduates of the school.

- Prepare a class presentation using three students. Each will research one of the three schools in the Northeastern part of the United States established in 1873: Bellevue Hospital Training School, Massachusetts Hospital Training School, and Connecticut Training School. Stress the contributions made by the schools to nursing education.

- Determine the amount of federal funds received by your school in the past five years and discuss how this money was used.

REVIEW

A.   Multiple Choice. Select the best answer.

1.   Many early schools of nursing in this country were patterned after
a. the school at Kaiserswerth.
b. the training of nurses by religious orders.
c. the St. Thomas Hospital.
d. the Nightingale system.

2.   The Brown Report, in 1948, recommended
a. training of practical nurses.
b. the development of associate degree programs.
c. the closing of diploma schools.
d. that the hospitals should license nurses.

3.   Three nursing schools opened in 1873 as a result of
a. recommendation made by the American Medical Association.
b. Louisa Lee Schuyler's committee report.
c. the Civil War.
d. the influence of Dr. Gill Wylie.

4.   The first nursing programs were
a. one year in length.
b. three years in length.
c. federally funded.
d. affiliated with federal hospitals.

5. The first standards for nursing school curricula in the United States
    were published in 1917 by
    a. the American Nurses' Association.
    b. the National League for Nursing Education.
    c. Mary Agnes Snively.
    d. the American Society of Superintendents of Nursing Schools.

6. The first federal funding for nursing schools was
    a. the result of the first Nurse Training Act.
    b. provided by the Lanham Act.
    c. provided by the Bolton Act.
    d. prior to World War II.

7. Accreditation of nursing schools was first done by
    a. the Committee on the Grading of Nursing Schools.
    b. the Division of Nursing Education, U.S. Public Health Service.
    c. the National League for Nursing Education.
    d. the American Nurses' Association.

8. As a result of the World War II demand for more nurses,
    a. the Cadet Corps was established.
    b. nursing schools reduced their programs to two and one-half years.
    c. federal funding was provided for nursing education.
    d. all the above.

9. The affiliation of nursing schools with institutions of higher learning
    was recommended by
    a. the Winslow-Goldmark Report.
    b. Florence Nightingale.
    c. the National Nurse Planning Committee.
    d. all the above.

10. One of the earliest American nursing textbooks was
    a. written by Linda Richards.
    b. *The New Haven Manual of Nursing.*
    c. *Fundamentals of Nursing.*
    d. developed by the American Hospital Association.

B. Briefly answer the following questions.

1. What was unique about Florence Nightingale's approach which still
    applies to the preparation of nurses.

2. What were four of the most significant recommendations of the
    Brown Report?

chapter 8
THE HISTORICAL DEVELOPMENT OF SPECIALIZATION

STUDENT OBJECTIVES

- Identify changes in society and technology which brought about the development of nursing specialties.
- Describe the five divisions of nursing practice.
- State the major goals of rehabilitation nursing.

Prior to the period of modern nursing and the influence of Florence Nightingale upon the role of the nurse, little thought was given to the concept of nursing specialties. The nurse tended to the basic needs of the patient, no matter what disease or medical problem necessitated nursing care.

At the turn of the century England passed a Nurse Registration Act and the United States passed state nurse practice acts. These played a large part in determining the role of the nurse. In the early decades of the twentieth century hospitals began to separate patients into specialized areas according to medical diagnoses. Nurses staffed these clinical areas. Students in the 1930s and 1940s often served as head nurses on clinical units during their senior year and were assigned to the operating and delivery rooms. Until World War II, however, the majority of nurses were employed as hospital nurses, public health nurses and private duty nurses. Nursing administration and education were really within the realm of hospital nursing. Scientific and medical advances made during and after the war drastically changed medicine and nursing. The body of knowledge became so vast that specialization became a necessity in order to further expand and utilize that knowledge. New demands were made on the health care professionals by industry, government, and society in general.

New jobs were rapidly created, many of which required advanced preparation in special areas. Nursing education developed in response to these needs.

The American Nurses' Association now recognizes five divisions of nursing practice:

- Psychiatric and Mental Health Nursing
- Maternal and Child Health Nursing
- Geriatric Nursing
- Community Health Nursing
- Medical-Surgical Nursing

The Bylaws provide that a division on practice can be established when a substantial number of nurses are practicing in an area which has a well-defined, unique body of nursing knowledge and skills and/or the existence of a significant health problem which requires the practice of nursing.

PSYCHIATRIC NURSING

Nurses have become aware that patients are not merely injured bodies or carriers of disease; they are individual human beings. Nurses also realize that as individuals, patients respond in an emotional way to being sick or injured. Because of this awareness, nurses have demanded that academic preparation include experiences and formal instruction which would enhance their understanding of human behavior. All basic nursing curricula include personality development, nurse-patient relationships, therapeutic nursing techniques, and neurotic and psychotic reactions. The successful completion of such formal basic courses is necessary for a nurse to practice effectively in all health care settings. A psychiatric nurse specialist is prepared at the graduate level, in master's or doctoral programs.

Historical Background

Many centuries were necessary to develop an understanding of mental illness and its relationship to mental health. In ancient times, people believed that the bodies of the mentally ill were inhabited by demons and evil spirits. Treatment consisted of physical tortures designed to drive the demons from the body. Some believed Satan had taken control of the soul and that the priest, as God's representative, was the only person qualified to cure the afflicted individual. In the Middle Ages mental illness was thought to be induced by witches who performed magic and cast spells on people. Witches were burned or hanged.

The mentally ill were thrown into prison and wrists, ankles, and sometimes even the neck were chained.

Bethlehem Hospital, a general hospital located outside London, became an exclusive hospital for the mentally ill in 1377. Bedlam, as it was usually called, was the first such hospital in Britain and the second mental institution in all of Europe. Mental hospitals, which were called insane or lunatic asylums, were not established for the care of the patient but for the protection and convenience of the community. Bedlam Hospital nursing personnel were not chosen for their nursing ability, but rather for the amount of physical strength they possessed. Patients were treated like animals, half starved, and kept in filthy surroundings. People believed that the mentally ill could not feel heat, cold, or even pain. Methods of fright and torture were used to drive out the madness. This was a primitive form of shock therapy. Patients who responded to treatment were required to go out into the streets to beg for alms to cover living expenses. They wore metal bands on their arms in order to be identified by the public. Violent patients were kept in chains and cells.

Psychiatric Nursing in the United States

The first psychiatric training school in the United States was begun in 1882 at the McLean Hospital in Belmont, Massachusetts. Students were awarded a certificate at the completion of the course. In 1886, the McLean Hospital affiliated with the Massachusetts General Hospital Training School. Nursing students received course credit by completing the senior year at McLean.

Men who fought during World War II witnessed massive destruction of life and property. Many soldiers suffered severe mental disturbances as the result of their experiences; following the war the need for mental health facilities became a serious problem. For several years after the war, the number of mental health programs grew tremendously in response to the demonstrated need. The World Federation for Mental Health, with headquarters in London, was established in 1948. The American Nurses' Association and the International Council of Nurses were a part of this program, dedicated to the promotion of mental health in all parts of the world.

Advanced courses in mental health and psychiatric nursing have been available in the United States since 1946. In 1935 the existing diploma schools of nursing were not required to offer psychiatric nursing and, consequently, only fifty percent of the schools included it in the curriculum. In 1950 the National League for Nursing published the results of a study which indicated a need for special training for psychiatric nursing. Therefore, a psychiatric nursing examination was added in 1952 to those required for state registration.

Psychiatric Nursing is a specialized area of nursing practice employing theories of human behavior as its scientific aspect and purposeful use of self as its art. It is directed toward both preventive and corrective impacts upon mental illness and is concerned with the promotion of optimal mental health for society, the community and those individuals and families who live within it. The dependent area of Psychiatric Nursing Practice is implementation of physicians' orders. The independent areas are assessment of nursing needs and development and implementation of nursing care plans, including initiation, development and termination of therapeutic relationships between nurses and patients. Psychiatric Nursing is practiced largely in collaboration and coordination with those in a variety of other disciplines who are working concomitantly with the patient. Thus, a high degree of interdependence with colleagues from other professions is inherent.

The Practice of Psychiatric Nursing is characterized by those aspects of clinical nursing care that involve interpersonal relationships with individuals and groups as well as a variety of other activities. These activities include: providing a therapeutic milieu, concerned largely with the sociopsychologic aspects of patients' environments; working with patients concerning the here-and-now living problems they confront; accepting and using the surrogate parent role; teaching with specific reference to emotional health as evidenced by various behavioral patterns; assuming the role of social agent concerned with improvement and promotion of recreational, occupational and social competence; providing leadership and clinical assistance to other nursing personnel. Joint planning or cooperative and collaborative efforts with other professionals are an essential part of providing nursing service. Most psychiatric settings employ an interdisciplinary team approach which requires highly coordinated and frequently interdependent planning.

Direct nursing care functions may involve individual psychotherapy, group psychotherapy, family therapy and sociotherapy. Psychiatric Nurses engaged in these therapies may employ a variety of approaches, particularly in the rapidly emerging area of sociotherapy and community mental health. With the national trend toward community mental health, Psychiatric Nurses are more and more involved in providing services aimed toward prevention of mental illness and reinforcement of healthy adaptions in addition to corrective and rehabilitative services.

The indirect nursing care roles of the Psychiatric Nurse are those of administrator with emphasis on leadership functions; as well as clinical teaching; director of staff development and training in a clinical facility; consultant or resource person, and researcher. In some of these indirect care roles, nurses will also be involved in providing direct nursing care services to improve their own clinical skills and to serve as role models. All of these roles require coordinative and collaborative efforts with other disciplines.

Fig. 8-1   Psychiatric-Mental Health Nursing Practice as defined by the Executive Committee and Standards Committee of the American Nurses' Association Division on Psychiatric-Mental Health Nursing Practice

The antiquated, prisonlike mental hospitals of the past have today been replaced by community mental health agencies and institutions which provide treatment in a therapeutic environment. Such facilities are staffed by psychiatrists, psychologists, psychiatric nurses, social workers, vocational and occupational therapists and other allied health professionals.

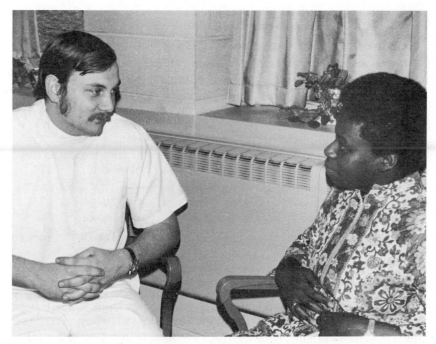

Fig. 8-2 The nurse establishes a therapeutic relationship with a patient.

MATERNAL AND CHILD HEALTH NURSING

This nursing specialty is directed toward individuals, their families and community during the childbearing and childrearing phases. Standards of Nursing Practice were developed by the Executive Committee and Standards Committee of the American Nurses' Association Division on Maternal-Child Health Nursing Practice, figure 8-3, page 130. Maternal and child health nursing is based upon principles and concepts drawn from the biological and social sciences. Such nursing care may be rendered in hospitals, home, school, community, independently or in collaboration with a physician.

Obstetrical Nursing

Obstetrics is the study of human reproduction. Some believe the origin of the word is *obstetrix*, which is Latin for midwife. In early civilization, mothers helped their daughters within the home. Some women were more skilled and experienced and were called upon to assist other women in labor; they became specialists and were called *midwives*. Physicians left this branch of medical science to the midwives and provided no prenatal care other than to treat an

Maternal and Child Health Nursing Practice is aimed at:

1. Promoting and maintaining optimal health of each individual and the family unit.
2. Improving and/or supporting family solidarity.
3. Early identification and treatment of vulnerable families.
4. Preventing environmental conditions which block attainment of optimal health.
5. Prevention and early detection of deviations from health.
6. Reducing stresses which interfere with optimal functioning.
7. Assisting the family to understand and/or cope with the developmental and traumatic situations which occur during childbearing and childrearing.
8. Facilitating survival, recovery and growth when the individual is ill or needs health care.
9. Reducing reproductive wastage occuring at any point on the continuum.
10. Continuously improving the quality of care in Maternal and Child Health Nursing Practice.
11. Reducing inequalities in the delivery of health care services.

Fig. 8-3 Objectives Developed by the Executive Committee and the Standards Committee of the American Nurses' Association Division on Maternal-Child Health Nursing Practice.

illness not associated with pregnancy. Although men, for many centuries, played no role in the delivery process, the Old Testament tells of the father being assigned the role of identification and subsequent acknowledgement of his newborn child.

In 400 B.C. Hippocrates studied some of the complications of pregnancy such as the convulsions of *eclampsia* (a condition related to hypertension and excretion of protein in the urine) and *breech presentation* (the buttocks are the presenting anatomy at birth). In the first and second centuries A.D., Celsus and Soranus developed the technique of removing the baby of a dying mother through an abdominal incision. This procedure was called *lex caesarea* which meant "the law of Caesar's land," first mentioned in the *Lex Regia of Numa Pompilius*. The myth that Julius Caesar entered the world abdominally has been discredited. However, even today, the surgical procedure is called a *caesarean section*. Soranus also introduced a procedure to induce labor prior to the due date. He wrote the oldest known textbook for midwives. About the year 1050 A.D., a woman named Trotula from Salerno, Italy taught midwives and wrote a book entitled, *Diseases of Women, Before, During and After Delivery*.

Early American folklore depicts the Indian woman having a difficult delivery being aided by the medicine man; he used fear tactics in an attempt to precipitate the birth of the baby. Another method involved tying the expectant mother to a stake or ladder device and shaking the baby out of her womb.

In 1828 a Philadelphia physician, Dr. Joseph Warrington, established a nursing course for the care of obstetrical patients. By 1832, a planned course of instruction was in operation and in 1851 the society known as Philadelphia Lying In Charity For Attending Indigent Women In Their Own Homes was founded. Physicians taught courses in obstetrics for nurses in 1861 at the Woman's Hospital of Philadelphia and in 1872 at the New England Hospital for Women. Obstetrical nursing care in the late nineteenth century was provided at the Boston Lying-In Hospital; according to records, the first nurse was hired in February 1873 for three dollars a week. She was a hardworking *Sairy Gamp.*

Not until 1877 did the physicians trust the nurse to administer medications. In 1901, the Instructive Nursing Association in Boston sent nurses to the Boston Lying-In Hospital to visit the expectant mothers. Other states adopted this policy and nurses began to visit pregnant women in their homes.

Originally, obstetrics in the United States consisted of the physician who delivered the baby as a specialty service; the obstetrical nurses who did hospital nursing; and public health nurses who provided labor, delivery, and postpartum nursing care. Acceptance of the nurse-midwife in America was slow. In 1955, the American College of Nurse Midwives was formed for the purpose of setting

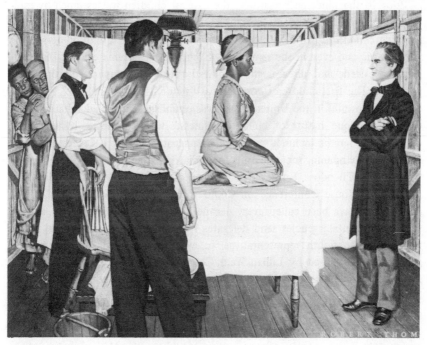

Fig. 8-4 J. Marion Sims: Gynecologic Surgeon. (Courtesy Parke, Davis and Company ©1961)

up standards of practice and education in addition to a national certification examination. This group was finally recognized by the American College of Obstetricians and Gynecologists in 1970. Today, the nurse-midwife plays a vital role on the health team. She is qualified to practice independently in normal pregnancies and is capable of identifying complications which need physician referral.

One of the most-remembered midwives in early America was Anne Hutchinson, after whom the Hutchinson River Parkway (near New York City) has been named. She was of invaluable service as a midwife in the mid-seventeenth century in Boston, Massachusetts. She died during an Indian raid in Pelham, New York. Another well-remembered pioneer of midwifery was Mary Breckenridge. She was a public health nurse who studied midwifery in England, and then, in 1920, organized the Frontier Nursing Service in Hyden, Kentucky. Mary Breckenridge rode into the Appalachian Mountains on horseback, as that was the only way the badly-needed maternity care could be provided.

Pediatric Nursing

Prior to the nineteenth century, the care of children was assumed by midwives, grandmothers, and mothers. The word *pediatric* is derived from Greek, meaning *child care*. In early hospitals children were placed with adults on the same wards and even in the same bed. Eventually it became evident that children had needs and diseases that required them to be separated from adult patients. The first children's hospital was founded in Paris in 1802. The first children's hospital in the United States was established in Philadelphia in 1855. Once the unique nature of childhood illnesses was recognized, basic nursing education programs included pediatrics as a separate course. General hospitals cooperated by opening separate units for pediatric patients.

In 1909, Theodore Roosevelt, President of the United States, called the first White House Conference on Children and Youth. Since then, similar conferences have been called every decade by the president in office. Private and governmental agencies send delegates from local, state, and federal levels, in addition to youth representatives, to evaluate the needs of the younger generation. Proposed by Lillian Wald, Congress created the Children's Bureau in 1912. The nursing division of the Children's Bureau administers federal health programs related to maternal and child health, handicapped children, and child welfare.

Current trends in nursing education combine obstetrical and pediatric nursing under the general classification of maternal-child health. However, the unique needs of pediatric and obstetrical patients make it necessary to separate them in the health care facility. Thus, the clinical experience is usually separated into pediatric and obstetrical nursing. A registered nurse is qualified to practice in obstetrics and pediatrics. Nurses who wish to develop their expertise may take additional courses at the baccalaureate and master's level. Nurse-midwives are registered nurses who acquire the knowledge and technical skills necessary for competent practice, through advanced educational programs recognized by the American College of Nurse-Midwifery.

GERIATRIC NURSING

Reduced infant mortality and the control of communicable disease has increased the life span by nearly fifty years since 1900. As a result, there are many more older people. Today there are over twenty million persons over age sixty-five and that number is growing. This older population, which is about ten percent of the total population in the United States, has unique needs and problems. The first organized efforts to deal with the problems of the aged were the establishment of the American Geriatrics Society and the Gerontological Society, Inc. in the 1940s. In 1950, the first National Conference on Aging was held in Washington, D.C., which led to the federal Committee on Aging. The Federal Council on Aging which was established in 1956, now coordinates the efforts of all state and local organizations. In 1961, The National Council on Aging, a voluntary organization, was established. Membership is open to all who share an interest in the elderly and it has become a very active and success-ful organization. Since the founding of the N.C.O.A. there has been much legis-lation designed to provide services and programs for the aged.

The geriatric patient is a person sixty-five years of age or over. The age of sixty-five is used, not because of the actual physiological, psychological, or sociological changes, but because it is the age of retirement in the United States. The 1935 Social Security Act and private retirement plans have defined sixty-five as the transition between middle and old age. Generally, the statistics indicate that persons sixty-five and over constitute a group sufficiently different from others, that the distinction is well founded.

The scientific study of the aging process is called *gerontology*. In the past twenty years research on aging has provided many new theories and concepts, all of which have contributed to a better understanding of the physiological and psychological changes which accompany aging. Separate from biological aging, but closely related to it, are the many cultural factors which influence the aging process. The growing body of knowledge was in itself an impetus which led to specialization in medicine and nursing.

Because medical and nursing sciences have contributed to the expanding longevity, there is a moral responsibility to ensure the quality of this longer

Nursing practice is a direct service, goal directed and adaptable to the needs of the individual, family and community during health and illness.

Geriatric Nursing is concerned with the assessment of the nursing needs of older people; planning and implementing nursing care to meet these needs, and evaluating the effectiveness of such care to achieve and maintain a level of wellness consistent with the limitations imposed by the aging process.

There are primary factors which make the nursing of older persons different. Among these factors are: the chronological age and the effect of the aging process; the multiplicity of an older person's losses; social, economic, psychologic and biologic factors; the frequently atypical response of the aged to disease, coupled with the different forms disease entities may assume in the aged person; the accumulative disabling effect of multiple chronic illnesses and/or degenerative process; cultural values associated with aging and social attitudes toward the aged.

Fig. 8-5 Statement of the Executive Committee and the Standards Committee of the American Nurses' Association Division on Geriatric Nursing Practice.

existence. Nursing has assumed the major responsibility for assisting the aged of our society in living optimally. Geriatrics has become a nursing specialty in the past decade.

All nurses who work with the elderly must have an understanding of the basic theoretical concepts of aging, and must be able to apply principles drawn from these theories in planning and implementing nursing care. Nurses who work in facilities which primarily provide services for the elderly, have the responsibility to expand their knowledge of aging and the unique needs of the geriatric patient. Nurses who direct the nursing practice of others caring for geriatric patients should have advanced educational preparation in geriatric nursing at the graduate level.

COMMUNITY HEALTH NURSING

History is replete with examples of rules established by civilizations to promote health and prevent disease. The Babylonian *Code of Hammurabi*, Egyptian records, the health codes of Moses, and Aesculapian rituals all contain evidence that public health was a very genuine concern. Public health as a body of knowledge was made possible by the scientific discoveries and contributions made in the seventeenth and eighteenth centuries. As science developed it became possible to maintain health and prevent disease. Society began to see the need for specific legislation to protect the public from those things which contributed to sickness and poor health. This concern for public health has developed into a responsibility of the government, to assure that all individuals receive adequate health care.

The deaconesses of the early Christian church went about in their communities caring for the sick and poor. Such services were seen as valuable

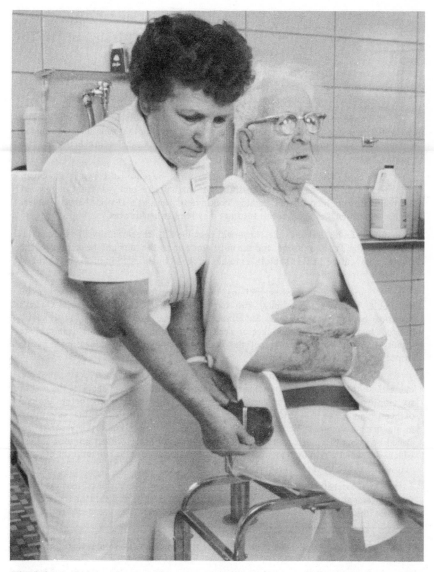

Fig. 8-6 A geriatric nurse provides nursing care designed to meet the needs of her elderly patient.

contributions and the Church encouraged women to assume such responsibilities. However, this approach to health care was abandoned with the increase in monasticism during the Middle Ages.

The Sisters of Charity, organized by St. Vincent de Paul in the seventeenth century, resurrected the idea of visiting the homes of the poor and sick. The

REGULATIONS FOR THE TRAINING OF
NURSES FOR THE SICK POOR,
AND THEIR SUBSEQUENT ENGAGEMENT

1. A Nurse desiring to be trained in District Nursing must have previously received at least two years' training in a large general Hospital, approved by the Committee, and bring satisfactory testimonials as to capacity and conduct.

2. If considered by the Superintendent likely to prove suitable for District Nursing, she will be received on trial for one month. If at the end of that time she is considered suitable, she will continue her course of training, with technical class instruction for five months longer.

3. The Nurse will, at the end of her month of trial, be required to sign an agreement with the Queen Victoria's Jubilee Institute that she will, for one year from the date of the completion of her District training, continue to work as a District Nurse wherever the District Council of the Queen's Institute may require her services.

4. While under training, the Nurse will be subject to the authority of the Superintendent of the Training Home, and she must conform to the rules and regulations of the Home. She will be further subject, as to her work, to the inspection of the Inspector of the Queen's Institute.

5. If, during the time of her training, the Nurse be found inefficient, or otherwise unsuitable, her engagement may, with the consent of the Inspector of the Queen's Institute, be terminated by the Superintendent of the Training Home, at a week's notice. In the case of misconduct or neglect of duty she will be liable to immediate dismissal by the Superintendent of the Training Home, with the concurrence of the Inspector of the Queen's Institute.

6. During her six months' training she will receive a payment of £12 10s., payable, one-half at the end of three months from admission, and the remainder at the end of six months; but should her engagement be terminated from any cause before the end of her training, she will not, without the consent of the Queen's Institute, be entitled to any part payment. She will be provided with a full board, laundry, a separate furnished bedroom or cubicle, with a sitting room in common, as well as a uniform dress, which she will be required to wear at all times when on duty. The uniform must be considered the property of the Institute.

7. On the satisfactory completion of her training, the Nurse will be recommended for engagement as a District Nurse, under some Association affiliated to the Queen's Institute, the salary usually commencing at £30 per annum.

Fig. 8-7   Florence Nightingale's description of the responsibilities of the District Nurses

sisters had no formal courses in nursing or public health. It was Florence Nightingale who recognized the need for formal training of nurses and saw the need of members of the community for home health services. The purpose of Miss Nightingale's school of nursing was to prepare nurses to work in hospitals and to care for the sick poor in their own homes as District Nurses. A District Nurse was a graduate of the Nightingale School who had six months of additional formal instruction.

In the United States, public health nursing was developed by Lillian Wald, who founded the Henry Street Settlement House and what is now the Visiting Nurse Service of New York. Miss Wald lectured on public health nursing at the Columbia University Department of Nursing Education. Miss Wald was also the first president of the National Organization for Public Health Nursing, which has had a great influence on the growth of public health nursing in this country. Adelaide Nutting, like Florence Nightingale, felt that public health nurses required postgraduate education.

Community health nursing today is a combination of nursing practice and application of public health principles directed at the promotion and maintenance of health of the society. Community health nursing involves care of individuals, families, and groups which together constitute the total population. The dimensions of that practice are influenced by the socioeconomic levels, the cultural environment, technical and scientific growth and the changing relationships between professional health workers. The goal of community health nursing is to help individuals maintain optimal health through health education, prevention of disease and provision of nursing and rehabilitative services. Community health nurses are employed by community, county, state and federal health care agencies, school districts, and industry.

Graduates of baccalaureate, associate degree, diploma, and practical schools of nursing are employed by health care agencies. Baccalaureate nursing programs provide the professional education for the community health nurse. Master's preparation in public health, education, and administration is often required for supervisors, clinical specialists, educators, and administrators in

---

Community Health Nursing is a synthesis of nursing practice and public health practice applied to promoting and preserving the health of populations. The nature of this practice is general and comprehensive. It is not limited to a particular age or diagnostic group. It is continuing, not episodic. The dominant responsibility is to the population as a whole. Therefore, nursing directed to individuals, families or groups contributes to the health of the total population. Health promotion, health maintenance, health education, coordination and continuity of care are utilized in a holistic approach to the family, group and community. The nurse's actions acknowledge the need for comprehensive health planning, recognize the influences of social and ecological issues, give attention to populations at risk and utilize the dynamic forces which influence change.

In Community Health Nursing Practice the consumer is the client or patient. Consumers include individuals, groups and the community as a whole. For example, the consumer may be a single individual, family (interpreted in the broadest sense), a school population, an industrial population or selected at-risk segments of the population. Professional practitioners of nursing bear primary responsibility and accountability for the nursing care consumers receive.

Fig. 8-8 Definition developed by the Executive Committee and the Standards Committee of the American Nurses' Association Division on Community Health Nursing Practice

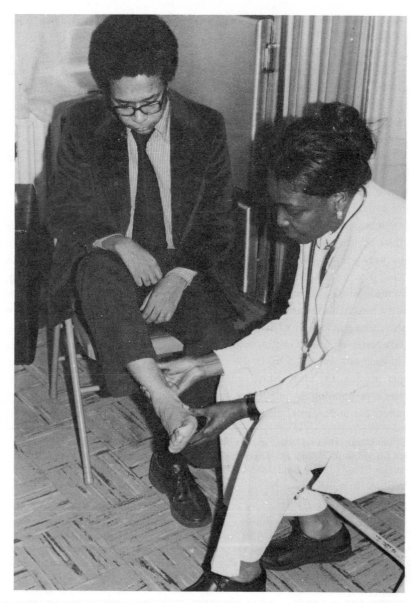

Fig. 8-9 The community health nurse gathers data in order to plan comprehensive care.

community health nursing. The PRIMEX project, funded by the National Center for Health Services Research and Development, prepares nurses to work with physicians to provide health services in all types of community settings. An academic degree is not required for admission to a PRIMEX program.

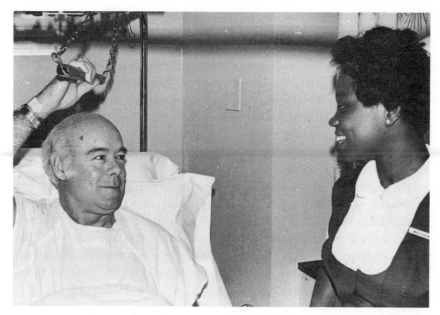

Fig. 8-10 The patient with a pathology of the musculoskeletal system requires nursing care which incorporates the principles of orthopedics.

MEDICAL-SURGICAL NURSING

Medical-surgical nursing is commonly defined as the nursing care of adults with suspected or diagnosed pathology of physiological function. It encompasses such a large scope that the trend is to subdivide medical-surgical nursing into other specialty areas such as orthopedic nursing, cardiovascular nursing, *oncological* (cancer) nursing, etc. The historical development of this specialty parallels the development of medical science and nursing. It has always been the central core of medicine and nursing, and only recently have the other specialties been developed.

Currently, all basic nursing programs prepare nurses to practice medical-surgical nursing. Advanced preparation at the master's and doctoral levels is necessary if the nurse wishes to develop expertise and acquire in-depth knowledge in particular aspects or subdivisions of the specialty.

NURSES IN REHABILITATION

Throughout history man has been concerned about the restoration of the disabled to functional roles in society. Original methods were primitive and results were not very satisfactory. Due to early beliefs that the person had been invaded by some evil spirit, treatment consisted of religious ceremonies.

The goal of early physicians was to cure the patient by eradication of the disease or disability rather than the preservation and restoration of optimal levels of functioning.   Such thinking hindered advancements in this field of health care.

The groundwork for modern rehabilitation therapy was laid in 1850 when services were developed to help crippled children. After World War I the need for physical reconstruction of maimed bodies became evident. The World War II period reinforced this thinking.   An Army Medical Corps colonel, Dr. Howard Rusk, the *Father of Rehabilitation* made great strides in developing the programs which currently return many dependent persons to an independent way of life. He referred to this as the third phase of medicine.

The major goals of rehabilitation are to eliminate or reduce the disability, and to educate and assist the patient to reach his maximum potential within the limitations of his disability. Every effort is made to restore the disabled person to his greatest physical, psychological, social, and economic potential.   The multidisciplinary approach is used to assess the unique problems of the patient, who at all times is treated as an individual human being, with specific short-term and long-term goals.   Rehabilitation cannot be accomplished without team

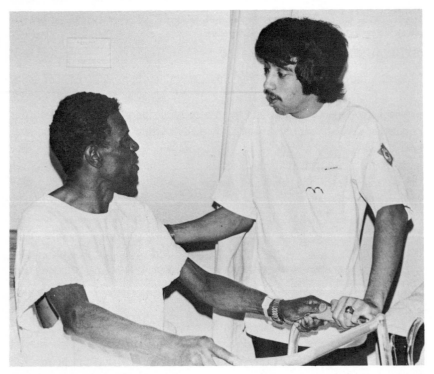

Fig. 8-11   A clinical specialist in rehabilitation teaches the patient how to get out of bed.

effort, not only of nursing personnel but also other allied health and social service professionals.   There must be integration and good communication among the team members if the goals are to be attained, figure 8-12.

The National Rehabilitation Training Institute is a nonprofit organization designed to provide education and training in all aspects of rehabilitation. The Institute offers lectures, workshops, seminars, and consultation by outstanding national leaders. Some of the workshops carry continuing education credits. Rehabilitation nursing workshops include current trends in the delivery of rehabilitation nursing services, problem-oriented programs, procedure-centered topics, and daily living activities. Community health nurses, extended care facilities, and rehabilitation center personnel find these programs most beneficial.

Nurses can specialize in rehabilitation by completing programs at the master's level.   A clinical specialist in rehabilitation is often employed by hospitals,

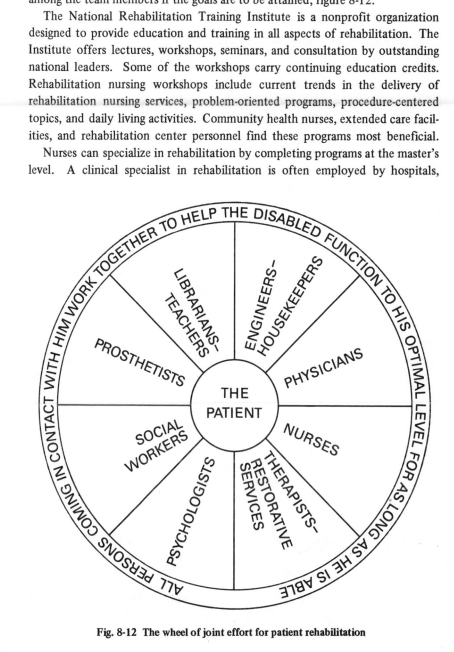

Fig. 8-12 The wheel of joint effort for patient rehabilitation

community health agencies, nursing homes, and extended care facilities to assist nurses and other health professionals in incorporating the principles of rehabilitation in the planning of health care.

STANDARDS OF NURSING PRACTICE

In 1974 the House of Delegates and Board of Directors of the American Nurses' Association established the development of standards of nursing practice as a priority. These standards were designed to support and assist the individual nurse in the performance of professional roles. All nurses are individually accountable for the quality of their practice and have the responsibility to utilize these standards to assure quality nursing and health care. The standards of the five divisions of practice are available in booklet form through the American Nurses' Association, 2420 Pershing Road, Kansas City, Missouri, 64108.

SUMMARY

The tremendous advances made in science, medicine, and technology after World War II necessitated the trend of specialization. Specialization in nursing led to the development of new curricula in basic nursing education and the establishment of new programs in graduate education, which were necessary for adequate preparation of nurse specialists. The ANA now recognizes five specialties in nursing practice; that number will grow in response to the demonstrated existence of additional specialties. In 1974, the ANA developed standards of practice for each of the existing five divisions on practice.

SUGGESTED ACTIVITIES

- Obtain permission to attend a staff meeting in the rehabilitation center or nursing home where you are assigned as a student. Observe the input of health care personnel in the total care of the patient.

- List all the clinical areas in the hospital to which you are assigned for clinical experience, and list the functions of the nursing staff. Compare duties among the clinical areas.

- Draw a chart showing the clinical areas you feel should be in a general hospital. Keep in mind the generalization of the term, medical-surgical. Be as specific as you can.

REVIEW

A. Multiple Choice. Select the best answer.

1. The first school in the United States to offer a psychiatric nursing course was
   a. Bellevue Hospital.
   c. Bethlehem Hospital.
   b. McLean Hospital.
   d. the Children's Bureau.

2. A nonprofit organization which provides continuing education and training programs for nurses in rehabilitation is
   a. the Rockefeller Foundation.
   b. the Department of Health, Education and Welfare.
   c. The National Rehabilitation Training Institute.
   d. The Rusk Foundation.

3. The World War II Army doctor who referred to rehabilitation as the third phase of medicine is
   a. Howard Rusk.
   c. J. M. Sims.
   b. Gerald Hirschberg.
   d. none of these.

4. The first children's hospital in the United States was
   a. established in Philadelphia in 1855.
   b. founded by Abraham Jacobi.
   c. created by an Act of Congress.
   d. founded by nurses.

5. Anne Hutchinson is remembered for
   a. her work in the Appalachian Mountains, assisting mothers during delivery.
   b. her contributions in establishing the first pediatric unit in a Boston hospital.
   c. her services as a midwife in Boston prior to the American Revolution.
   d. her contributions as founder of the American College of Nurse-Midwifery.

6. The most recent nursing specialty to be recognized is
   a. psychiatric-mental health nursing.
   b. rehabilitation nursing.
   c. public health nursing.
   d. geriatric nursing.

7. The voluntary organization established to promote interest in and services for the aged is
   a. The Federal Council on Aging.
   b. the National Conference on Aging.
   c. the National Council on Aging.
   d. Senior Citizens, Inc.

8. Sixty-five has been arbitrarily chosen as the transition from middle age to old age because
   a. persons sixty-five and over show certain physiological changes.
   b. persons sixty-five and over usually want to retire.
   c. after sixty-five, individuals have different interests.
   d. none of the above.

9. The American Nurses' Association has established standards of nursing practice
   a. in order to judge the competency of its membership.
   b. in order to evaluate the quality of its services.
   c. in order to protect the health care consumer.
   d. all of the above.

10. In 1952, in order to qualify for state registration and licensure, a nurse
    a. had to have public health experience.
    b. had to complete a course in psychiatric nursing.
    c. had to take advanced courses in psychiatry.
    d. had to spend at least three months in a psychiatric hospital.

B. Briefly answer the following questions.

1. List the five divisions on practice of the American Nurses' Association.

2. Briefly define the term "rehabilitation."

SECTION 3
EDUCATION FOR NURSES

chapter 9
THE RN:
DIPLOMA SCHOOLS
AND ASSOCIATE
DEGREE PROGRAMS

STUDENT OBJECTIVES

- Explain the historical development of associate degree programs.

- Identify current trends in nursing education relative to the diploma and associate degree programs.

- Identify those factors which have contributed to a decline in diploma school nursing education.

Beginning in 1873, nursing schools developed in hospitals in response to the need of hospitals for trained nurses. The three-year diploma schools developed in the 1920s, as an upgrading of early nursing education. The first associate degree programs in nursing were established in the 1950s, three years after the Brown Report recommended the development of two-year collegiate nursing programs. The diploma and associate degree programs have provided the basic nursing education for the majority of nurses registered to practice in the United States.

THE DIPLOMA SCHOOL OF NURSING

Diploma schools were established in hospitals across the country and, therefore, each program developed to meet the particular needs of the hospital. Initially, there was no standardization. Each school had its own admission criteria, curriculum, standards, and philosophy. Through the efforts of the National League for Nursing (known earlier as the National League of Nursing Education), and the influence of the Winslow-Goldmark study, uniform standards were developed. The accreditation of nursing schools by the NLN and the requirements set up by the federal government for funding led to the implementation of the standards. However, within these standards, there was considerable room for flexibility. Diploma school programs may only be described in a general way because all programs had individual characteristics.

The Faculty

The school faculty was headed by a director, who sometimes functioned as the director of nursing services in the hospital. However, it was considered advantageous to have a director responsible solely for the school of nursing. The educational director was usually responsible to the director of nursing service in the hospital. The number of faculty members depended upon school enrollment. Many of the instructors were graduates of the school. Although skilled in nursing functions, they had no academic preparation for teaching. Each school operated its own library and the librarian was a member of the school faculty. Often there was a counselor, a director of student health, and a social

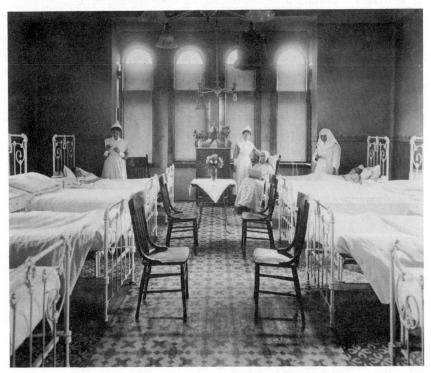

Fig. 9-1 A typical ward scene in the early twentieth century

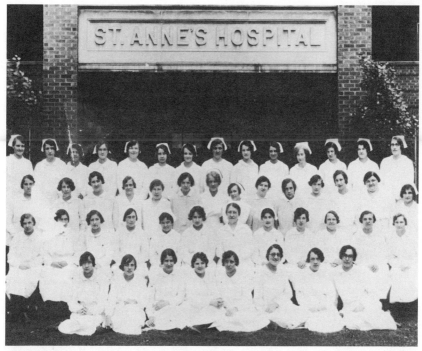

Fig. 9-2 Diploma nursing school students. Underclassmen were distinguished by their black stockings and lack of a black band on the cap.

director on the staff. Members of the medical staff were usually hired to give lectures on their clinical specialties. Supervisors or clinical instructors supervised the clinical experiences of students.

The Students

The length of the program was three years and there were four classifications of students. During the first six months (or probationary period) students were referred to as preclinical students or *probies*. For the second six months, the students were freshmen. Second year students were juniors, and third year students were seniors. In some schools, students received stipends for services rendered in the course of their training program. Amounts may have varied with specific hospitals but freshmen received less than the juniors, and they in turn received less than seniors. Students were required to live in residences on or near the hospital grounds. Living in the nurses' residence required a great deal of adjustment for most students. Juniors were often assigned the role of a *Big Sister* to an incoming preclinical student. Orientation to the rules,

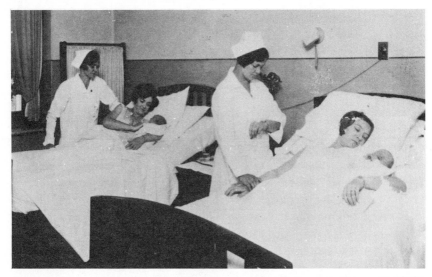

Fig. 9-3   Diploma school students spent three months on the postpartum unit of the hospital.

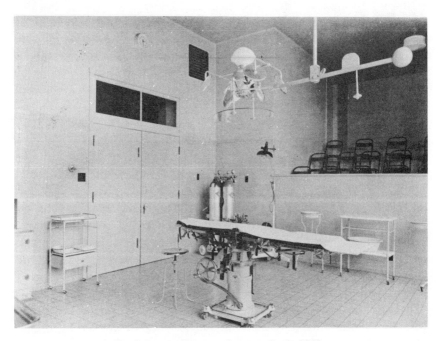

Fig. 9-4   A typical operating room in the 1920s

regulations, routines and other aspects of student life was achieved through this association, and it alleviated much of the anxiety involved in adjustment to a new way of life.

The Curriculum

The diploma schools of nursing increased the number of courses considerably from what was required in the early training schools. It was believed that a multitude of courses were necessary in order to prepare a nurse who could meet all the needs of nursing service. The typical diploma program offered a curriculum which included courses in anatomy and physiology, nursing arts, chemistry for nurses, drugs and solutions, nutrition, microbiology, pathology, obstetrics, pediatrics, psychiatric nursing, medical nursing, surgical nursing, emergency and first aid, history of nursing, and a professional adjustments course.

Some schools considered laboratory and pharmacy experiences essential. Operating room duties provided a touch of glamour and excitement for some and fear and anxiety for others. When university affiliation was encouraged as an upgrading of education, college courses in philosophy, psychology, history or sociology were often added to the existing curriculum. Textbooks were limited to seven or eight.

The larger the hospital, the greater were the experiences and facilities available for clinical practice. Clinical experience was gained in all units of the hospital and all three shifts were covered by students. Frequently, students were assigned the morning and evening hours as split shifts with classes in between. Changing to an eight-hour day with an annual vacation caused older graduates

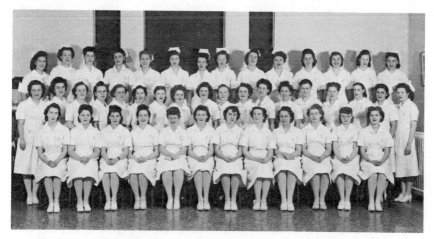

Fig. 9-5 A typical graduating class from a hospital nursing program in the 1940s

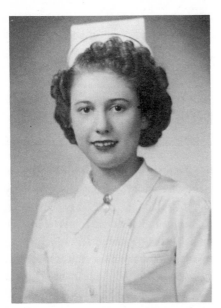

Fig. 9-6   Uniform pride: Starched uniform, school cap and pin of the new diploma school graduate.

to shake their heads in dismay. Students were sent on an affiliation for pediatrics, communicable disease or psychiatric nursing experiences if the hospital could not provide them.

Decline of the Hospital Diploma School

The diploma school was a practical and successful approach to nursing education for many years. As costs increased, hospitals found they could not afford to financially support their own schools. Today, diploma school nursing schools are on the decline. Many of them have closed or have made plans to phase out their programs. Others have affiliated themselves with federally funded public colleges and universities, and now offer programs leading to an associate or baccalaureate degree in nursing.

THE ASSOCIATE DEGREE PROGRAM IN NURSING

The associate degree in nursing is granted by many junior and community colleges. Liberal education and nursing education are combined to produce a nurse capable of functioning as a quality practitioner in the health care field. The period following World War II influenced the patterns of education because of the needs of the general public and the demand of many for more education and better health care.

The Division of Nursing Education of Teachers College, Columbia University, initiated and sponsored the Cooperative Research Project in Junior and Community College Education for Nursing. The project began in 1952 under the direction of Dr. Mildred Montag.

Prior to 1955 some community colleges offered prenursing courses in sciences and the liberal arts; these courses had transferable credit. Community college faculty occasionally were hired to teach one or more courses in a hospital school. The concept of placing nursing education totally in a junior college setting was received with much skepticism and concern. Graduates of the seven junior and community colleges and one hospital school which participated in the project, were successful on the licensing examination and in employment. This tended to promote wider acceptance of this new approach to nursing education.

The Cooperative Research Project

The five-year Cooperative Research Project was made possible by an anonymous grant of $110,000 in 1952. Since the community college was concerned with meeting the service needs of the community, a nursing program logically belonged in that setting. The purpose of this project was to describe the development of the associate degree nursing program, evaluate its graduates, and to determine its implications for the future of nursing.

At the time of this study it was assumed that there would be a growing demand for nurses. The project was an attempt to meet the needs of society by preparing nurses in a shorter time than was required in hospital diploma programs. The hospital schools of nursing (85 percent of all schools of nursing) saw a decline in student enrollment annually, beginning in 1956. Conversely, the number of junior-community college students rose steadily. Students were attracted to this type of education because of its low tuition and costs, the close proximity to their homes, and the removal of the requirement to live in a nurses' residence. The emphasis was on education, not service in that students were not required to relieve nursing personnel on the hospital units on weekends and holidays.

The graduates of the community college program were to be prepared to function as bedside nurses in staff level positions, under supervision. They would be eligible to write the registered nurse licensing examination and receive an associate degree from the junior-community college.

The First Participating Colleges. The decision was made to develop the nursing programs in well-established community colleges. This allowed for savings of funds and a wide variation among types of institutions. By 1957, there were at least as many associate degree nursing programs operating outside, as well as within, this particular project. The participating colleges were selected on the basis of the following:

- There was an interest in departing from the traditional approach to nursing education.

- An educational institution rather than a hospital would sponsor the program.

- There was general acceptance of the concept by the community and college faculty.

- There was evidence that an adequate theoretical and clinical curriculum existed.

- Learning experiences were available in community agencies.

- There was legislative approval of the program.

- There was community assurance of job opportunities for program graduates.

The seven participating in the project were located in six states: New York, New Jersey, Michigan, Utah, California, and Virginia. The colleges selected were:

- Orange County Community College, Middletown, New York

- Farleigh Dickinson College, Rutherford, New Jersey

- Henry Ford Community College, Dearborn, Michigan

- Weber College, Ogden, Utah

- Pasadena City College, Pasadena, California

- Virginia Intermont College, Bristol, Virginia

- Virginia State College, Norfolk, Virginia

Upon the advice of the advisory committee, a hospital program was to be included as a participant, providing that: (1) the program was owned and operated by a hospital; (2) a two-year program, in lieu of the traditional three-year program, would be developed to prepare the graduate for state licensure; (3) the school would be philosophically committed to nursing education rather than service; and (4) the curriculum and faculty were adequate. The hospital selected was Monmouth Memorial in Long Branch, New Jersey. In the eight programs, the average number of faculty members was five. The need for more and better-educated faculty was evident and this need continued through the seventies.

Differences between the community college basic nursing program and the hospital program were: the length (two years instead of three) because of emphasis on educational experiences rather than hospital service; the governing body; the supervision of faculty; and the 811 participating students who enjoyed college status. There were some changes in curriculum as degrees were earned (therefore, requirements were different).

Some of the student differences were: the age of community college students was older; students were allowed to marry if admitted single, married women were allowed to enter initially; and residency was not required since students

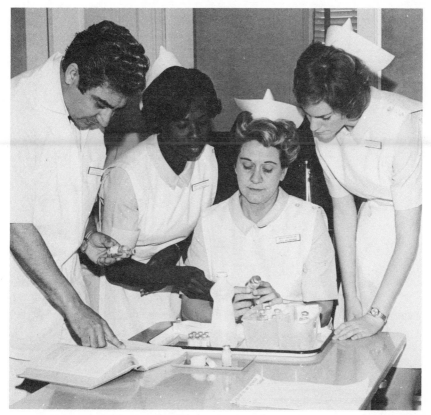

Fig. 9-7 Associate degree students apply theoretical principle to the practical application.

lived within commuting distances of the college. Three percent of the 811 students were males; mainly former hospital corpsmen who would not have enrolled in other types of nursing programs.

Although all of the participating programs were two-year community college programs, differences in curriculum content and faculty probably created the variation in scores achieved, on the State Board Test Pool Examination, by graduates of the project.

Project Graduates

Graduates tended toward general duty or staff nurse positions in hospitals, usually those in which clinical experience had been given them as students. Nursing service administrators were unaware of the orientation needs of this new graduate nurse. The accelerated program, with minimal clinical experience

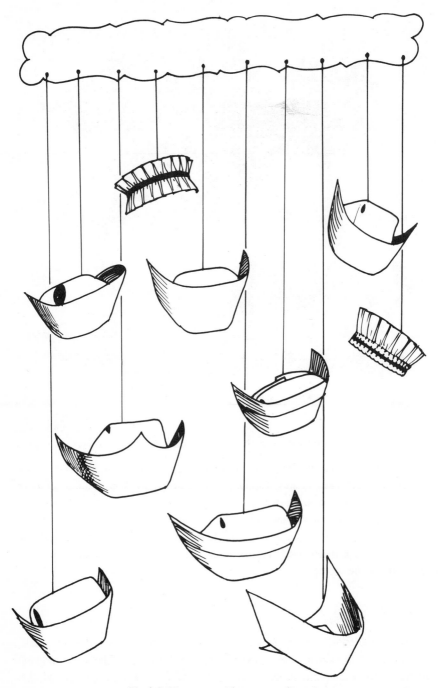

Fig. 9-8 Many caps with one commitment

and responsibility, necessitated at least three weeks of on-the-job experience and a planned orientation program for associate degree graduates. Such programs were not provided by most hospitals and the advent of the associate degree nurse was the impetus which led to the development of more effective orientation and in-service programs.

Although prepared to function as bedside nurses giving primary care, many associate degree graduates were placed into supervisory positions. At first, this involved merely relieving a head nurse or supervisor on vacation. The new graduates experienced mixed emotions concerning their educational experience. Nursing service directors also varied in their acceptance of the associate degree graduate. Lack of adequate orientation appears to be one of the major problems encountered by the new graduate; also, in-service programs are not always effective or available.

In 1956, there were approximately twenty-five associate degree programs which were state-approved; in 1967, there were over 281 approved programs. By 1971, the National League for Nursing had accredited 491 programs. There can be little doubt that the trend in nursing education is to provide basic nursing education in community colleges. In order to provide assistance in the transition, and aid to those academic institutions interested in starting a program, the NLN appointed a consultant on junior college education and published *Guiding Principles for Junior College Participation in Nursing Education.*

SUMMARY

For nearly half a century, most nurses were trained in hospital diploma schools of nursing. In that period, nursing education developed higher standards and better practitioners than ever before. Beginning in the 1950s the trend has been to provide basic nursing education in the two-year college. This has led to the decline in the numbers of diploma schools of nursing and a tremendous growth in the numbers of associate degree nursing programs.

SUGGESTED ACTIVITIES

- Prepare a panel presentation with one person doing additional research on each of the approaches to nursing education discussed in this chapter.
- Trace the history of the associate degree program in your institution. Cite changes in curriculum, clinical assignments, etc.
- Find out which hospitals in your county currently have an approved diploma program and which hospitals phased out programs in the past. Investigate the reasons and the date of discontinuance.

REVIEW

A. Multiple Choice. Select the best answer.

1. The director of the Cooperative Research Project in Junior and Community College Education for Nursing was
   a. Dr. Esther L. Brown.   c. Ruth Matheney.
   b. Dr. Mildred Montag.   d. none of these.

2. Standardization of nursing education in the early diploma schools was brought about by
   a. the study done by Winslow and Goldmark.
   b. the guidelines established by the National League of Nursing Education.
   c. the process of accreditation.
   d. all of the above.

3. As diploma schools began to affiliate with universities and colleges
   a. tuition went up.
   b. nursing courses were taught on the university campus.
   c. the nursing curriculum was shortened.
   d. courses in psychology, sociology and philosophy were added.

4. The decline in diploma nursing schools began
   a. after World War II.   c. about the year 1956.
   b. about the year 1960.   d. none of these.

5. The most common hospital affiliation for nursing students enrolled in three-year programs was
   a. maternity nursing.   c. psychiatric nursing.
   b. pediatric nursing.   d. b and c.

6. The project to study the associate degree program in nursing
   a. involved seven junior and community colleges.
   b. was funded by a grant from the Rockefeller Foundation.
   c. involved seven diploma schools of nursing.
   d. all of the above.

7. The variations found in State Board scores of the graduates of community colleges participating in the study were due to
   a. small number of participants.
   b. differences in admission criteria.
   c. differences in curriculum and faculty.
   d. b and c.

8. The problem(s) most frequently encountered by new graduates of associate degree programs is lack of
   a. adequate supervision.
   b. adequate orientation and in-service programs.
   c. acceptance by other nurses.
   d. all of the above.

9. Graduates of associate degree programs are prepared
   a. to give primary nursing care.
   b. to relieve the head nurse.
   c. to teach nursing in-service courses.
   d. none of the above.

10. The purpose of the diploma school was primarily to
    a. provide sound basic nursing education.
    b. prepare nurses who could meet the needs of the community.
    c. provide the hospital with trained nurses.
    d. prepare nurses who could pass the licensing examination.

B. Briefly answer the following questions.

1. Give three reasons why students were attracted to the associate degree program in lieu of the hospital school diploma program.

2. Explain why many diploma schools of nursing have either closed, made plans to phase out their program, or reorganized with college or university affiliation.

chapter 10
THE RN: BACCALAUREATE, MASTER, AND DOCTORAL PROGRAMS

STUDENT OBJECTIVES

- Explain the historical development of collegiate nursing education.
- Identify the general trends of baccalaureate nursing education.
- Identify the primary objectives of graduate nursing programs.

The baccalaureate degree nursing program is offered in a senior college or university in a special division or department of nursing. Each program is subject to the policies of the institution and establishes its own requirements for admission. The program must be approved by the state in which the school is located in order for the graduates to be eligible to take the examination for licensure as a registered nurse. Programs may apply for review for accreditation by the National League for Nursing. Graduate nursing programs leading to a master's degree or doctoral degree prepare nurses for administrative, teaching, consultant, research, and practitioner positions; all of these require specialized, in-depth knowledge and skills. Nurses with graduate education are needed to promote excellence and to provide leadership in nursing.

HISTORICAL DEVELOPMENT OF COLLEGIATE NURSING PROGRAMS

According to the Federal Bureau of Education, the number of schools of nursing increased from 432 to 1,755 between the years 1899 to 1920. Hospitals were increasing rapidly and so were nursing schools. Hospitals could not expand without an increase in the number of graduate nurses to staff the hospitals. In an effort to produce more nurses, the screening of applicants became deficient

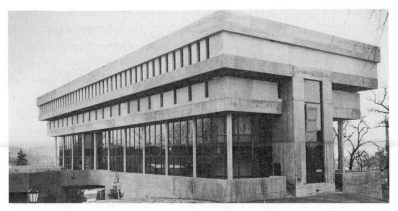

Fig. 10-1 The College of Nursing, State University of Iowa

and persons not suitable for nursing were often admitted. Faculty were not prepared to provide the instruction students needed. Graduate courses offered to those persons having inadequate academic preparation proved unsatisfactory. However, the preliminary courses offered by Rebecca Strong in Glasgow, Scotland in 1893 and Adelaide Nutting at Johns Hopkins in 1901 did alleviate many of the inadequacies in their particular schools.

As early as 1905, training schools were affiliated with major universities. Originally, the intent of such a merger was for the provision of science courses. Mercy Hospital in Chicago, Illinois affiliated with Northwestern University in 1889 for such purposes. Nursing graduates shared commencement ceremonies with the university graduates. This situation has existed through the years to the present time.

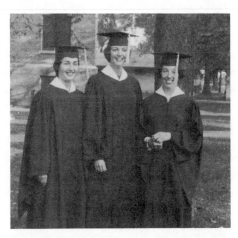

Fig. 10-2 Candidates for a B.S. degree in nursing

Teachers College, Columbia University, which was founded in 1887, was considered highly progressive. A high degree of professionalism also prevailed. In 1893, the college became an official department of the university. Many non-academic fields were in a dearth for quality educators to prepare leaders in the educational roles open in programs of instruction. Nursing was among those careers and Teachers College provided an excellent setting for nursing education at the collegiate level.

Teachers College was the first institution to recognize the need for nurses, assigned to the instruction of nursing students to be academically prepared for their important role in nursing. The one-year course in hospital economics established in 1899, was extended in 1905 to a two-year program. Two of the most remarkable women in nursing, Isabel Hampton Robb and Mary Adelaide Nutting, who brought about the economics course, later developed the Department of Nursing and Health at Teachers College in 1910. In 1912, courses in district nursing and health protection were offered for administrators, teachers, and public health nurses. Public health nursing was the first of the nursing specialties to encourage graduate education. One major problem of postgraduate education was that the courses did not carry academic credit. These courses were offered to graduates of diploma school programs who desired additional training in a clinical specialty in order to qualify for roles as supervisors, head nurses, or instructors in given areas. These programs generally lasted four to six months and consisted of lectures combined with on-the-job training.

At the turn of the twentieth century, universities were reluctant to accept professional schools as part of their tradition-bound institutions. University students were considered to be the scholarly students who delved into the realms of the humanities, mathematics, or history of the world. Nursing curricula was not accepted as appropriate for higher education. Rather, it was thought nurses were to be trained to perform skills, not educated in principles and theory. Nurses, however, thought differently. Articles appearing in issues of the professional journals during the early part of this century made reference to the value of well-educated persons performing nursing functions. The need for intelligent, as well as physically strong, dexterous women in the field, was recognized. As early as 1913, the editor of the *American Journal of Nursing* predicted the nurse would function as the co-worker of the physician. If nurses were going to assume duties beyond the custodial care and comfort of the patient, further educational preparation was a necessity. The need for a good theoretical background in the sciences was necessary. The ideal setting for this newly conceived curricula was the university or college.

In 1909, the University of Minnesota nursing program was established. Although based in the university setting, the program was not a baccalaureate program but operated as a superior three-year hospital school, preparing students for R.N. licensure. Students were subservient to physicians and were required to perform hospital service as payment for the education they received. In 1919, the University of Minnesota instituted an undergraduate baccalaureate nursing program.

Most of the early baccalaureate programs were five years in length and that was the norm until the 1950s. The five-year program was basically the three-year nursing school curriculum with the addition of two years of liberal arts. It has taken a number of years to develop an integrated professional curriculum. It has also been difficult to prepare enough nursing educators who were qualified to teach in such programs.

Even though the concept of collegiate education was gradually accepted, the growth of collegiate schools was steady but not rapid. A mere decade ago, there were in operation approximately five hospital diploma schools for every undergraduate program in existence. In 1919, there were 8 baccalaureate programs; in 1974, the number had grown to 313.

The Association of Collegiate Schools of Nursing was organized in 1934. The first major task of the association was to clearly cite the differences between basic degree and diploma programs. Margaret Bridgman, a dean at Skidmore College, served as an adviser on nursing education to institutions of higher education. She later served as a consultant to the National League for Nursing Department of Baccalaureate and Higher Degree Programs. She wrote *Collegiate Education in Nursing* which was published by the Russell Sage Foundation in 1953. Other authors provided similar expertise through publications which helped guide the development of baccalaureate education of nurses. In 1960, the NLN Department of Baccalaureate and Higher Degree Programs published *Criteria for Baccalaureate and Masters Programs in Nursing.*

ISSUES AND TRENDS IN BACCALAUREATE NURSING EDUCATION

In 1965, 35 percent of the NLN accredited baccalaureate programs were four academic years in length. Forty-two percent were four academic years plus one or two summer sessions and 23 percent were longer. By 1971, 57 percent were four years in length, 39 percent required one or two summer sessions in addition to the four academic years and only 4 percent were longer.

One of the serious problems created by the advent of the collegiate nursing program was the obstacle that confronted the diploma graduate who wished to obtain a baccalaureate degree. The baccalaureate degree has become widely accepted as a necessary requirement for supervisory positions in nursing. The diploma graduate with substantial experience often found that her training

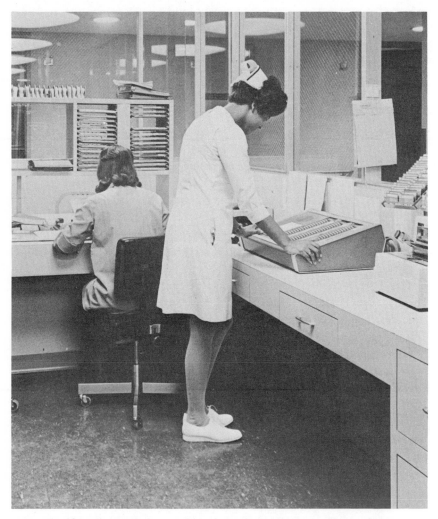

Fig. 10-3 Many supervisory positions in nursing require a baccalaureate degree.

was not acknowledged by institutions of higher education and thus she again had to take courses, for college credit, which covered material she already knew. Such repitition was costly and demoralizing.

Currently, the number of registered nurses enrolling in baccalaureate programs on both full- and part-time basis is increasing. Based upon NLN annual surveys, there were 1,377 nursing education programs preparing individuals for licensure in 1972. Included in these were 293 baccalaureate programs, 82 percent of which offered some form of advanced placement or career mobility for graduate nurses. Graduates of R.N. programs, whether diploma or associate

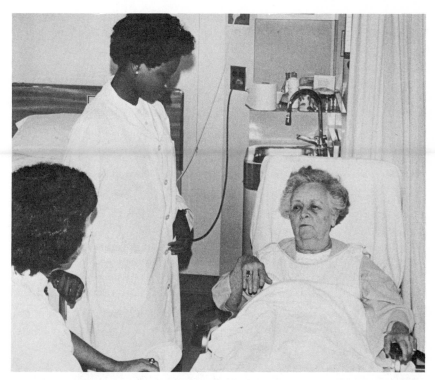

Fig. 10-4 Two baccalaureate nursing students collect data by interviewing the patient.

degree, who wish to obtain a baccalaureate degree in nursing, should seek information relative to career mobility. Reference material such as the NLN's *Directory of Career Mobility Opportunities in Nursing Education* should be reviewed before the college or university is selected. Serious investigation of open curriculum opportunities is advisable to avoid unnecessary repetition of courses. The open curriculum policy varies with each school and a directory is helpful to identify the school which will provide the ultimate credit for an applicant either by transfer or examination.

One of the most innovative basic baccalaureate programs is the evening program offered at Hunter College-Bellevue School of Nursing. The program, begun in 1974 under an HEW grant, is offered three evenings a week and affords an opportunity to persons engaged in full-time careers in other fields of employment, to pursue a baccalaureate degree in nursing.

HISTORICAL DEVELOPMENT OF GRADUATE NURSING EDUCATION

Organized master's level education began in the last quarter of the nineteenth century. Patterns for master's work were based mainly on the German programs,

SCHOOL	YEAR
Yale 1872	
Harvard 1872	
Columbia 1864	
Johns Hopkins 1867	
Clark 1887	
Catholic University of America 1889	

Fig. 10-5 In the United States, graduate programs in nursing originated during the late 1800s.

where the leaders of American higher education either spent time as graduate students or as observers of the system. Prior to World War I, American scholars went to the European countries for advanced study. Today students from all parts of the world seek education in our institutions of higher learning.

The need for graduate programs in nursing became apparent as the demand for better-educated faculty increased. As more schools of nursing sought to upgrade their programs, the pressure was placed on instructors to seek advanced preparation in education and clinical nursing specialties. The number of nurses desiring graduate education grew, and this encouraged the growth (in numbers) of graduate programs.

One of the early graduate programs for nurses was The Catholic University of America in Washington, D.C.; courses in nursing education were offered for the first time in 1932. In 1935, the Board of Trustees granted approval for the conferring of a master's degree in nursing education.

Criteria for graduate programs were developed by the National League for Nursing in 1952, and were published in the *Report of Work Conference on Graduate Nurse Education*. This report advocated nursing specialization at the master's degree level. In 1954, the administrators of graduate programs developed guidelines for the improvement of existing programs and to aid in the development of new advanced degree programs. This led to the 1957 publication of guidelines for the *Development of Educational Programs in Nursing Which Lead to a Masters Degree*.

NEW GRADUATE PROGRAMS IN NURSING

In 1961, there were forty-three master's programs in nursing. That number continues to grow, as does the variety of programs. In 1974, the University of Arizona College of Nursing was the first to offer a program leading to a master's degree in medical-surgical nursing, which prepares a pulmonary nursing practitioner. The American Lung Association is offering limited funding for the

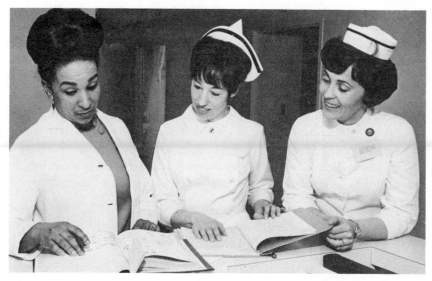

Fig. 10-6 Two graduate nursing students confer with their instructor about data they are collecting for their thesis.

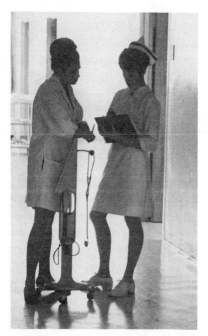

Fig. 10-7 The nurse with a master's degree shares her expertise with the nursing staff.

postgraduate semester, which focuses on pulmonary function. The New York Medical College will grant a Master of Science in Nursing to students who have received a baccalaureate degree in another field. The University of Missouri-Kansas City started a Master of Science degree program in nursing in the spring semester, 1974. The program requires three semesters as a full-time student or five semesters part-time. The first students majored as pediatric nurse practitioners. A major is also offered in the nursing care of adult medical patients. A unique graduate program open to nurses with a bachelor's degree, is the health science/anthropology program at the University of Kansas Medical Center. The program is one to two years in length and the major focus of study is on health care delivery from the consumer's point of view.

HISTORY OF DOCTORAL PROGRAMS IN NURSING

Nineteenth century German universities introduced the doctoral degree to North America, where the same degree requirements were adopted. In 1861, Yale University awarded the first doctorate (Ph.D.) in this country. The rigid requirements for this degree have remained static and there is general uniformity among universities. Generally, the doctorate cannot be obtained in less than three full years devoted to intense scholarly study and original research.

The first four doctoral degree programs led to a Ph.D., Ed.D., or D.Sc. in Nursing degree with emphasis on research, clinical nursing, allied sciences, and philosophy. The four universities granting these degrees were Boston University, New York University, Teachers College of Columbia University, and the University of Pittsburgh.

In 1972 there were six such programs while nine schools offered nurse scientist doctoral programs. The nurse scientist is prepared in another discipline such as biology, psychology, or sociology in addition to nursing. Nurses also complete doctoral programs in disciplines other than nursing.

In January, 1974, the first students enrolled in the Ph.D. program at the University of Texas School of Nursing. The new program offers a doctorate in nursing and requires a minimum of 57 semester hours beyond the master's degree. An opportunity is provided for advanced study in nursing in addition to education, administration, research, behavioral and physical sciences.

In September, 1975, the University of Illinois College of Nursing instituted a Ph.D. program in nursing. The primary program objective is the development of research and theory in the field of nursing. Major areas of investigation by the doctoral students are related to nursing practice, administration, and nursing education. Students must be capable of independent research under the supervision of an assigned faculty adviser. The university received a $40,699, one-year grant, from the United States Public Health Service Division of Nursing in 1974. This grant enabled three nursing faculty members to conduct the program planning.

The W. K. Kellogg Foundation in 1974 sponsored a doctoral program at the University of British Columbia in Vancouver, B.C., Canada. The program offers training to health professionals for careers as continuing education specialists. The doctoral program is two years in length.

The Rush College of Nursing and Allied Health Sciences was awarded a two-year grant of $100,000 to establish a Center for Clinical Nursing Research as the foundation for a doctoral degree program begun in 1975. The college opened in 1973, offering a four-year baccalaureate degree in nursing. Eleven colleges and midwestern universities in five states were affiliated with this program.

Even though the number of nurses achieving the doctorate degree today is increasing, the need for doctorate faculty in the higher education programs will not be met in the immediate future. The National League for Nursing does not accredit doctoral programs but does provide information in the publication, *Doctoral Programs in Nursing.*

SUMMARY

Early in the twentieth century interest began to grow in placing nursing education in the college or university setting. Initially, it was thought that graduates of nursing schools who desired additional training should be allowed to take courses, without credit, at the college level. In an effort to upgrade their programs, nursing schools added science courses, taught by university faculty, to their curricula. Gradually, educators began to talk about developing programs leading to a baccalaureate degree in nursing. Placing nursing education in institutions of higher education met with considerable resistance and created problems which still face the profession today. Nursing leaders have begun to realize the need to be less traditional and rigid in degree requirements. Both master and doctoral programs are growing in numbers because many schools are requiring faculty to obtain advanced education. Although the original goal of graduate education for nurses was to prepare qualified faculty to meet the improved status of basic nursing education programs, degree-seeking nurses are becoming involved in research, administration, and leadership. The rapid gains in scientific knowledge, increased specialization, changing health care needs, and methods of health care delivery, have created a need for nurses with postgraduate preparation.

SUGGESTED ACTIVITIES

- Search the literature and read at least three articles based on research findings related to current issues in collegiate nursing education.

- Correlate the various functions of nursing with the educational preparation you believe should be achieved for quality performance. Compare your chart with the requirements specified in your State Nursing Act.

- Survey school catalogs available in your nursing office, lab or library and make a list of schools and types of programs open to nurses beyond the basic nursing program.

REVIEW

A.   Multiple Choice. Select the best answer.

1.   The first nursing program in a university setting was
  a. established in 1909 at the University of Minnesota.
  b. offered at Teachers College, Columbia University.
  c. designed to prepare administrators and educators in nursing.
  d. none of the above.

2.   Doctoral programs in the United States are accredited by
  a. The National League for Nursing.
  b. The American Nurses' Association.
  c. The Department of Health, Education and Welfare.
  d. none of the above.

3.   The first nursing specialty which required graduate education was
  a. psychiatric nursing.   c. pediatric nursing.
  b. public health nursing.   d. geriatric nursing.

4.   The early baccalaureate programs in nursing were
  a. five years in length.
  b. integrated nursing and liberal arts studies.
  c. part-time programs.
  d. funded by the federal government.

5.   To earn a doctoral degree in nursing
  a. a nurse usually must spend a minimum of one year doing original research.
  b. a nurse must study a discipline other than nursing.
  c. generally requires three years of study and original research.
  d. a nurse can choose from four doctoral programs.

6. One of the problems which came about as a result of baccalaureate nursing education was
   a. the lack of adequately prepared faculty.
   b. the inability to integrate nursing and liberal arts courses.
   c. the failure of baccalaureate programs to provide credit for nursing education received in diploma programs.
   d. all the above.

7. The trend in baccalaureate education today is
   a. to offer advanced placement for graduate nurses.
   b. the development of five-year programs.
   c. to prepare nurse researchers.
   d. none of the above.

8. A program leading to a baccalaureate degree in nursing designed for persons who have full-time jobs is offered by
   a. the University of Arizona.
   b. Teachers College.
   c. Hunter College-Bellevue School of Nursing.
   d. New York Medical College.

9. Baccalaureate and graduate programs in nursing are accredited by
   a. the State Department of Registration.
   b. the NLN.
   c. the ANA.
   d. The Association of Collegiate Schools of Nursing.

10. The European country after which graduate education in America was patterned is
    a. England.   c. Germany.
    b. France.   d. Austria.

B. Briefly answer the following questions.

1. What specific need brought about the interest in collegiate nursing education?

2. Generally, what are the primary objectives of graduate nursing programs?

chapter 11
THE LPN: VOCATIONAL EDUCATION

STUDENT OBJECTIVES

- Explain the historical development of practical nursing.

- Identify the administrative controlling bodies of practical nursing programs.

- Explain the role of the LPN as a member of the health care team.

About the time of World War II, it was discovered that schools of nursing could not meet the demand for nurses through the existing three-year programs. During the war years the American Red Cross recruited and prepared nonprofessional nurses who were utilized mainly in hospitals and public health agencies. This method of supplementing nursing resources proved successful and it was felt by many that there was a permanent place in nursing for the nonprofessional nurse.

The concept of practical nursing is not a new one by any means; the practical nurse has been at the patient's bedside for many years. The friend of the family or the neighbor who came to a home to offer assistance in caring for a sick or injured person was, in a sense, a practical nurse. Some of these self-taught practical nurses were still functioning until as late as 1970. During the era in which they functioned, they made a contribution because of the experience and skill acquired over the years. Some of them even had a state license, granted by waiver, although they were never enrolled in an approved practical nurse training program. On the other hand, the trend in the fifties was to establish approved schools with a program designed to train practical nurses in all of the basic areas prescribed in the required curriculum developed by the National

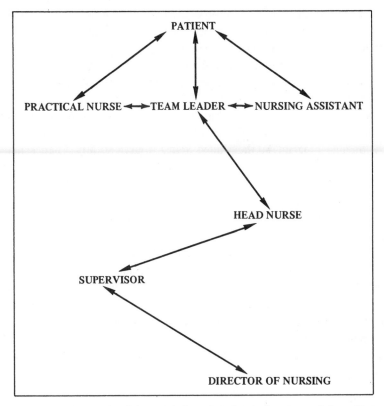

Fig. 11-1 Relationship of the practical nurse to the nursing team and the patient

Committee on Practical Nurse Education under the auspices of the United States Office of Education.

Practical nursing was established to provide the nation with nonprofessional persons prepared to provide bedside nursing care to the patient. This tends to relieve the professional nurse of many of the routine procedures so that she/he may assume the responsibilities of more skilled nursing care.

OVERVIEW OF PRACTICAL NURSING HISTORY

Before 1860 nursing services in America were provided by practical nurses who gained their knowledge by experience. In 1873, the first professional nursing schools were established. However, there was no formal training available for practical nurses until the end of the nineteenth century.

The Young Women's Christian Association (Y.W.C.A.) was based upon the religious beliefs of the Evangelical church. It originated in England, Germany, and Switzerland. With the advent of the Industrial Revolution in 1850, young girls ventured to the big cities for new careers. The Y.W.C.A. housed many of the girls who sought employment far from their own homes. Many of them were untrained and could not compete for the jobs available. The Y.W.C.A. undertook the offering of classes in domestic chores and cooking. It is assumed that basic home nursing and child care instruction was also included in these courses.

The Y.W.C.A. course for practical nursing began around 1892, in Brooklyn, New York. The course was financed by Miss Lucinda Ballard. Credit for this early training program in the United States is given to Mrs. Charles Judson, President of the Brooklyn Y.W.C.A., who served as program director, and her friend, Mrs. Katharine A. Adams, an instructor from the American Red Cross Society. The course was approximately three months in length and its purpose was to train practical nurses who could care for invalids, the elderly, and children. Students were referred to as *attendants.* The Ballard School of Practical Nursing was very successful until it was closed in 1948. A similar program was established in Boston by the Massachusetts Emergency and Hygiene Association in 1892. In 1907, the Brattleboro School for Practical Nurses was opened in Vermont. All of these programs centered on home nursing care with emphasis on simple cooking and household duties which included the laundry. Few of the early schools provided hospital experience. When they were affiliated with a hospital, students were given a stipend in return for services rendered.

Red Cross Nurse's Aides

At the time the early practical nursing programs were preparing women for home nursing, the American Red Cross undertook the training of lay women, in 1908, to provide nursing care for their own families. During World War I it became evident that a program was needed to train nonprofessional persons to care for the wounded and sick in Army hospitals. Jane Delano, the Director of Red Cross nursing, planned the course of instruction. She and other nursing leaders of that era, including Annie W. Goodrich, were not in favor of using nurse's aides or practical nurses to work in military hospitals. During World War II, however, the need for the Red Cross nurse's aide was acute. A planned curriculum was developed in 1942; it consisted of thirty-four hours of lecture and forty-five hours of supervised clinical experience in the hospital setting. A one-hour examination was given and each participant was required to take the Red Cross First Aid Course. Those who completed the course were utilized in industry, schools, hospitals, outpatient clinics, and public health agencies.

Controls on Practical Nursing Education and Practice

Prior to World War II practical nurse education was aimed at preparing a home nurse. Wide variation among programs existed until the programs were placed in educational institutions; were conducted by state departments of education under the division of vocational education; or were controlled by state legislation and state agencies. In 1914, the state of Mississippi enacted a law controlling the preparation of the practical nurse in that state. The Minneapolis Girls' Vocational High School established the first practical nurse program in a vocational school in 1919. By 1945 there were eight states whose programs were recognized by the State Boards of Nurse Examiners. Gradually, the programs in approved schools throughout the country became increasingly uniform.

It became necessary to stop untrained people from functioning as practical nurses. Just as the states set up laws to regulate the preparation and practice of professional nursing, the states individually established laws for practical nursing. By 1955 some states had mandatory laws regarding licensure of practical nurses and all but a few states had some type of licensure law. In instances where licensing laws had not yet been enacted, employing institutions gave preference to the practical nurses who had been prepared in approved schools. Consequently, it became important that preparation be obtained in an approved practical nurse training program and that the nurse realize the significance of obtaining licensure as soon as possible after successful completion of the course.

The Early Curriculum

The general objective of the early practical nurse training program was to give effective theoretical and clinical training that would result in a mastery of the skills and related knowledge required to perform the duties assigned to the graduate practical nurse.

Usually school authorities were required to determine the length of the program before considering the organization, financing, staffing, and recruitment. However, it was suggested that sound experimentation be carried on as early as possible in order to determine a desirable time minimum. There were many factors involved in the determination of the length of time required for a satisfactory program. One of the principal factors was the precedent established by the schools which had been operating for several years. Another factor was the viewpoint held that if the program exceeded one year, many older, more mature persons would hesitate to take the course due to the loss of earning power during the learning period. It was generally recommended that not less than one year, or approximately 2000 hours, should be allotted for a satisfactory program.

Division, Section, or Unit		Percent	
	Total	100.0	
DIVISION A –	BASIC NURSING SKILLS AND RELATED INSTRUCTION	72.0	Total
Section I	Meeting the health needs of apparently well individuals and families.	3.0	
Section II	Meeting the nursing needs of the mildly ill and of the convalescent patient	35.0	
Section III	Meeting of the nursing needs of the patient with long term illness or disabling conditions . .	19.0	
Section IV	Meeting the nursing needs of the mother and infant	11.0	
Section V	Meeting the common emergency needs of individuals and families.	4.0	
DIVISION B –	CONCURRENT UNITS OF INSTRUCTION . .	28.0	Total
Unit I	Basic homemaking skills and related instruction.	14.6	Total of Unit
	(Meal planning and preparation, including special diets	10.0	
	Care of the home	3.0	
	Care of flowers and plants in the sickroom . . .	0.6	
	Care of linen)	1.0	
Unit II	Basic related subjects	13.4	Total of Unit
	(Body structure and function	5.0	
	The life span)	8.4	

Fig. 11-2 Practical nursing curriculum – 1950

Approximately one-third of the total training period was devoted to pre-clinical classroom and laboratory instruction. The remaining two-thirds of the total time was devoted to clinical experience in approved institutions, and whenever possible, to some nursing experience in home situations.

The outline in figure 11-2 was the suggested program of instruction which was prepared in 1950 by a curriculum committee of the United States Office of Education. It served as a guide for instructors concerned with the training of practical nurses.

The Faculty

The instructor concerned with the teaching of the student practical nurse in the preclinical classroom situation was employed by the public school system and devoted full time to the preclinical classroom and laboratory instruction. Educational qualifications were high and experience in teaching was required. An instructor in a practical nurse program in a public school system was required to meet the state's minimum requirements for a teaching certificate. Faculty members in the practical nurse training program had to understand the common administrative practices and organizational patterns peculiar to this type of program. It was also considered important that the nurse who sought a career in practical nurse education understand the characteristics of the public education system. The clinical teacher-supervisor was employed as a full-time member of the school of nursing faculty in the institution offering clinical experience to the student practical nurse.

Availability of Employment

The graduate of approved schools of practical nurse training did not find any difficulty in securing employment. Hospitals, health agencies, nursing

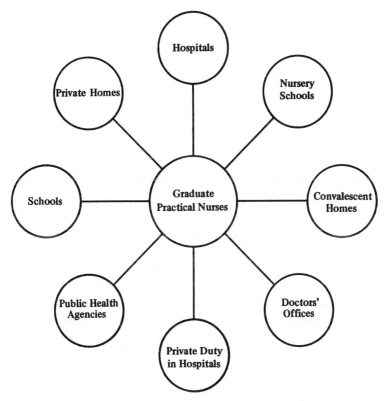

Fig. 11-3 Areas of employment represented by graduate practical nurses in 1950

homes, and private individuals were eager to obtain the services of the practical nurse. Salaries were not stabilized but generally the early graduate earned approximately two-thirds to three-fourths of the salary received by registered professional nurses on the staff nurse level. Generally speaking, the salary of the licensed practical nurse compared favorably with that of women with comparable training.

Acceptance of the Practical Nurse

In 1947 the Joint Committee on Auxiliary Nursing Service published a pamphlet entitled *Practical Nurses and Auxiliary Workers for the Care of the Sick.* This committee was composed of appointed representatives of six national nursing associations. It was pointed out in the pamphlet that it was necessary to recognize the specific functions of assistant nursing personnel. Many individual professional nurses, however, appeared unable to accept the nonprofessional person in the nursing situation. There were some who even spoke disparagingly of the use of assistant personnel in caring for the sick. Some professional nurses expressed sincere concern about the quality of patient care the nonprofessional would be capable of giving, while other nurses were fearful of their own future. Practical nursing has progressed through a series of role definitions and in 1957 the American Nurses' Association (A.N.A.) and the National Federation of Licensed Practical Nurses, Inc. (N.F.L.P.N.) attempted to clearly define the functions of the practical nurse. Today there is a better understanding of the role and functions of the practical nurse, who has been accepted as a member of the nursing team.

RECENT TRENDS IN PRACTICAL NURSING
EDUCATION AND PRACTICE

The health occupations have increased tremendously in number and kind. Nursing has changed considerably in response to the development of new health care workers, technological advances, specialization, and the changing health care needs in the community. Practical nursing education also reflects these changes and has demonstrated an awareness of the need for uniform standards and a curriculum which will prepare a technically competent health care worker.

Classification and Accreditation

The National League for Nursing classifies programs as adult education if they are conducted for adults and not as part of a high school curriculum. High school programs are offered to high school students and lead concurrently to a high school diploma. Programs offered to high school students, but requiring additional time for completion, are called high school extended programs. Graduates of all state-approved programs are eligible to write the licensing examination for practical nursing. In 1973, there were 1,214 schools that conducted 1,306 programs preparing practical nurses.

Current administrative control of practical nursing schools may be: secondary schools; trade, technical or vocational schools; adult education centers; senior colleges or universities; junior or community colleges; hospitals; independent agencies; or government agencies. Their principal source of financial support is either public or private.

In the United States, the first public school practical nursing program accredited by the National League for Nursing was the Chicago Public Schools program in 1966. The number of accredited programs has grown consistently since them.

Program Objectives

The faculty of each practical nursing program develops its own philosophy. The program should be consistent with the philosophy of the parent institution. Believing in this philosophy, the faculty should plan the program to meet the educational needs of the student. The program should be flexible so as to allow development of the individual potential. Learning is a continuous process. Therefore, the program should be developed from the simple to the complex while the student develops knowledge through study and experience. Nursing is designed to meet the physical, psychological, and sociological needs of the patient; the students should study and practice patient-centered nursing care of all age groups.

Statements of objectives might specify that, upon completion of the course, the graduate will be expected:

- To function as a licensed practical nurse under the supervision of the registered nurse, licensed physician, or licensed dentist;.

- To use acquired knowledge and skills to meet effectively the physical and emotional, social, and spiritual needs of the patient;

- To teach health and prevention of disease as a member of the health team and the community;

- To have an awareness of the continuing changes in society, medical science, and technology;

- To identify the contributions made by local and national organizations which represent the interests of practical nurses;

- To recognize the need for continual personal and educational growth.

The ultimate purpose of a practical nursing program is to implement a program of study for men and women who desire a career as a licensed practical nurse. The program should be designed to develop the student's knowledge of nursing in order to facilitate participation in the care of the sick and injured, the rehabilitation of the disabled, the maintenance of health, and the prevention of disease.

The Curriculum

Curriculum patterns vary from state to state and even among schools within a given state. Most, however, are one year in length; if it is offered in a community college, the curriculum tends to follow the school calendar. The former trend of dividing the curriculum into two periods, preclinical and clinical, is now considered educationally unsound. Theory and clinical experience should be correlated. The individual program may include elective courses in behavioral sciences and humanities.

Generally the fall or first semester is an introduction to basic nursing and communication skills essential in meeting physical and emotional needs of the patient. Lecture, laboratory, and clincial experience may be conducted by team teaching. Basic concepts of body structure and function, nutrition, fundamentals of nursing, mental health, and personal and vocational relationships are studied.

The spring or second semester is an integrated study of medical and surgical nursing, including diet therapy, pharmacology and gerontology. Utilizing the problem-solving approach, the student applies knowledge and skill in practice of comprehensive nursing care.

A third session during the summer could be an emphasis on maternal-child health, as a concentrated course, integrating principles of growth and development and community health. Advanced study in personal and vocational relationships would prepare the student for the role of a licensed practical nurse.

The Faculty

The faculty is carefully selected on the basis of education and nursing expertise. Generally, baccalaureate and master's degrees are preferred, in addition

FACULTY SUPERVISION	FALL SEMESTER	SPRING SEMESTER	SUMMER SESSION
	12 weeks - 10 hrs/week (2 1/2 hrs/day - 4 days/week)	16 weeks - 15 hrs/week (3 hrs/day - 5 days/week)	8 weeks - 15 hrs/week (3 hrs/day - 5 days/week)
Instructor 1	HOSPITAL #1 Medical Unit	HOSPITAL #1 Medical-Surgical Unit	HOSPITAL #1 OB Unit / HOSPITAL #1 Pediatric Unit
	4 weeks Section III / 4 weeks Section I / 4 weeks Section II	4 weeks Section I / 4 weeks Section II / 4 weeks Section III	4 weeks Section I / 4 weeks Section I
			NURSING HOME #1
			4 weeks Section I
Instructor 2	HOSPITAL #2 Medical-Surgical Unit	HOSPITAL #2 Medical-Surgical Unit	HOSPITAL #2 OB Unit / HOSPITAL #2 Pediatric Unit
	4 weeks Section II / 4 weeks Section III / 4 weeks Section I	4 weeks Section II / 4 weeks Section III / 4 weeks Section I	4 weeks Section II / 4 weeks Section II
			NURSING HOME #2
			4 weeks Section II
Instructor 3	EXTENDED CARE FACILITY Semi-Skill Care Unit	HOSPITAL #3 Neurosurgery-Orthopedic Unit	HOSPITAL #3 OB Unit / HOSPITAL #3 Pediatric Unit
	4 weeks Section I / 4 weeks Section II / 4 weeks Section III	4 weeks Section III / 4 weeks Section II / 4 weeks Section I	4 weeks Section III / 4 weeks Section III
			NURSING HOME #3
			4 weeks Section III

2 students per 3 days - Central Service Department

1 student per 2 days - Recovery Room

1 student per day - Respiratory Care Department

1 student per day - Operating Room Observation

1 student per day - Physical Therapy Department

1 student per day - Occupational Therapy Department

Hours:

FALL – 8:30 to 11:00 A.M.
    M. T. W. Th.

SPRING – 9:00 A.M. to 12:00 P.M.
    M. T. W. Th. F.

SUMMER – 8:00 to 11:00 A.M.
    M. T. W. Th. F.

Fig. 11-4 Clinical experience plan for a practical nursing program

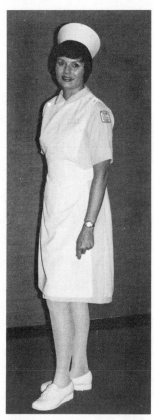

Fig. 11-5 A practical nursing student models her uniform.

to evidence of competent experience in nursing and successful teaching experience. In community college programs, nonnursing courses may be taught by nonnurses who have had preparation commensurate with their position.

Current Job Opportunities

The role of the Licensed Practical/Vocational Nurse (LPN, LVN) has had drastic changes from the early emphasis on simple nursing procedures and home care. In 1973, the U.S. Army offered practical nurses the opportunity to enlist for duty as clinical specialists with the Army Medical Service. The Army conducted nine state-approved schools for enlistees who were interested in becoming practical nurses. Graduates are eligible to take the state board licensure examination. The first of these schools was organized in 1954 at Walter Reed Medical Center. Applicants must enlist for three years and must complete four weeks of basic military training and eight weeks of basic corpsman training. Before attending the Clinical Specialist School there must be a record of six weeks' experience in the hospital setting. The program is a full calendar year and is basically equivalent to civilian state-approved school programs. In addition to the basic curriculum, techniques of instruction, techniques of management, and military medical science are covered. Unlike the civilian functions of the practical nurse, the administration of parenteral fluids and blood derivatives, and the application of simple casts and traction are considered appropriate assignments.

By 1971, licensed practical nurses were employed in a wide variety of positions which included all nursing services. Employment opportunities were available in all geographic areas. However, by 1975 it was noted that some geographic locations were meeting their budgeted vacancies with ease and the L.P.N. found some difficulty in securing the exact position desired. Rural areas, not in the vicinity of a practical nursing school, tended to be more in need of graduates.

Practical nurses are employed in general hospitals, psychiatric and mental health facilities, institutions for the mentally retarded, doctors' offices, blood bank clinics, private duty, public health agencies, extended care and skilled care centers, tuberculosis sanitariums, and in industry. Increasing numbers of licensed practical nurses are functioning in roles with supervisory responsibilities.

SUMMARY

Nursing duties in America before 1860 were performed by practical nurses who gained their knowledge by experience. Organized practical nurse training began as early as 1892 when the first practical nurse program was organized at the Brooklyn Y.W.C.A. Today practical nurse education is generally received in public secondary schools or community/junior colleges. The general objective of a practical nursing program is to give effective theoretical and clinical education that will result in a mastery of the skills and related knowledge required to perform the duties assigned to the graduate practical nurse. The time allotted for a satisfactory program is generally one full year of concentrated study and learning experiences. Generally the graduate of an approved school of practical nursing will not find any difficulty in securing employment. The salary of the licensed practical nurse is usually three-fourth that of the registered professional nurse on the staff nurse level. Career ladder opportunities have facilitated the upward mobility of licensed practical nurses who aspire to careers as registered nurses.

SUGGESTED ACTIVITIES

- Visit a local hospital or health agency which employs licensed practical nurses. Find out how the practical nurse functions in that setting. Compare your findings with the functions of a registered nurse in the same setting.

- In a panel presentation, discuss how a licensed practical nurse would function on an adult medical-surgical unit that has the following approaches: team nursing, primary nursing, and functional nursing.

- Compare the clinical experience in a practical nursing program (see figure 11-4) with the clinical experience in your program.

REVIEW

A.   Multiple Choice. Select the best answer.

1.   In 1892, Mrs. Charles Judson and Mrs. Katharine A. Adams organized a practical nurse training program in
   a. Kaiserswerth, Germany.   c. Philadelphia, Pennsylvania.
   b. St. Catherines, Canada.   d. Brooklyn, New York.

2. The average length of an approved full-time practical nursing program today is
   a. one year.   c. three years.
   b. two years.   d. four years.

3. A one-year program which trains clinical specialists who can administer blood and apply casts is
   a. offered in many vocational schools.
   b. typical of practical nursing programs.
   c. offered at New York Hospital.
   d. offered by the U.S. Army.

4. The Minneapolis Girls' Vocational High School established the first practical nursing program in a
   a. two-year college.   c. hospital school of nursing.
   b. high school extended program.   d. vocational school.

5. The first public school practical nursing program to be accredited by the National League for Nursing was the
   a. Boston public schools program.
   b. Chicago public schools program.
   c. Brattleboro public schools program.
   d. Philadelphia public schools program.

B. Match the dates in Column II to the correct statement in Column I.

Column I	Column II
1. Brattleboro School for Practical Nurses established.	a. 1860
	b. 1873
2. Practical nursing programs recognized by State Board of Nurse Examiners in eight states.	c. 1892
	d. 1907
3. Law controlling the preparation of the practical nurse enacted in Mississippi.	e. 1914
	f. 1919
4. Mandatory laws regarding licensure of practical nurses enacted by many states.	g. 1945
	h. 1955
5. First professional schools of nursing organized in the United States.	i. 1966
6. First practical nurse program established in a vocational school.	j. 1973
7. Organized practical nurse training began at Brooklyn Y.W.C.A.	

8. Prior to this date practical nurses were self-taught.

9. Practical nurse programs conducted in 1,214 schools.

10. First public school practical nurse program in the United States accredited by NLN.

C. Briefly answer the following questions.

1. Why was practical nursing established?

2. Why was it necessary to license practical nurses?

3. List six administrative controlling bodies of the practical nursing programs.

chapter 12
TECHNICAL vs. PROFESSIONAL NURSING

STUDENT OBJECTIVES

- Explain the positions of the national nursing organizations on technical and professional education and practice.
- Define the roles of the technical and professional nurse.
- Explain why the blurring of the roles of technical and professional nurses has become an issue.

There is no question that nursing is an occupation. But there is considerable difference of opinion as to whether nursing is a professional occupation or a technical one. The problem is compounded by virtue of the fact that there are at present three kinds of educational programs which prepare nurses to be eligible for licensure as registered nurses. Are the graduates of all three programs considered professionals? Are the graduates of the collegiate programs *professionals,* and diploma and associate degree students *technicians?* Where does the licensed practical nurse belong? There is no apparent consensus. Nurse educators feel there is a need for a clear understanding so that employers can appropriately utilize graduates from all programs; also, the distinction is necessary so that the quality of nursing practice can be improved rather than be maintained.

PROFESSIONALISM

Experts in the social sciences are considered the authorities on what makes an occupation a profession. Although there is some variation in actual criteria, it is generally agreed that:

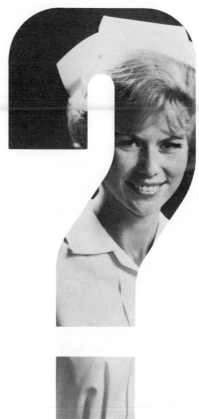

- Professional status is achieved when an occupation involves a unique practice which carries great individual responsibility and is based upon theoretical knowledge.

- The privilege to practice is granted only after the individual has completed a standardized program of highly specialized education and has demonstrated an ability to meet the standards for practice.

- The body of specialized knowledge is continually developed and evaluated through research.

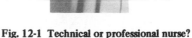

Fig. 12-1 Technical or professional nurse?

- The members are self-organized and collectively assume the responsibility of establishing standards for education and practice; they continually evaluate the quality of services provided in order to protect the individual members and the public.

Does nursing meet all the criteria and is it a profession? The professional organizations refer to nursing as a profession. Current nursing leaders and publications discuss the profession of nursing. In Illinois and New York (and in a growing number of other states) individuals are licensed to practice as *professional* nurses. It would seem that if nursing is not a profession, it is certainly approaching that status.

This statement sets forth Standards of Nursing Practice developed by the Congress for Nursing Practice.

WHY STANDARDS OF PRACTICE?

"A professional association is an organization of practitioners who judge one another as professionally competent and who have banded together to perform social functions which they cannot perform in their separate capacity as individuals."[1]

A professional association, because of its nature, must provide measures to judge the competency of its membership and to evaluate the quality of its services. Studies show that the tendency for self-organization has been found to be characteristic of professions and the establishment and implementation of standards characteristic of the organization. Mary Follet points out that professional associations have one function above all others:

"The members do not come together merely for the pleasure of meeting others of the same occupation; nor do they meet primarily to increase their pecuniary gain; although this may be one of the objects. They join in order to better perform their functions. They meet:

To establish standards.

To maintain standards.

To improve standards.

To keep members up to standards.

To educate the public to appreciate standards.

To protect the public from those individuals who have not attained standards or willfully do not follow them.

To protect individual members of the profession from each other."[2]

A profession's concern for the quality of its service constitutes the heart of its responsibility to the public. The more expertise required to perform the service, the greater is society's dependence upon those who carry it out. A profession must seek control of its practice in order to guarantee the quality of its service to the public. Behind that guarantee are the standards of the profession that provide the assurance that the guarantee will be met. This is essential both for the protection of the public and the profession itself. A profession that does not maintain the confidence of the public will soon cease to be a social force.

In recognition of the importance of standards of professional practice and the need to guarantee quality service, the various Divisions on Practice have each formulated a set of standards. The American Nurses' Association recognizes that as standards are implemented in practice settings and as the scope of nursing practice enlarges and the theoretical basis upon which this practice rests becomes more sharply delineated, ongoing revision of the standards of professional practice will be warranted.

Congress for Nursing Practice

1. Merton, Robert K. "The Functions of the Professional Association," American Journal of Nursing, Vol. 58 (January, 1958), p. 50.
2. Dynamic Administration, The Collected Papers of Mary Follet, edited by Henry C. Metcalf and L. Urwick, New York: Harper & Brothers, 1942, p. 136.

Fig. 12-2 The American Nurses' Association believes nursing is a profession.

PROFESSIONAL NURSING

The definition of nursing as contained in the Nurse Practice Act of New York State gives nursing professional status. The legal definition, signed into law on March 15, 1972, established a precedent in nursing legislation: *The practice of the profession of nursing as a registered professional nurse is defined as diagnosing and treating human responses to actual or potential health problems through such services as casefinding, health teaching, health counseling, and provision or care supportive to or restorative of life and well-being, and executing medical regimens prescribed by a licensed or otherwise legally authorized physician or dentist. A nursing regimen shall be consistent with and shall not vary any existing medical regimen.*

In order to be licensed in New York to practice professional nursing, the applicant must have received an education and a diploma or degree in professional nursing in a state-approved school. In other words, graduates of the associate degree, diploma, and baccalaureate degree are all licensed as registered nurses and all practice professional nursing in New York. Regardless of the type of preparation, the graduates take the same state board examination; upon the successful completion of the examination, they are licensed as registered nurses in all states throughout the country. All registered nurses can become members of the professional organizations.

Although there is no differentiation between technical and professional nurses in terms of licensure, there is definitely a trend to define the professional nurse as a graduate of an approved baccalaureate school of nursing, who has successfully passed the state licensing examination required for registration. Therefore, *professional education* would take place in a four-year university or senior college. Baccalaureate programs generally require 120-124 credit hours with approximately 50 hours in the nursing major and the remaining hours in liberal arts and the sciences.

In October of 1974, the voting body of the New York State Nurses' Association adopted a Resolution on Entry Into Professional Practice; this has led to the development of statutory language which, if passed by the state legislative bodies, would make it mandatory by 1985 for all applicants for licensure as a registered

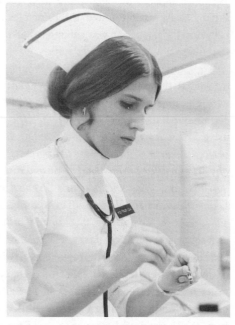

Fig. 12-3 Does the nurse in a specialty area need professional or technical education?

nurse in New York to have a minimum of a baccalaureate degree in nursing. The rationale for this proposed legislation is: *That it has long been recognized that, as a professional endeavor, nursing practice must be based upon a minimum of baccalaureate education. It is necessary now to resolve the persistent confusion created by the existence of multiple kinds of basic nursing education programs leading to licensure as a registered professional nurse.*

TECHNICAL NURSING

Technological progress has necessitated the need to prepare the technician. The technical worker maintains a middle position between the professional person, who has the responsibility to make major desicions based on in-depth knowledge and expertise, and the skilled worker who has had on-the-job training.

Technical education initially was designed for the preparation of technicians for industry, with concentration on science and mathematics. The rapid growth of community colleges in the past decade has created vast opportunities for the preparation of a large variety of technical workers.

When nursing programs were established in community colleges, it was generally accepted that these programs would provide *technical* education. Technical nursing included more than good manual dexterity and mastery of skills. It also incorporated the principles and theories of the biophysical and behavioral sciences. It was assumed that the technical nurse would work under the supervision of *professional* nurses.

The Council of Associate Degree Programs of the National League for Nursing developed the following definition: *The technical nurse is a registered nurse with an associate degree in nursing licensed for the practice of nursing who carries out nursing and other therapeutic measures with a high degree of skill, using principles from an ever-expanding body of science. The technical nurse performs nursing functions with patients who are under the supervision of a physician and/or professional nurse and assists in planning the day-to-day care of patients, evaluating the patient's physical and emotional reactions to therapy, taking measures to alleviate distress, using treatment modalities with knowledge and precision, and supervising other workers in the technical aspects of care.*

Technical education takes place, therefore, in the junior or community college. Associate degree programs are two years in length and usually consist of sixty-eight credit hours. Half of these credits are in nursing courses and the other half are earned in courses in liberal arts and the sciences. Most of the courses offer transferable college credits. Based on a 1976 survey of its members, the Council of Associate Degree Programs announced that the membership approved the use of the term, *associate degree nurse* over *technical nurse.*

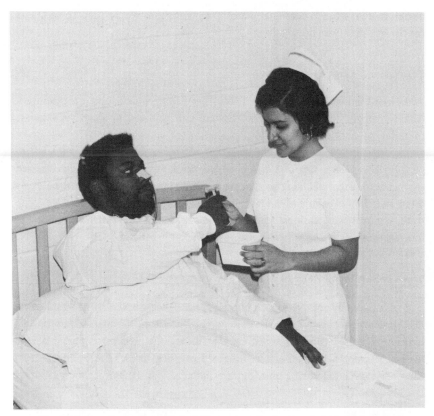

Fig. 12-4 Does the nurse at the bedside need professional or technical education?

GROUP POSITION STATEMENTS

Professional organizations and labor groups have attempted to categorize nurses by identifying education and skill levels of graduates of the various types of nursing education programs. There is no unanimous agreement on a single definition of the terms. Included here are positions of several major groups.

The American Nurses' Association

The American Nurses' Association (ANA) published a position paper on nursing education in 1965 after a fifteen-year study. The ANA promotes the baccalaureate degree program as the basic education for *professional nurses.* Registered nurses who graduated from associate degree and diploma programs, therefore, would be termed *technical nurses.* The ANA supports the concept that the minimum preparation for the technical nurse should be an associate degree in nursing.   Vocational education institutions would prepare assistants for the health service occupations.

The National League for Nursing

At the biennial convention in 1965, the membership adopted a resolution which strongly supports the trend toward college-based programs in nursing. In order to continue the professionalization of nursing, the NLN will make a concerted effort to define the *different programs for personnel prepared to perform complementary but different functions.*   The resolution also stressed the need for local planning so that recruitment into all programs will be expedited and the needs of the community will be met. It further encouraged local, state, regional, and national planning to allow for the development and maintenance of a balance of nursing personnel from all programs.

The National Labor Relations Board

In May 1975, the National Labor Relations Board (NLRB) in Washington, D.C. ruled that licensed, registered nurses constitute a separate appropriate bargaining unit.   This was based on the finding that registered nurses have a distinct community of interest.   Licensed practical nurses are excluded from the professional bargaining unit, but are included in a technical unit with other

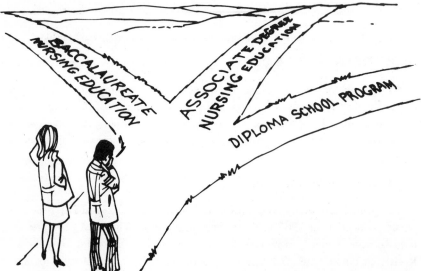

Fig. 12-5   The future nurse has several alternatives in choosing a basic nursing education program.

technical health workers. Therefore, under the auspices of the NLRB all registered nurses are considered professional employees and licensed practical nurses are technical employees.

National Student Nurses' Association

In the mid-seventies, the Board of Directors of the National Student Nurses' Association issued a statement opposing the use of the terms *technical* and *professional.* They felt that the term *technical* connoted a less-qualified nurse on the par with laborers. The NSNA recognizes the different levels of nurse practitioners and the varying types of educational programs. It is their contention that the duties performed by the Associate Degree Nursing graduate are above a technical level and the term, therefore, appears to be inappropriate.

SUMMARY

The purpose of this chapter was to discuss the differences of opinion regarding technical and professional nursing. The issue is a complex one and has led to heated discussions, meetings, seminars, and studies. Many questions remain unanswered, but the trends are becoming increasingly clear. The technical nurse is educated in an associate degree program and the professional nurse is educated in a baccalaureate degree program. Nursing practice is regulated in its scope by the nurse practice acts of each state. Each program prepares a nurse to function in specific roles which are commensurate with the level of education attained. These roles are different, but each is dependent upon and complementary to the other.

SUGGESTED ACTIVITIES

- Compare school catalog listings of curricula and course descriptions of a diploma program, associate degree in nursing program, and a baccalaureate degree nursing program.

- Interview one student enrolled presently in each of the three types of programs. Ascertain what their previous education and experiences were and what their goals are in nursing, after graduation.

- Write your own personal definition of a technical nurse and a professional nurse in light of your own philosophy.

REVIEW

A.   Multiple Choice. Select the best answer.

1.   Which state Nurse Practice Act set a precedent for nursing legislation?
      a. California.   c. New York.
      b. Illinois.   d. Florida.

2.   A technician is
      a. a skilled worker who has had on-the-job training.
      b. a person who can make major decisions based upon in-depth knowledge.
      c. trained in math and science.
      d. a semiprofessional who maintains a middle position between the professional and the skilled worker.

3.   When associate degree programs in nursing were first established it ·was expected that they would provide
      a. professional education.
      b. semiprofessional education.
      c. technical education.
      d. the same kind of education as the diploma school.

4.   The organization which advocates a baccalaureate degree as the basic requirement for professional nursing is
      a. The American Nurses' Association.
      b. The National League for Nursing.
      c. The Council of Associate Degree and Baccalaureate Degree Programs.
      d. none of the above.

5.   The organization which advocates a baccalaureate degree as the minimum education for licensure as a registered nurse is
      a. The American Nurses' Association.
      b. The National League for Nursing.
      c. The New York State Nurses' Association.
      d. none of the above.

6.   The position of the National League for Nursing
      a. included support for college-based nursing programs.
      b. encouraged regional planning for recruitment of nurses into all programs.
      c. included awareness of the need to define the different programs in nursing.
      d. all of the above.

7. According to the NLRB, an associate degree nurse is
   a. not eligible to be in a collective bargaining unit.
   b. a technical employee.
   c. a professional employee.
   d. a and b.

8. The National Student Nurses' Association position states that
   a. the members opposed using the terms *technical* and *professional.*
   b. there were no differences between graduates of associate degree, diploma, or baccalaureate nursing programs.
   c. graduates of associate degree programs function at the same level as technicians, but the term is inappropriate.
   d. none of the above.

9. The American Nurses' Association position concerning the practical nurse is
   a. the L.P.N. is a technical nurse.
   b. the L.P.N. should be trained in two-year associate degree programs.
   c. the practical nurse is an assistant to the registered nurse.
   d. the practical nurse needs on-the-job training only.

10. If the proposed changes are made in the New York Nurse Practice Act, associate degree graduates
    a. could not be licensed as registered nurses in New York.
    b. would still be licensed as registered nurses, but would be technical rather than professional nurses.
    c. would be licensed as a registered professional nurse.
    d. none of the above.

B. Briefly answer the following questions.

1. List the characteristics of a profession.

2. How does the Council of Associate Degree Programs of the National League for Nursing define technical nurse?

SECTION 4
HEALTH CARE AND THE CONSUMER

chapter 13
CONTEMPORARY
HEALTH CARE

STUDENT OBJECTIVES

- Identify major trends which are influencing health care in the United States.

- Describe services provided by nontraditional health care facilities.

- Identify the major factors which have brought about changes in the distribution of health care services.

Society is never static; it is always in the process of change. Change is occurring more rapidly than ever and the changes taking place have had a tremendous impact on health care and the distribution of health care services. Consumer participation in planning the distribution and delivery of health care has increased appreciably in recent years. The hospital is no longer the single provider of health care. The responsibility for health care and its delivery has been assumed by a growing number of public and private agencies at the national, state, and local levels, and by many diversified health professionals. The purpose of this chapter is to identify the conditions and trends which are changing the health care system, the measures which have been taken to affect change at the community and national levels, and the dimensions and characteristics of contemporary health care.

TRENDS INFLUENCING HEALTH CARE

The major trends influencing health care services and their distribution are:

- Health care is becoming increasingly specialized and complex.

- Health care workers need more education in the collegiate setting.

- Federal funding of education in the health fields has increased.

- Auxiliary workers are needed to extend the services of educated health care specialists.

- There is an increased utilization of electronic data processing equipment in health care facilities.

- The growing cost of health care has necessitated federal assistance.

- The consumer has demanded the establishment of new health services and facilities which focus on the maintenance of health rather than on the treatment of illness.

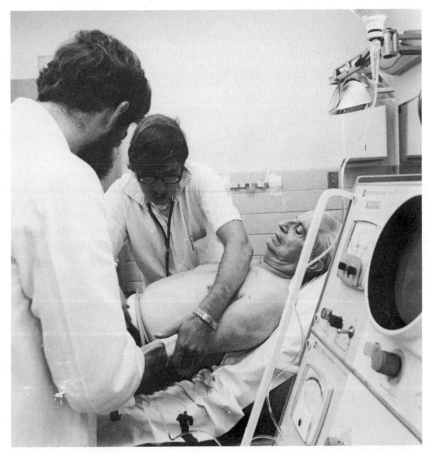

Fig. 13-1 New methods of diagnosis and treatment have brought about highly specialized health occupations.

The explosion of scientific knowledge during and after World War II has brought about tremendous growth and advances in the behavioral and biological sciences and in the development of *technology* (application of scientific principles in a practical manner). Advances have facilitated rapid growth and change in medical treatment and diagnosis, and the evolution of highly specialized health occupations. Collectively, these changes have made health care much more complex.

Collegiate Education

It became obvious that individuals involved in health care needed more education and more specialized training. As a result of scientific advances and

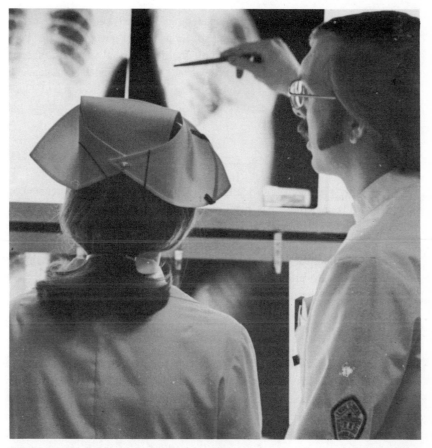

Fig. 13-2 Many paramedical health care workers, including nurses and radiological technicians, are prepared in community college programs.

the evolution of specialized health occupations, there has been: (1) an increase in the level of education for health workers, (2) a growth in specialized education in institutions of higher learning, and (3) an increase in the kinds of technical and professional health workers. The junior-community colleges have become increasingly involved in the education and preparation of *paramedical specialists* (persons who supplement the work of highly trained medical professionals), for example, laboratory technicians and x-ray technicians. The senior colleges and universities have increased the numbers and types of health career programs which prepare health care professionals such as doctors, nurses, social workers, physical therapists, and hospital administrators.

Federal Funding

The cost of education has skyrocketed and placed collegiate education beyond the means of the average student. The federal government has been forced to assume a growing responsibility for the financial support of technical and professional education in the health fields. Federal assistance is provided through scholarships, traineeships and loans to individuals. Federal subsidization of schools is accomplished through project, construction and research grants, and capitation.

Auxiliary Workers

Along with the increased numbers of allied health workers prepared in collegiate programs, there has been a demand for auxiliary workers who are skilled and semiskilled, and who provide supportive services in health care facilities; nursing assistants, ward clerks, laboratory technicians, and secretaries are examples of auxiliary workers. Many of the functions formerly associated with the professional health worker have been assigned to these assistants in order to extend the services of the health care team.

Computerization

The complexity of health care has created a need for better communication and coordination. The data collected relating to the health care of patients, research, and the operation of health care facilities has become immense and unmanageable. In an effort to process and better utilize the accumulated data, concepts of *cybernetics* (science involving comparative study of automatic control systems) and *computer technology* (the use of machines to process data) have been applied in hospitals and other health care institutions. Com-

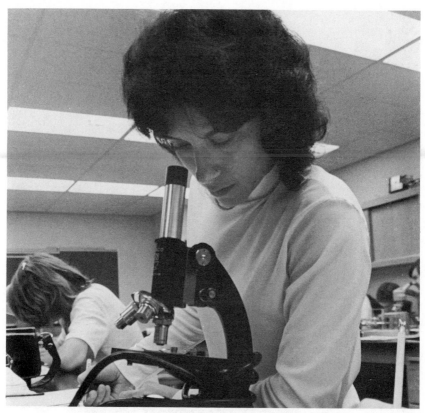

Fig. 13-3 Medical lab technician studying blood sample

puter systems were first used in 1957 by hospitals to assist with accounting, payroll, and insurance records. Later, computers processed laboratory data, admission and discharge data, medication records, and service requests. The use of electronic data processing equipment has grown to include automation of laboratory procedures, patient monitoring, electrocardiograph analysis, automated nurse staffing, automated patient histories, and automated medication systems, to mention just a few. The effects and effectiveness of a computer-assisted health care system have yet to be fully realized and evaluated.

Costs of Health Care

The cost of health care is considerable and still growing. Most middle-class citizens are covered by some type of health insurance which makes it possible to afford health care. *Medicare* is a federal program which provides hospital and medical insurance protection for people over sixty-five. *Medicaid* is a

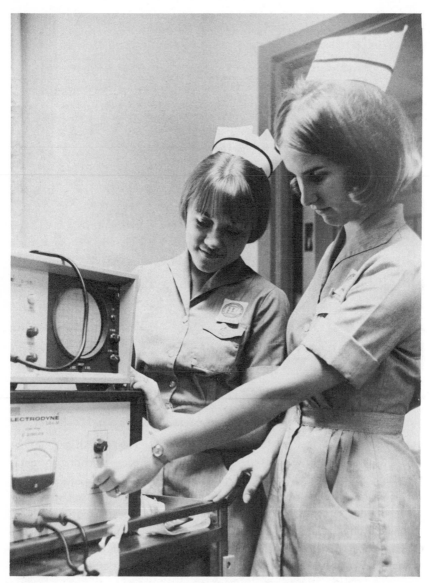

Fig. 13-4 Two nursing students learn to work with electronic equipment.

federal and state program which provides medical assistance for persons receiving public assistance. There is a growing interest in a national health insurance program which would enable all citizens to obtain health insurance. With increased government funding, there are increased government controls. It is apparent that such controls have promoted better health care facilities.

The Health Care Consumer

The public, or health care consumer, has become increasingly aware of health care through health education programs and exposure to the mass media. There has been an increase in the utilization of existing health care facilities. The consumer has become better informed and much more critical of health services. No longer is the consumer content to have access to what is provided; the consumer demands what services are to be provided and how they should be distributed. The focus is no longer on the treatment of illness but on the maintenance of health. The influence of the consumer has led to the development of new health services and facilities which meet the needs of the public more effectively. Therefore, more health care personnel are employed in nonhospital health facilities.

OTHER FACTORS INFLUENCING HEALTH CARE

In addition to current trends, there are other factors and conditions which have had an impact on organized health care. They are:

- Changes in patterns of illness
- Family planning and abortion
- Abuse of chemical substances
- Inflation
- The energy crisis
- Federal legislation

Patterns of Illness

More people are living to reach old age; therefore, there is a large new group of people who have unique needs and illnesses. The aged are more prone to develop chronic, degenerative diseases. This puts pressure on the health care system to provide facilities which are designed to treat and care for persons with disabling, long-term illnesses. Treatment of patients with chronic illnesses in the hospital is expensive and unnecessary; however, there are too few extended care facilities to meet the current needs.

The prevention of communicable diseases has become so successful that institutions established for treatment have become obsolete and unnecessary. Polio, smallpox and diphtheria all have declined in incidence.

Diseases associated with environmental conditions are on the increase. Heart disease, cancer, and kidney disease are leaders in cause of death. Diagnosis

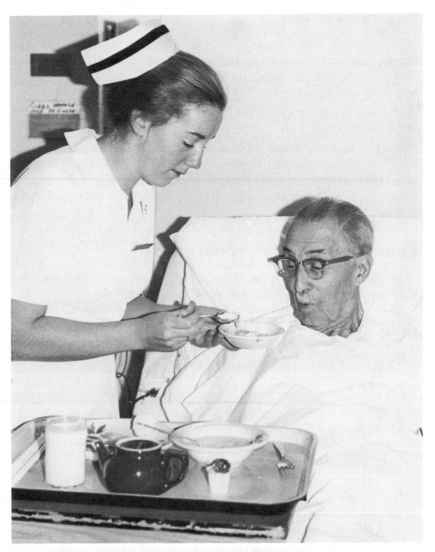

Fig. 13-5 Chronic, long-term illnesses are among the leading health problems.

and treatment of these three diseases requires the effort of many health workers and researchers and consumes a phenomenal amount of public dollars.

Because there is an increased incidence of disabling disease, there is also a growing interest in and need for rehabilitation services and associated health services, such as physical therapy, occupational therapy, speech therapy, and vocational rehabilitation. Rehabilitation is no longer seen as a service for the rich but as a right of every disabled citizen.

Family Planning and Abortion

The movement toward family planning came with the development of more effective means of birth control. Now such services are available in many communities. The effects of the proliferation of family planning have been seen in the reduction in the number of births. Hospital obstetric and pediatric units have felt the impact and many units have been closed to avoid financial loss.

The legalization of abortion in most states has brought about an increased demand for termination of pregnancy. This has necessitated the development of facilities and specialized health care workers. On the other side of the coin, advances in knowledge about conception have brought about the development of fertility clinics. Couples who previously could not have children are now able to produce offspring, due to the services provided by such clinics.

Abuse of Chemical Substances

Drug and alcohol use and abuse has become an increasingly serious problem in the United States. Many scientists and health professionals are involved

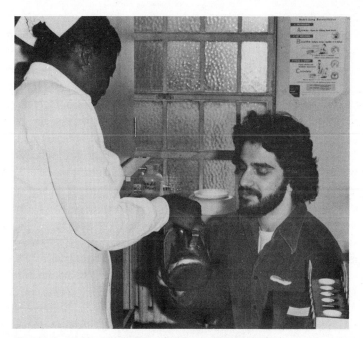

Fig. 13-6 There are a growing number of facilities designed to help the individual with problems other than physical illness.

in the national problem of drug and alcohol use, research, and rehabilitation. The study and treatment of substance abuse is costly and requires an inter-disciplinary approach in nontraditional community settings.

Inflation

Although the U.S. Labor Department releases monthly bulletins which list current prices, unemployment statistics, the cost of living, and the value of the American dollar, the true picture is not generally understood. But as the overall cost of living rises, the costs of health care also increase. However, cutting the health care budget may adversely affect the quality or quantity of health services. Comprehensive health planning at the state and local levels is necessary to determine priorities and to make recommendations as to how to contain costs while maintaining a quality health care system. Such planning can prevent duplication of expensive services and facilities. It can also prevent slipshod management practices such as employing poorly prepared personnel, at low wages, to replace skilled professional personnel.

Energy Crisis

Federal fuel allocation regulations may be a major concern for both the providers and consumers of health care. Most hospitals and other health care facilities have disposed of the rubber, stainless steel, and glass items previously used in nursing and medical procedures and utilize disposable plastic equipment instead. The use of disposable equipment has eliminated the need for cleaning, sterilization, packaging, and storage which required much labor. If disposable plastics were no longer produced, many hospitals and nursing homes would experience great difficulty in returning to the former procedures.

In areas where heating and lighting powers are reduced during periods of "brownouts," the functioning of some lifesaving machinery may be impaired. The patient whose very life depends upon a heart-lung or kidney machine may be concerned over power allocation cuts that may affect the efficiency of the equipment; however, most life-sustaining equipment have special generators which are not affected by cutbacks in power.

A gasoline shortage can have serious impact on health care delivery if nurses, physicians, and other allied health personnel are unable to obtain gasoline to drive to the institutionalized patient, or if consumers are unable to drive to health care facilities. Gas shortages may delay delivery of necessary hospital supplies. Ambulance service might be curtailed without adequate fuel supplies. The state of Maryland has led the country in the establishment of an emergency plan for such a fuel crisis situation.

Federal Legislation

At the federal and state level there is considerable legislation which affects health care. It would be impossible to cite all such legislation in this text. However, there is legislation which broadly affects health care. The National Health Planning and Resources Development Act of 1974 is such legislation. The Act calls for planning activities at the local or regional level which result in the development of Health Systems Plans. The Act also calls for the development of an overall State Health Plan which includes all planning related to mental health, mental retardation, alcohol abuse, drug abuse, immunization, and family planning programs, currently being supported with federal funds. The local planning groups are called Health Systems Agencies (HSA). The functions of HSA and state agencies will be melded into one overall process resulting in a planning document which is applicable for all purposes. The HSA are expected to implement the planning goals of federally funded projects, and to recommend capital improvement of health facilities, legislative action, licensure of institutions, and establishment of rates for institutional providers of health services (the latter is optional with each state). The State Health Plan will represent state health planning programs and health goals, in conjunction with the local plans of each HSA. This plan therefore becomes the official guidance document for the HSA and state. The plan is to be sent to the Department of Health, Education and Welfare. It remains to be seen if such legislation can provide for integrated regional planning and improved health care.

THE CHANGING HOSPITAL SYSTEM

The early hospital was a simple institution which provided food and shelter for the sick, in the spirit of Christian charity. Gradually hospitals became the centers of medical knowledge and contributed greatly to the expansion of that knowledge. Hospitals were supported by gifts and donations and run by religious groups.

The modern hospital has changed considerably but still retains some of its original purposes and characteristics. Hospitals have developed in response to the needs of its clients and advancements in medicine and technology. No longer does the hospital provide only facilities and services for the ill. It also provides specialized services related to prevention of illness, maintenance of health, diagnosis of pathology, treatment, and rehabilitation. The hospital is also an educational institution which provides experience for the growing number of health care workers and carries out research in all aspects of health care. In order to carry out these functions, the hospital has to employ a large number of professional, technical,

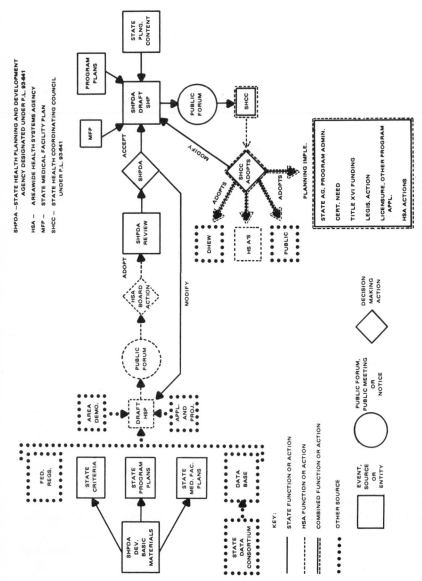

Fig. 13-7 The implementation of the National Health Planning and Resources Development Act of 1974

and skilled health care workers. The physical plant is complex, unique and expensive to build and operate. Most large hospitals are located in urban areas where manpower and resources are most readily available. The rate at which diagnostic and therapeutic techniques are introduced leads to rapid obsolescence of equipment, facilities, and skills. Thus, the hospital undergoes considerable change in short periods of time. Most hospitals no longer receive enough income from gifts and donations to keep them solvent. Many patients cannot pay the full cost of the hospital services they receive and the hospital is forced to absorb the loss. All of these factors have contributed to the rising cost of hospital services.

Hospital Costs

Expenses incurred by hospitals in the treatment of patients are referred to as *hospital costs.* In order to evaluate all types of costs, it is necessary to measure them according to a defined unit. Hospitals cannot measure the outcome of services effectively due to the nature of its product. Hospital output, therefore, is measured in terms of patient days, which is simply each twenty-four hour period of time during which hospital services are provided to each hospitalized person.

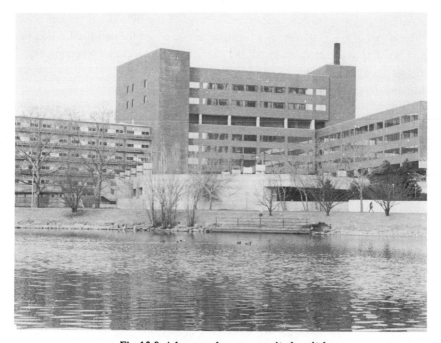

Fig. 13-8 A large modern community hospital

According to the National Hospital Panel Survey in 1967, the average cost per day in community hospitals was $53.14 and in 1972 it was $96.77, an increase of 82.1 percent. In 1972 the patient received 32.7 percent more laboratory tests than in 1967 and new types of equipment such as dialysis machines appeared on the hospital scene.

Inflation has contributed to increased hospital costs in numerous ways, such as annual increases in wages of personnel, cost of equipment and supplies, and replacement of obsolete methods and equipment. In hospitals the hourly wages of nonsupervisory personnel increased by 73.7 percent from 1966 to 1973. New health care occupations are being formed as a result of research and technical progress. An example is the newly formed departments of inhalation therapy with their trained and skilled respiratory care therapists, expensive equipment, and maintenance costs.

Another factor in the cost increase is related to the physician who takes advantage of the increased availability of diagnostic services. Today, a patient rightly expects that every possible measure be undertaken to ensure a correct diagnosis and cure.

Increased demand for hospital care has been brought about by extensive public and private health insurance coverage. Approximately 90 percent of Americans were covered by hospitalization insurance in 1971. Even though a patient generally pays a deductible portion of the bill, called the net price, the amount is minimal. Another factor which increased the demand for hospital services was the introduction of the Medicare and Medicaid programs aimed at two groups in society most likely to have poor health—persons over sixty-five and the poor, respectively.

Hospital outlay of funds is normally beyond that which is internally available; therefore, external sources of capital funding or financing are utilized. Three sources are employed: private grants, government grants, and long-term commercial borrowing. Commercial borrowing by hospitals has been growing rapidly through the purchase of bonds or mortgages with high interest rates, resulting in the rise of hospital costs.

Cost Controls

Several House Committee members voted against government control of hospitals, but they also proposed legislation to prohibit physicians, hospitals, and nursing homes from making unreasonable charges. However, all controls are generally ineffective at this time. The consumers of health care services will no doubt be watching hospital costs very closely in the future. The American Hospital Association is making an attempt to restrain hospitals in matters relative to price increase. Hospitals suffered tremendous losses during the period that the Economic Stabilization Program Act of 1971 was enforced as an economic control on the health care industry.

Hospital Classification

Classification of hospitals is made according to control or ownership, and the type of services rendered. The military, United States Public Health Service, and Veterans Administration hospitals are controlled by the federal government. The state, city, and county hospitals are controlled by the local governments. Government-operated hospitals usually have large bed capacities. Privately controlled hospitals are owned by churches, fraternal orders, business corporations, or individuals. Hospitals which operate for a profit are called *proprietary*, although the majority are voluntary nonprofit organizations. General hospitals provide care for patients with all types of illnesses. Special hospitals offer services in a specialty area; examples of such hospitals are a children's hospital or psychiatric-mental health facility.

Accreditation

Minimal standards must be met by the hospital in order to receive accreditation. The agency charged with evaluating and inspecting hospitals and insuring that standards are met is The Joint Commission of Accreditation of Hospitals (JCAH). Representatives on this team are selected from the American College of Physicians, American College of Surgeons, American Medical Association and the American Hospital Association. Hospitals are required to ensure quality care for all patients. All hospitals (as of July, 1975) are required to submit evidence of accountability, through ongoing patient care evaluation, to the Joint Commission for Accreditation of Hospitals.

HEALTH CARE DISTRIBUTION

There is a need for health care facilities other than the traditional hospital as the patterns of illness change. Today, the emphasis is on extended care facilities, rehabilitation centers, and institutions which provide long-term custodial care. Also, many citizens who live in remote, rural areas do not have access to health care facilities because most hospitals are in urban areas. The need for local health care facilities to provide comprehensive services and the manner in which they are made available to the consumer is changing. The growing number of nontraditional health care facilities reflect this trend.

A brief look at contemporary health care would indicate that health care, in one form or another, is provided by almost every established institution in society. Industrial plants and businesses provide health services. Churches sponsor blood pressure clinics. Civic groups hold preventive health care programs. Television stations run programs on every aspect of health and illness. Children receive health care supervision from nursery school through high school and college. Large corporations, as a public service, carry out activities to promote health.

Private, Nonprofit Health Organizations

There are a multitude of privately funded, nonprofit associations which provide health care services. Examples of such organizations would be the Epilepsy Foundation of America, the Multiple Sclerosis Association, the Leukemia Foundation, the American Heart Association, American Cancer Society, and the Society for the Prevention of Blindness. Services rendered vary from the issuance of bracelets—which identify an individual as a diabetic—to public education, drug discount rates, transportation, planned recreational activities, and benefits derived from research.

Department of Health, Education, and Welfare (DHEW)

The U.S. Department of Health, Education, and Welfare was established in 1953. It has affected the life of every American. The agencies which function under the auspices of DHEW include the Public Health Service, Social Security Administration, Social and Rehabilitation Services, and the Office of Education.

The Public Health Service administers Environmental Health Services, Health Services and Mental Health Administration, Food and Drug Administration, and National Institutes of Health. The Social Security Administration is comprised of six bureaus: (1) Data Processing and Accounts, (2) Disability Insurance, (3) District Office Operations, (4) Health Insurance (Medicare), (5) Hearing and Appeals, and (6) Retirement and Survivors' Insurance.

The Social and Rehabilitation Services agency is concerned with juvenile delinquency, youth development, and problems of the aged. The Office of Education is composed of bureaus for (1) elementary and secondary education, (2) adult vocational and technical education, (3) education for the handicapped, (4) higher education, (5) educational personnel development, (6) libraries and educational technology, and (7) other centers for research, development, and planning in education.

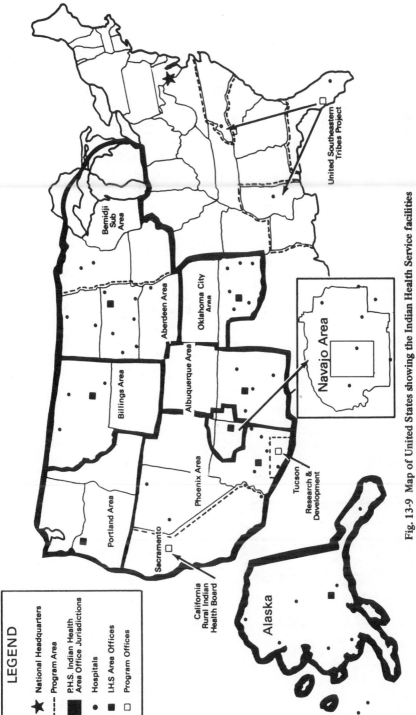

Fig. 13-9 Map of United States showing the Indian Health Service facilities

LEGEND

★ National Headquarters
- - - Program Area
- - - P.H.S. Indian Health Area Office Jurisdictions
■ Hospitals
• I.H.S Area Offices
▪ Program Offices
□

Bemidji Sub Area

Aberdeen Area

Oklahoma City Area

Billings Area

Albuquerque Area

Portland Area

Phoenix Area

Sacramento

California Rural Indian Health Board

Tucson

Research & Development

Navajo Area

United Southeastern Tribes Project

Alaska

Indian Health. Attention is being focused on the serious health care problems of the American Indian. Legislative recommendations include budgetary allocations to bring the level of health services for Indians up to at least minimal standards.

One of the biggest problems is the shortage of physicians to staff the Indian Health Services Hospitals. Prior to the expiration of the Doctor Draft Act in June, 1973, physicians served their two-year military obligation by staffing the Indian Health Service facilities. An example of one facility is in northern Arizona where the first Indian-owned and operated health care system evolved from Project HOPE. This Navajo Indian reservation has almost 200,000 residents; they are dependent upon a handful of nurse practitioners for health care. Many of the nurses who staff the hospital, the extended care facility, and the Public Health Service field clinics are Navajo Indians.

One of the outstanding nurses who is providing professional leadership is Ruth Begay, figure 13-10. Ms. Begay, a registered nurse and Navajo Indian, is on the staff of the Project HOPE, Wide Ruins Family Health Center. As a family nurse practitioner she has worked to improve the quality of health care on the reservation and is the first Indian nurse to become a member of the American Nurses' Association Council of Family Nurse Practitioners and Clinicians. She was involved in the organization of District 20 of the Arizona Nurses' Association in an effort to promote better health care for the Navajo families.

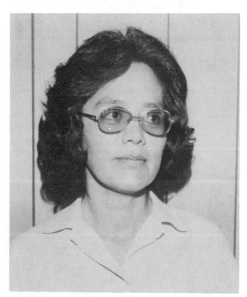

Fig. 13-10 Ruth Begay, R.N., was the first Indian nurse to become a member of the ANA Council of Family Nurse Practitioners and Clinicians.

Free Clinics. A new development in the health care system is the establishment of free clinics. Approximately 200 of these clinics served poverty groups throughout the country in 1974. Health care is brought to the people in their own environment so as to reach those who would not seek the traditional sources of health care.

Many services are available and the free clinic seems to be the answer to meeting the health care needs of many. Set up in vacated stores, church basements, and walk-up flats, the free clinic is more apt to attract persons who hesitate to bring their medical problems to conventionally operated hospitals and clinics. Persons seeking help may need more than medical or dental care. Some clinics have a psychologist, social worker, or lawyer on the staff. Referrals for more extensive health care are made when indicated.

Some clinics are funded by official agencies such as public health departments of the U.S. Department of Health, Education, and Welfare. Others are totally dependent upon volunteer personnel, equipment that has been donated, and small individual monetary donations.

Persons visiting the free clinic find the atmosphere at a level which permits them to identify with the decor, language, culture, and environment to which they are accustomed. Staff personnel are committed to this type of health care delivery and the patient is able to participate in his health care because of good interpersonal relationships. The first free clinics began in 1967 and the number of new clinics is on the increase. They have made a definite impact on the health care delivery system and play an important role in meeting the health needs of the poor.

School Health

Some school systems have a well-defined program which utilizes the nurse practitioner working in collaboration with a physician, psychologist, social worker, and learning disabilities teacher. Hearing losses, dental needs, and visual problems are some of the problems detected by the teacher-nurse.

Referrals from teachers, administrators or families of school children are received by the teacher-nurse assigned to the school district. It is her responsibility to explore the problem. The major goal is to remedy the physical, emotional, or social disability that may be interfering with learning. After assessment is completed, solutions to the problem are developed by the professional team in the school system; this allows the student to obtain optimal benefits from the educational experience.

Clinical observations of a nurse practitioner, Mary Ann Lewis, suggested that children demonstrated more interest in their own health when they were actively involved in the processes related to their own care.[1] A study which was conducted in Los Angeles has implications for nursing as well as children's health services. The study centered around the processes by which children develop health-related beliefs and behaviors and how such behaviors are affected

---

[1]Mary Ann Lewis, "Child-Initiated Care," *American Journal of Nursing,* 74 (April 1974), pp. 652-655.

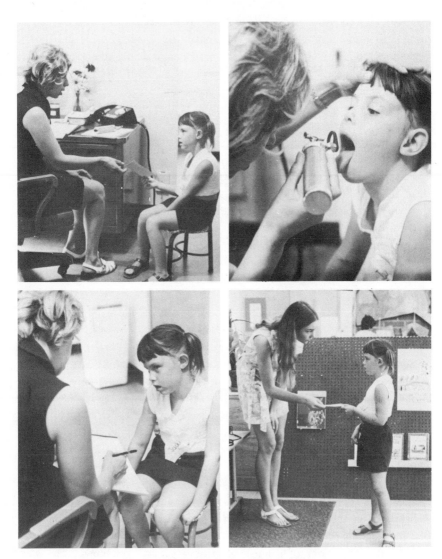

Fig. 13-11 Child and nurse discuss treatment

by a system which allows children to (1) initiate their own care and (2) be involved in the decision-making processes related to their own health problems. At the University Elementary School at UCLA a child-initiated care system has been established (free of adults); children are involved actively in making decisions about the nature of care, as well as the disposition of their health problems. Concepts of social learning and reinforcement theory underlie the nursing intervention employed. Data from the studies of the impact of this system (which continues in operation) indicate that it does have effects on the health-related beliefs of children as well as their behavior in seeking care.

Mental Health Facilities

The traditional psychiatric hospitals and private psychiatrists and psychologists cannot possibly meet the needs for mental health services. The trend has been to develop local mental health clinics which offer the services of psychiatrists, psychologists, social workers, psychiatric nurses, family therapists, and so forth. Emergency help is rendered to persons with acute mental disorders as well as to persons with chronic emotional problems. Short-term counseling and psychotherapy are usually provided. Programs are planned to deal with school problems, family problems, marital problems, problems of drug and alcohol abuse, and problems of the adolescent. Night clinics and suicide prevention centers are often established when a need exists.

Many nontraditional facilities have been established to meet the needs of local areas. An example of such a facility is a psychiatric day-care center which was developed in a sparsely populated rural area in Michigan. Lacking funds to support a psychiatric day-care center, a psychiatric nursing consultant found lay volunteers and facilities in a community church and set up a program designed to maintain and support persons referred by the local hospital psychiatric service and the community mental health center outpatient service. The nurse spent two hours one day a week as a group therapist. She also acted as a consultant to the volunteers. The program met its objectives successfully; it has grown from one group and one volunteer to three groups and thirty volunteers.

FORM OF THERAPY	PERSONS INVOLVED	TIME INVOLVEMENT	SESSION FREQUENCY
Individual	1 individual; 1 therapist	30 - 50 minutes	1 - 4 times per month
Family	Several or all members of a family; 1 - 2 therapists	45 - 60 minutes	2 - 4 times per month
Marital	Marriage partners; 1 therapist	45 - 60 minutes	2 - 4 times per month
Group	4 - 8 individuals; 1 - 2 therapists	60 - 90 minutes	1 - 4 times per month

Fig. 13-12 Factors to consider when planning therapy in a mental health facility

The Health Maintenance Organization

The Health Maintenance Organization, commonly referred to as an HMO has evolved as a system of health care delivery. It takes into account the current trends and problems affecting health care in the United States. The major objectives are to improve the delivery of health care and to reduce its cost. These objectives are expected to be achieved through the prevention of disease, maintenance of health, and early diagnosis and treatment. Generally, a *Health Maintenance Organization* (HMO) can be defined as an organized system of health care which provides comprehensive services to subscribers for a prepaid, fixed fee. In other words, the HMO is prepaid group practice and one-stop health care.

Without a system like the HMO, the burden for obtaining needed health care rests with the patient. The level of care the patient obtains is related to his sophistication and ability to find what he thinks he needs. Such an approach leads to great variations in the quality of care provided and it fails to deliver preventive care. The HMO would provide continuity of care and guarantee access to the care needed. The early detection of disease and subsequent early treatment will help prevent the need for costly hospitalization. Effective management of most chronic diseases can be better achieved by providing continuing comprehensive care outside of the hospital; this action may prevent the need for hospitalization and radical treatment. In the HMO setting, health care teaching can also be more easily integrated with medical treatment and supervision, all of which are necessary in the management of chronic illness.

The HMO staff includes family physicians, physicians representing the existing specialties, and allied health care professionals and technicians. Together they form a health care team. The consumer will have access to his own physician. If referral is necessary, it is done within the organization of the HMO. The HMO provides physician coverage twenty-four hours a day, every day of the year. The HMO has the facilities, staff, and equipment to provide comprehensive diagnostic and curative health services which reflect new scientific and medical advances. This pooling of equipment and resources not only assures quality but also helps to control costs. The HMO provides both outpatient and hospital services. The costs of hospitalization are high; therefore, the emphasis of the HMO is to prevent the need for hospital services. The HMO profits from wellness and economy rather than from sickness and duplication of effort. The consumer benefits are obvious.

The HMO also prevents the fragmentation of services and health records. All individual health histories and records are maintained in one compact file which is available to each member of the health team. This unit medical record permits health care intervention to be firmly based on previous knowledge obtained about the patient. This continuity of records provides a resource for research and a guide for the maintenance or restoration of health.

The following is a list of services which the HMO would provide for a fixed fee:

1. All visits to the family physician and all other physician services, including consultation and referral.

2. Inpatient and outpatient hospital services.

3. Emergency health services.

4. Mental health services.

5. Medical treatment and referral services for the abuse or addiction to alcohol and drugs.

6. Diagnostic laboratory services.

7. Diagnostic and therapeutic radiological services.

8. Home health services.

9. Preventive health services including family planning services, fertility services, preventive dental care, and examinations to detect vision problems.

10. Social services and health education.

Other services, such as prescriptions and full dental services, might be provided at an additional cost.

In addition to being an effective and efficient method of health care delivery, the HMO is likely to promote quality and efficiency in the health care industry as a whole. The HMO, in the effort to reduce health care costs, provides competition for existing health care facilities. In order to attract the health care consumer, other facilities will have to provide services of equal quality and cost. In this sense, the HMO has been called a vehicle for reforming the health care industry. However, administrators and policymakers of health care facilities do not see the HMO as such and acknowledges it only as an alternative approach to health care delivery. This position may effectively prevent legislators, and the public generally, from setting priorities: the facilitation of HMO development, and conditions which would encourage serious competition with the traditional health care facilities.

SUMMARY

It is apparent that one of the serious problems with health care delivery in this advanced, industrialized, and specialized society is the inability to rapidly adopt and finance new approaches of health care delivery to cope with the changing patterns of disease and health needs. The traditional approach to health care focused on curative services for the sick, which were provided in the hospital setting. There is a growing awareness of the inadequacy of such an approach; this has led to proposals of a variety of programs and new approaches. The theme of all such proposals is that every citizen has the right to health care. The providers and consumers of contemporary health care are still faced with the problem of how to convert the desire and right for preventive and curative care for all, into a system which provides it.

SUGGESTED ACTIVITIES

- Visit a free clinic in a nearby community and report to the class on the physical setup, services rendered, quality and quantity of staff, and types of patients provided for.

- Interview a staff member of the local county public health department to collect data concerning services provided in the community and assess future potential needs and programs.

- Make a list of the nontraditional health care facilities in the area. Identify the characteristics of each one and the services they provide.

- Have a discussion about the problems members of the class have had, as health care consumers, in obtaining access to appropriate health care.

REVIEW

A.   Multiple Choice. Select the best answer.

1.   Medicare can be defined as
   a. a state program which provides medical assistance for persons receiving public assistance.
   b. a federal program which provides medical assistance for persons receiving public assistance.
   c. a state program which provides hospital and medical insurance protection for persons over sixty-five.
   d. a federal program which provides hospital and medical insurance protection for persons over sixty-five.

2.   The science involving comparative study of automatic control systems is called
   a. computer technology.   c. systems theory.
   b. electronic data processing.   d. cybernetics.

3. Individuals seeking a health career can obtain federal financing through
   a. scholarships.   c. traineeships.
   b. federal loans.   d. all of these.

4. Changes in the patterns of illness include
   a. an increase in chronic, degenerative diseases.
   b. an increase in communicable diseases, particularly upper respiratory.
   c. a decrease in diseases caused by environmental conditions.
   d. none of the above.

5. A state health plan, as described in the National Health Planning and Resources Development Act of 1974, would
   a. be developed by all HSA in the state.
   b. cover all programs currently receiving federal funding.
   c. be an official guidance document.
   d. all of the above.

6. Characteristic of the modern hospital is the fact that
   a. hospitals are centers of medical knowledge and contribute to the expansion of that knowledge.
   b. the majority of hospital income comes from gifts, donations and direct patient payment.
   c. hospitals are focusing on preventive health services rather than curative services.
   d. all the above.

7. Hospitals are classified by
   a. size and location.
   b. services provided and type of ownership.
   c. size and services provided.
   d. size and type of ownership.

8. Hospitals are accredited by
   a. the American Hospital Association and American Medical Association.
   b. the American College of Physicians.
   c. The American College of Surgeons and the American Medical Association.
   d. none of the above.

9. Characteristics of an HMO include
   a. focus on prevention, early diagnosis, and treatment.
   b. provision of curative services with hospital care.
   c. access to medical care twenty-four hours a day.
   d. all of the above.

10. The greatest advantage of a continuous, single unit medical record is
    a. that it eliminates the need to write away for patient histories.
    b. intervention is based upon sound knowledge about the patient.
    c. it is less expensive to maintain.
    d. all the above.

B. Briefly answer the following questions.

1. List the services which would probably be provided by the HMO.

2. List major trends which are influencing contemporary health care.

chapter 14
THE HEALTH
CARE CONSUMER

STUDENT OBJECTIVES

- Identify the rights of the health care consumer.

- Recognize controls and guidelines applied to protect the health care consumer.

- Describe the steps involved in a patient care audit for quality assurance.

- Explain the purpose of Professional Standards Review Organizations.

Since the beginning of organized health care, the majority of the burden for obtaining health care has rested with the individual patient. There have been no health care professionals or government agencies to assume the responsibility for seeing that the appropriate kind of health care is provided. There has been no guarantee of quality. The deficiencies in the health care system have brought about ever-increasing costs and the omission of needed health care services. The public has grown weary of this expensive, inefficient non-system and is demanding that something be done to improve accessibility and quality and to reduce costs. The consumer is becoming increasingly aware of his rights to such care and is willing to participate in bringing it about. This public mandate has forced the federal government to take steps to improve health care and its delivery. It has also forced health care institutions and professionals to take a long, hard look at the quality and delivery of health services.

In the sixties, consumers began to organize themselves in order to make their concerns and needs heard. The consumer felt he was the victim of unnecessary environmental pollution, poor planning, fraudulent advertising, unhealthy industrial competition, untested food additives and drugs, planned obsolescence, and a multitude of other business and institutional practices. The consumer began to expose the perpetrators of such practices and demanded that the federal government enforce more strict regulation and control to assure the consumer of quality, safety, and honesty.

The health care industry was also the focus of concern. Consumers exposed the deficiencies and inequities of the health care system and demanded that the industry be accountable to the public for the quality of services, the way in which services are provided, and the cost of those services. The consumers also felt that many of their rights were being abrogated by institutions and individuals within the system.

In 1973, at a workshop conducted by the National Association of Health Services Executives, and Kings County Hospital Center in Brooklyn, New York, patients' rights were discussed. The major concern of the community participants was the area of research. Minority groups feared being treated as experimental subjects in New York City hospitals. They believed that adequate information pertaining to the rights of the patient should be clearly explained and understood by both the patient and hospital personnel and that, in addition, these rights must be enforced.

The public is becoming increasingly concerned about their legal rights in relationship to research. Many lawsuits have been filed with the courts in several states where patients were part of an experimental program. These patients claimed ignorance of the methods of the research project and were not satisfied with the effects of the experimentation. No human being can be used as a research subject without voluntary consent. The patient has the right to withdraw consent at any stage of the experiment and has the right to expect that the researcher is well qualified and will not deliberately proceed with the project if any ill effects might occur. Animal testing prior to human testing is imperative in order to determine safety of the project.

Another highly controversial dilemma is the issue of *euthanasia* (the practice of killing as an act of mercy) and the right to die. There is no consensus of agreement on either issue, both of which have even reached the point of court ruling in specific cases. Medical, legal, and religious groups have difficulty in accepting the views of each other. This is mainly because of each person's unique understanding and interpretation of the meaning of life and death.

POSITION OF THE AMERICAN HOSPITAL ASSOCIATION

The American Hospital Association (AHA) began to see the value of becoming a consumer advocate and has made considerable effort to project itself

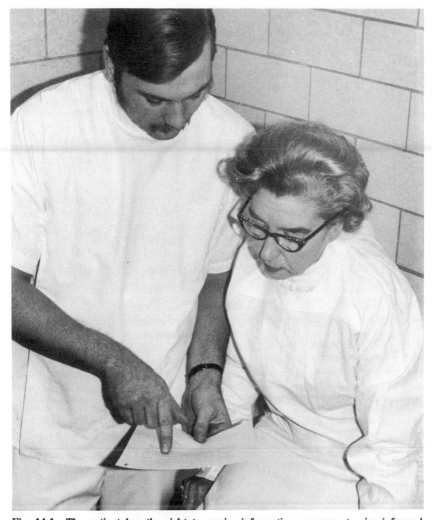

Fig. 14-1 The patient has the right to receive information necessary to give informed consent before any procedure or treatment is undertaken.

as such. In 1973 the House of Delegates of the AHA approved a statement called *A Patient's Bill of Rights,* figure 14-2, pages 228 and 229. The statement has been widely distributed and has received the support of the consumers and professional health organizations.

POSITION OF THE AMERICAN NURSES' ASSOCIATION

The purpose and platform of the ANA reflect the organization's concern with patient's rights. The ANA has assumed the responsibility for assuring the public

A PATIENT'S BILL OF RIGHTS

The American Hospital Association Board of Trustees' Committee on Health Care for the Disadvantaged, which has been a consistent advocate on behalf of consumers of health care services, developed the Statement on a Patient's Bill of Rights, which was approved by the AHA House of Delegates February 6, 1973. The statement was published in several forms, one of which was the S74 leaflet in the Association's S series. The S74 leaflet is now superseded by this reprinting of the statement.

The American Hospital Association presents a Patient's Bill of Rights with the expectation that observance of these rights will contribute to more effective patient care and greater satisfaction for the patient, his physician, and the hospital organization. Further, the Association presents these rights in the expectation that they will be supported by the hospital on behalf of its patients, as an integral part of the healing process. It is recognized that a personal relationship between the physician and the patient is essential for the provision of proper medical care. The traditional physician-patient relationship takes on a new dimension when care is rendered within an organizational structure. Legal precedent has established that the institution itself also has a responsibility to the patient. It is in recognition of these factors that these rights are affirmed.

1. The patient has the right to considerate and respectful care.

2. The patient has the right to obtain from his physician complete current information concerning his diagnosis, treatment, and prognosis in terms the patient can be reasonably expected to understand.

When it is not medically advisable to give such information to the patient, the information should be made available to an appropriate person in his behalf. He has the right to know, by name, the physician responsible for coordinating his care.

3. The patient has the right to receive from his physician information necessary to give informed consent prior to the start of any procedure and/or treatment. Except in emergencies, such information for informed consent should include but not necessarily be limited to the specific procedure and/or treatment, the medically significant risks involved, and the probable duration of incapacitation. Where medically significant alternatives for care or treatment exist, or when the patient requests information concerning medical alternatives, ·the patient has the right to such information. The patient also has the right to know the name of the person responsible for the procedures and/or treatment.

4. The patient has the right to refuse treatment to the extent permitted by law and to be informed of the medical consequences of his action.

Fig. 14-2 A patient's bill of rights   (Continued)

5. The patient has the right to every consideration of his privacy concerning his own medical care program. Case discussion, consultation, examination, and treatment are confidential and should be conducted discreetly. Those not directly involved in his care must have the permission of the patient to be present.

6. The patient has the right to expect that all communications and records pertaining to his care should be treated as confidential.

7. The patient has the right to expect that within its capacity a hospital must make reasonable response to the request of a patient for services. The hospital must provide evaluation, service, and/or referral as indicated by the urgency of the case. When medically permissible, a patient may be transferred to another facility only after he has received complete information and explanation concerning the needs for and alternatives to such a transfer. The institution to which the patient is to be transferred must first have accepted the patient for transfer.

8. The patient has the right to obtain information as to any relationship of his hospital to other health care and educational institutions insofar as his care is concerned. The patient has the right to obtain information as to the existence of any professional relationships among individuals, by name, who are treating him.

9. The patient has the right to be advised if the hospital proposes to engage in or perform human experimentation affecting his care or treatment. The patient has the right to refuse to participate in such research projects.

10. The patient has the right to expect reasonable continuity of care. He has the right to know in advance what appointment times and physicians are available and where. The patient has the right to expect that the hospital will provide a mechanism whereby he is informed by his physician or a delegate of the physician of the patient's continuing health care requirements following discharge.

11. The patient has the right to examine and receive an explanation of his bill regardless of source of payment.

12. The patient has the right to know what hospital rules and regulations apply to his conduct as a patient.

No catalog of rights can guarantee for the patient the kind of treatment he has a right to expect. A hospital has many functions to perform, including the prevention and treatment of disease, the education of both health professionals and patients, and the conduct of clinical research. All these activities must be conducted with an overriding concern for the patient, and, above all, the recognition of his dignity as a human being. Success in achieving this recognition assures success in the defense of the rights of the patient.

Fig. 14-2 A patient's bill of rights

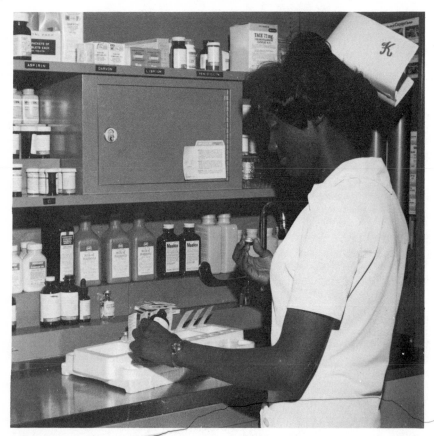

Fig. 14-3 The patient has the right to expect that nursing personnel are qualified to provide the necessary nursing services.

of the quality of nursing practice. The association also supports the position that every patient must be afforded safe and comprehensive care and that the patient has the right to make decisions concerning his own care. The ANA also actively supports federal legislation which is in the best interests of the consumer and frequently ANA representatives testify at congressional hearings as consumer advocates. The ANA encourages and promotes many professional activities which are directly and indirectly related to the right of the health care consumer to expect high standards and accessibility of health care.

POSITION OF THE NATIONAL LEAGUE FOR NURSING

In 1959, the National League for Nursing issued a statement entitled *What People Can Expect of Modern Nursing Service.* In general, the statement declared that: (1) the patient has a right to expect nursing care that will help him achieve a maximum degree of health, (2) nursing personnel are qualified to provide the necessary nursing services. (3) nurses will be responsive and sensitive to his needs, (4) record keeping will be complete and confidential, (5) patient and family will receive necessary health education, and (6) community resources will be able to provide continuing services.

The National League for Nursing acknowledges the need for public involvement in their organizational structure. The league continues to have both individual and agency members; many members who are not nurses make valuable contributions to the profession. The accreditation of nursing education programs, an NLN activity, is done by nurses and knowledgeable public representatives.

CONSUMER EVALUATION

Channels of communication have been developed by the health care industry to allow the patient or his family to have a voice and recourse, if there are legitimate complaints about any aspect of health care. The Joint Commission on Accreditation of Hospitals (JCAH) welcomes comments by patients about the care received, cleanliness, and equipment used in hospitals. Every hospital administrator is obliged to give the date of the next evaluation survey by the JCHA team. The consumer is free to contact the JCAH and arrange for a public information interview.

A nonprofit group, the Consumer Commission on the Accreditation of Health Services located at 4 West 58th St., New York, New York 10019, may be contacted if a consumer has a justifiable complaint pertaining to hospital care. Hospitals who receive funding under the auspices of the Medicare program are required by law to submit to accreditation surveys by the Social Security Administration. Any consumer covered by Medicare or Medicaid, who has a complaint about the services provided or received in a facility, may contact the U.S. Social Security Administration regional office.

Many communities have established community review groups which are made up of private citizens interested in improving health care services and facilities. Such community groups publicize undesirable health care practices which are brought to their attention. On a more positive side, they also survey the health care needs of the community and often do comparative studies. From such data, sound recommendations can be made to the official planning agencies.

FEDERAL CONTROLS

Consumer concern about the inadequacy of health care grew into a public mandate. The federal government was forced to take steps to improve health care services, facilities, and delivery. The Department of Health, Education, and Welfare charged that the health industry lacks responsible leadership and has cautioned that in the absence of responsible leadership, government control of the industry is highly probable.

Health planning legislation, the establishment of wage and price controls on the health care industry, and appropriations of federal monies for health care programs and education are a few examples of concrete action taken by the government in response to consumer demands.

Consumer pressure was also partly responsible for the Social Security Amendments of 1972 which contains a number of provisions requiring the establishment of programs to monitor, review, and evaluate health care services. Once health care legislation is passed, the Department of Health, Education, and Welfare then develops proposed rules and regulations for the implementation of the law. These proposals are published in the Federal Register. Time is allowed for consumers and members of the health care industry to respond to the proposals. The responses and comments are then published in the Federal Register along with the final and binding DHEW rules and regulations. This system allows consumer input into the actual implementation of federal law.

Peer Review and Utilization Review

DHEW regulations mandate the establishment of hospital review committees which are charged with the responsibility of reviewing and evaluating medical care provided to patients covered by Medicare, Medicaid, and Title V (Maternal and Child Health). Hospital utilization review committees are expected to study and review the utilization of hospital facilities, the length of hospital stay, and the follow-up care; these are done in addition to study and review of diagnosis and treatment.

The regulations also stressed the importance of developing peer review mechanisms. The American Medical Association (AMA) has been very involved in the development of such programs. In 1972 the AMA published a two-volume *Peer Review Manual.* These volumes contain information concerning organizational frameworks, implementation, funding, legal aspects, and utilization review concepts. The concept of peer review has met with some resistance on the part of health care professionals who feel that professional practice cannot be evaluated by members of other professions. They are also concerned that the inflexible rules and regulations will force rigid, inflexible health care rather than care designed to meet the needs of individuals. The professionals resent the control of decision making which has always been considered in the realm of professional judgment. Generally, most honest health professionals will admit that mechanisms which prevent perpetuation of poor quality and self-interest are healthy and necessary. On the other hand, the public is very concerned because traditionally health care professionals have always protected one another. In the words of Dr. Marjorie Ramphal it "is like asking the cat to watch the milk."[1]

Two types of peer review have been developed. One is the individual peer review and the other is agency review. The *peer review* deals with the evaluation of professional practice of an individual by practicing members of the same profession. *Agency review* refers to the evaluation of patterns of health care provided to patients in a specific health care agency. The ANA has developed guidelines for the initiation of agency peer review. It is hoped that peer review will be used as a means of implementing the Standards for Nursing Practice. It is also recommended that the consumer be involved in the review process because it is the consumer that nursing has promised to serve.

Professional Standards Review Organizations (PSROs)

The 1972 Social Security Amendments also contained a provision which required the establishment of PSROs which have the responsibility to review the health care services provided to patients covered by Medicare, Medicaid, and Title V (Maternal and Child Health Care). these are reimbursed by the Social Security Administration. The PSROs were to be developed in regional areas designated by the Secretary of DHEW; the PSRO functions could be carried out by physician organizations. If, after January 1, 1976, there was no such physician organization in the region, the Secretary had the right to appoint a public or nonprofit agency to do the review. The PSROs receive federal funding for planning and operation.

Each PSRO is expected to first develop a system to review short-term hospitalization of Medicare, Medicaid, and Title V patients. Then a plan for review of long-term health care facilities is to be established. The purpose of the review is to assure that the services rendered to Medicare, Medicaid, and Title V patients were medically necessary, that they met professional standards, and that they were provided in the most economical and appropriate facility.

The PSRO provision caused considerable concern on the part of the AMA, which was uncertain of the impact of the program on the practice of medicine. However, the Advisory Committee on PSRO recognized the benefits of the program to the public since the AMA was to be involved in the planning and implementation of PSRO activities.

---

[1]Marjorie Ramphael, "Peer Review," *American Journal of Nursing,* 74 (Jan. 1974) pp. 63-67.

PSROs may develop programs which focus only on the cost and quality of medical care or they may grow to include the cost and quality of all health services. Of major concern to nurses is the strong possibility that the PSROs may develop as regulatory mechanisms, with the medical profession as the sole authority. Nurses and other health professionals feel that the PSRO would be most effective if its scope was broadened to include *all* health services and if more than one health professional participated in the review process. However, if nurses do not actively involve themselves in regulating the quality of nursing services, it seems inevitable that the medical profession will assume that responsibility.

What the Public Stands to Gain (or Lose)

Peer review, utilization review, and professional standards review have been required by federal law based on consumer pressure. The law provides for health professionals to regulate the cost and quality of health care in the best interests of the health care consumer. If the health professions fail to do this, the prophecy of DHEW official might well be realized; the government would be forced to assume control of the health care industry. It is always a possibility that any government control can lead to the establishment of rules and regulations which are not in the best interests of the consumer. Indeed there are many examples which would indicate such to be the case. Also, increased government control would undoubtedly minimize consumer participation, which in itself is detrimental. Furthermore, government control of health care does not guarantee high quality health care at lower costs.

THE PATIENT CARE AUDIT

The PSROs have been given the responsibility of evaluating the health care paid for through Medicare, Medicaid, and Maternal and Child Health programs. It has been recognized that there is a need for comprehensive review of all health care services. In 1970 the staff of the Joint Commission on Accreditation of Hospitals reviewed and revised its standards for hospital accreditation. The major change was the shift in focus from minimal to optimal care. In order to effectively evaluate care, an ongoing system of quality control was necessary in each hospital. The JCAH standards require such a system. JCHA staff and physicians developed a *retrospective medical care audit,* which is a tool the hospital can use to assure quality control. The American Hospital Association has included the audit in its Quality Assurance Program. The concept of the audit is closely related to peer and utilization review.

AUDIT STUDY IDENTIFICATION DATA SUMMARY

AUDIT STUDY TOPIC

No. Records Reviewed:

PATIENT DISTRIBUTION

Age Range	No. Patients	Sex	No. Patients	Other*	No. Patients
		Male			
		Female			

*Examples of Other include admitting diagnoses or problems, presence on admission of a specified complication, secondary diagnoses, referring or consulting physician or hospital.

PHYSICIAN/NURSING UNIT DISTRIBUTION

No. Physicians in Study: _____ No. Nursing Units in Study; Total: _____ Discharge: _____

MD No.	No. Patients	MD No.	No. Patients	Unit* No.	No. Patients	No. Discharges

*If patients were cared for on more than one nursing unit, the number of patients distributed will exceed the total number of patients in the study. However, the No. Discharges should equal the No. Records Reviewed.

Committee:	Committee Chairman:
Date:	Committee Assistant:

Fig. 14-4 Portion of a JCAH audit worksheet. (Courtesy of Joint Commission on Accreditation of Hospitals ©1974)

The *audit process* is meant to be an objective method of evaluation which also provides for the initiation and documentation of the need for constructive change. The process is started by listing critical factors related to a major disease entity. Such factors include: (1) the rationale for admission, diagnosis, and treatment; (2) patient outcomes in relation to the prevention or management of complications; and (3) the appropriateness of the rationale and management. Using predetermined criteria, the process is one of measurement rather than evaluation. This is essential if the process is to be objective and not subjective.

As with the PSROs, the focus of the audit has been *medical* care and the process has been carried out by physicians. However, nurses found the audit a useful tool and have begun to use it, in modified form, to review nursing care. The quality care/nursing audit committee at Mercy San Juan Hospital in Carmichael, California, has developed a successful audit model; it is used to review patient care, rather than nursing or medical care, and the same model is used by both the medical and nursing staffs. The audit process consists of ten steps:

1. Selection of a topic, which can be a diagnosis, symptom, or a nursing procedure.

2. Development of criteria which reflect the essential aspects of the topic.

3. Development of performance standards.

4. Peer evaluation of the criteria and standards.

5. Chart review.

6. Identification of variations.

7. Analysis of variations.

8. Development of solutions to correct poor performance.

9. Implementation of corrective action.

10. Evaluation and reaudit.

This process is completed in a fixed period of time, generally six months to a year. Elsewhere, nurses involved in the audit process have recommended a multidisciplinary audit which focuses on patient care. Such an approach would assure quality of health services provided by all members of the health team.

SUMMARY

The health care consumer has mandated the government to take action to improve the accessibility, quality, and cost of health care. The government

CARE OF PATIENTS WITH PNEUMONIA AS THE PRIMARY DIAGNOSIS

Patient # ____ Age ___ Sex ___ Admitted ____ Discharged ____ L.O.S. ___

ON THE PATIENT'S CHART, THERE SHALL BE EVIDENCE OF:

	Yes	No	Expected Compliance Level	Actual Compliance Level
1. Nursing assessment of patient's physical state *on admission and at least once daily thereafter—all* of the following:				
a. presence or absence of cough (if present, includes type & character; color & character of sputum, if present)	____			
b. presence or absence of respiratory distress	____			
c. presence or absence of wheezing, retractions, rales, or rhonchi	____			
d. general condition of patient (includes color of skin, diaphoresis, or pain)	0	____	95%	0%
2. Vital signs (TPR) indicating type and quality *on admission and at least once per shift until* afebrile (temp. less than 100° F. orally) for 24 hours *or* until respirations less than 24 for 24 hours	2	____	95%	8%
3. Nursing assessment of patient's psychological state *on admission and at least once daily during* hospitalization (such as crying, apprehensive, coping with condition)	7	____	90%	28%
4. Patient on I & O until afebrile (temp. less than 100° F. orally)	16	N/A 3	90%	73%
5. Prevention of immobilization by turning, ROM exercises, or ambulation *at least once per shift* throughout hospitalization	2	____	95%	8%
6. Encouragement of coughing, deep breathing, and/or expectoration of mucus *at least once per shift* throughout hospitalization (includes suctioning if patient can't expectorate)	1	____	95%	4%

Fig. 14-5 An example of a patient care audit

PNEUMONIA as the Primary Diagnosis

Analysis	Solutions

I. Problem – Criterion #1 – 0% compliance
  1. Staff may not realize importance of making these observations on admission.

    1. We feel that if an observation is significant to the care of the patient it should be charted. Stress this in a future workshop on charting.

  2. May be making the observations, but not charting them if they are not abnormal (negative charting).

    2. Relax criteria slightly by requiring "3 of the following."

    3. Develop a nursing history form for better charting on admission.

II. Problem – Criterion #2 – 8% compliance
  1. Ancillary personnel frequently admit the patient and probably do not note type and quality of vital signs because of inadequate training.

    1. Should ancillary personnel be assessing quality of vital signs? If so we must teach them how to do it.

  2. Ancillary personnel may report abnormal quality to team leader and the team leader may not be recording this in her notes.

    2. See I–1. Same applies.

III. Problem – Criterion #3 – 28% compliance
  1. Nursing personnel may not remember to assess psychological status unless it is extreme in nature.

    1. Stress importance at next Head Nurse meeting and in workshop on charting.

IV. Problem – Criterion #4 – 73% compliance
  1. Some nurses may wait for physician to order I & O. However Quality Care Committee feels this is a nursing judgment and no order is required when patient is febrile.

    1. Stress at next Head Nurse meeting.

V. Problem – Criterion #5 – 8% compliance
  1. Nurses will chart ambulation but usually won't chart turning if the patient is turning on his own.

    1. Stress importance of documenting how the patient's exercise needs are met. Will cover in nursing lecture on "Assessment."

  2. May not observe & document on night shift if patient is sleeping well.

    2. Change criterion to read "at least twice in 24 hours."

VI. Problem – Criterion #6 – 4% compliance
  1. If patient sleeps through the night, he probably will not be awakened to cough & deep breathe especially with mild cases of pneumonia.

    1. Change to read "at least twice in 24 hours."

Reaudit in 6 months.

Fig. 14-6 An example of audit analysis

responded to the public by passing legislation which created mechanisms which would allow health care professions to regulate the quality and cost of their services. These are done in the best interests of the consumer. The consumer remains skeptical about the ability of health professionals to adopt self-regulation which is not self-serving. However, professional associations and practicing health care professionals are clearly making an effort to meet the expectations of the consumer. There is a long way to go, but the initial planning and implementation of quality assurance programs has been completed in many health care facilities. The consumer has made his point. It is now up to the health care industry to see that the consumer is served.

SUGGESTED ACTIVITIES

- Locate the consumer interest groups in the local area and elicit their concerns about health care in the area.

- At the health care facilities which provide the clinical experience for nursing students, inquire as to what steps have been taken toward quality assurance.

- Locate the Professional Standards Review Organization in the region and determine its scope of operation and stage of development.

- Contact the State Nurses Association to see what steps have been taken to regulate the quality of nursing practice in the state.

REVIEW

A.   Multiple Choice. Select the best answer.

1. *A Patient's Bill of Rights* was developed by
   a. Health care consumers.
   b. The American Nurses' Association.
   c. The American Hospital Association.
   d. Ralph Nader.

2. Concern for the consumer is reflected by the American Nurses' Association in the development of
   a. the Quality Assurance Program.
   b. Standards of Practice.
   c. *A Patient's Bill of Rights.*
   d. all the above.

3. If the health care consumer has complaints about hospital care, he can best make them heard
   a. by contacting the JCAH.
   b. through his local PSRO.
   c. by contacting the Secretary of DHEW.
   d. by complaining to the hospital administrator.

4. Hospitals providing services which are reimbursed through the Medicare and Medicaid programs are subject to accreditation by
   a. The American Hospital Association.
   b. PSRO.
   c. Social Security Administration.
   d. none of the above.

5. The retrospective medical care audit
   a. was required by the 1972 Social Security Amendments.
   b. is a standard required by JCAH.
   c. is a tool developed by JCAH to provide a system of quality control.
   d. is done only on Medicare and Medicaid patients.

6. The current operations of PSROs came about as a result of
   a. consumer pressure for better health care.
   b. the 1972 Social Security Amendments.
   c. the development of DHEW regulations.
   d. all the above.

7. The PSRO reviews
   a. the health care of all patients hospitalized in the region.
   b. the rationale for hospital admission of Medicare and Medicaid patients.
   c. medical costs of all hospitals and health care facilities in the region.
   d. all the above.

8. Guidelines for the initiation of agency peer review have been developed by
   a. DHEW.   c. ANA.
   b. Social Security Administration.   d. JCAH.

9. Health professions have resisted the concept of peer review because
   a. it is too expensive.
   b. members don't want to subject professional judgment to critical analysis.
   c. members do not want federal control.
   d. members feel it cannot effectively upgrade quality.

10. The following can be considered a right of the patient:
    a. the right to refuse treatment.
    b. the right to euthanasia.
    c. the right to ignore hospital regulations.
    d. the right to refuse to pay for what he considers inferior service.

B. Briefly answer the following questions.

    1. State five rights of the patient as stated in the 1959 statement of the NLN.

    2. List the basic steps of the patient care audit process.

chapter 15
NEW ROLES AND NEW RESPONSIBILITIES FOR NURSES

STUDENT OBJECTIVES

- Explain the differences between episodic and distributive care.
- Identify the common characteristics of nurse practitioner roles.
- Explain the process of certification.
- Identify the major issues brought about by the development of non-traditional nursing roles.

For many years the role of the nurse has been geared to providing nursing services to institutions. For at least half of those many years nursing leaders have felt nurses were not meeting their full potential and that they could make much more valuable contributions to health care if given the opportunities. Consumer demand and the changes in health care services and delivery have brought about the long awaited opportunities. Nurses have recognized the need for new roles and have developed them. It would be impossible to discuss all these new roles in one short chapter. It must suffice to discuss the general trends of nursing practice, characteristics of new nursing roles, and the issues which both have generated.

In *An Abstract for Action,* a report by the National Commission for the Study of Nursing and Nursing Education, Jerome Lysaught recommended that health care delivery be classified under two general types: episodic and distributive. The focus of *episodic nursing practice* would be curative and restorative care of patients with acute and chronic illness, in a hospital or similar setting. The focus of *distributive care* would be health maintenance and prevention of illness, which generally takes place in community or emergency institutional settings.

NEW ROLES FOR NURSES IN EPISODIC CARE

The report of the National Commission for the Study of Nursing and Nursing Education stated that the functions of the nurse had increased to include assessment, intervention, and teaching. Such functions require knowledge in addition to technical skills. Using the nursing process, the nurse identifies the needs of the patient and makes prescriptions for nursing intervention based upon those needs. Thus, the role of the nurse has become much more sophisticated.

Specialized Technical Skills

Due to the complexity of modern diagnostic and therapeutic procedures, there is a growing demand for nurses with specialized technical skills and knowledge. Such expertise is necessary to make sound judgments concerning nursing

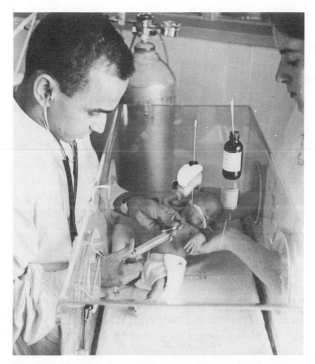

Fig. 15-1 There is a demand for nurses with specialized technical skills, such as nurses who work in a pediatric intensive care unit.

intervention in the care of patients in critical care areas of the hospital such as the coronary care unit, intensive care units, hemodialysis units, and so forth. The trend toward specialized care units is gaining momentum, which would indicate that there will be continued development of new roles for nursing in such settings.

Esther Lucile Brown in Part I of *Nursing Reconsidered – A Study of Change,* stated that nurses in special care units are highly skilled practitioners whose major concern is making decisions necessary to carry out technical functions. Dr. Brown points out that the quality of such practice is dependent on the nurse's awareness of what the patient is experiencing. The scope of such practice must include meeting the psychosocial needs of the patient and therapeutic use of the environment. The nurse in such settings has a tendency to identify with the physician, rather than to identify herself in a role which complements that of the physician.

Innovations in Nursing Service

During the sixties there was a growing interest in clinical nursing. Nurses began demanding that they be relieved of nonnursing responsibilities so that they might get back to the bedside. New personnel were hired to assume many of the tasks necessary in operating a hospital nursing unit. This allowed the nurse to become more involved in clinical nursing. There have been a number of hospitals where innovations have been made which facilitate and reward professional clinical practice.

Rachel Ayers, as the Director of Nursing at the City of Hope Medical Center near Los Angeles, developed a systematic plan for facilitating and rewarding clinical practice. Nurses receive promotions and salary increases as a result of demonstrated competence in clinical practice. Individual performance is evaluated at least once a year by the individual nurse, the immediate superior, the administrative nurse on the unit, and the coordinator of staff development. This approach also provides an incentive for continued educational growth, as some promotions require meeting educational requirements.

The late Lydia Hall designed and directed a health care facility which emphasized the importance of professional clinical practice. The purpose of Loeb Center for Nursing and Rehabilitation is to provide continuous quality nursing care which focuses on facilitation of healing, prevention of complications, promotion of health, and prevention of recurrences and new illnesses. Loeb Center is run by nurses. They are the primary therapeutic agents and coordinate the activities of all other health professionals. The Center admits patients who are referred by a physician who continues to provide medical care. These

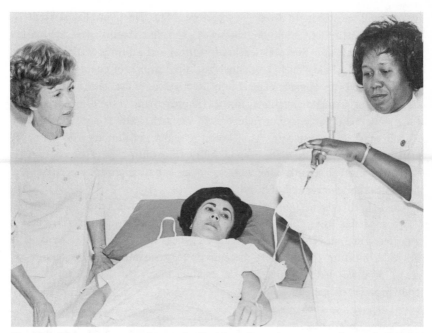

Fig. 15-2 There is a growing interest in clincial nursing and competence in practice is being rewarded.

patients are medically stable but require twenty-four hour supervision, have the potential to return to active community living and have the desire for admission and participation in the teaching-learning process. Loeb Center has demonstrated that through professional clinical practice, provided only by registered nurses, patients recover faster. Upon discharge, they are able to cope with their medical regimen and residual disabilities.

The Clinical Specialist

A relatively new role in nursing is that of the clinical specialist. The clinical specialist is usually prepared at the graduate level in a specialty, and her forte is clinical practice. Many clinical specialists are employed by facilities geared toward episodic care, although some do practice in community settings and are mainly concerned with distributive care. The unique characteristic of the clinical specialist is the relative autonomy and freedom of movement which allow her to develop her role as she sees the need for her expertise. Therefore, the roles of clinical specialists may vary considerably. The clinical specialist acts as a role model. She often carries a caseload of patients who have been referred to her (by physicians and other nurses), or those patients who she feels would most benefit from her expertise. She can be a change agent by influencing attitudes, modifying behavior, and introducing new approaches to clinical practice. She also teaches in formal and informal settings and provides an atmosphere which is conducive to the learning of concepts and skills. She also strives to upgrade clinical nursing practice by evaluating nursing practice, making recommendations for its improvement, establishing standards for practice and carrying out independent research. She is a resource person to colleagues and consumers. The clinical specialist collaborates with the physician and shares with him the responsibility for health care. She coordinates the efforts of all health care workers in an interdisciplinary approach that facilitates the achievement of health goals.

Of the effectiveness of the clinical specialist, Esther Lucile Brown says: "The impact of the . . . clinical specialist in the hospital setting has been of a degree that transcends their numbers. . . . these nurses . . . are responsible in no small measure for fostering the current reconsideration of the nature and scope of direct patient care, and for creating interest in clinical nursing as a truly professional pursuit."

The Nurse Anesthetist

Nurse anesthesia was first recognized as a nursing specialty early in the twentieth century. In an effort to establish uniform standards and quality, the National Association of Nurse Anesthetists (now the American Association of Nurse Anesthetists) was founded in 1931. In 1952 the Association was designated by DHEW as the official accrediting agency for schools of nurse anesthesia. Nurse anesthetists are certified by the Association upon completion of postgraduate study in an accredited school and successful completion of a national examination. Nurse anesthetists work with anesthesiologists in the hospital. If there is no anesthesiologist, they may work with the operating surgeon. Many work in group practice with other nurse anesthetists, while others independently contract services to one or more hospitals.

Nurse Coordinator for Data Processing

With the increased use of the computer in large health care facilities, the nurse has become involved with data processing. The nurse works in collaboration with other health professionals and experts in data processing in order to develop and implement nursing care applications particularly designed to facilitate clinical practice and communication. The nurse also participates in the development of integrated applications designed to benefit all health professionals, the health care facility, and the client.

NEW ROLES FOR NURSES IN DISTRIBUTIVE CARE

Health care services have been provided in community settings for many years, by county and state health departments, visiting nurses' associations, and other voluntary agencies. However, in recent years the numbers and kinds of health care services have increased markedly in response to the needs of the community. The focus has also shifted to primary care. *Primary care* refers to the concept that long-term health maintenance of individuals and families can best be achieved through a relationship with one health care professional. This professional is fully cognizant of their health-illness patterns, and is qualified to plan, implement, and coordinate all health services in collaboration with the consumer and members of the health care team. Nurses have assumed the role of primary health care provider in a multitude of settings, with as many titles, roles, and functions. The primary care nurse and the nurse-midwife are two such examples. Primary care nurses may be found in health care facilities which practice primary care nursing. A health professional follows the same patient(s) from admission to discharge and follow-up home referrals, when necessary. However, a new category, the nurse practitioner is emerging. She is the medical, pediatric, or family nurse practitioner. After a brief description of the nurse-midwife and the pediatric nurse in distributive care nursing, the preparation and responsibilities of nurse practitioners will be given in detail.

The Nurse-Midwife

Although the nurse-midwife is not a new role, the responsibilities of that role have changed. In a joint statement of the American College of Obstetricians and Gynecologists, and the American College of Nurse Midwives, the nurse-midwife is given the responsibility for the complete care and management of uncomplicated maternity patients.

The Pediatric Nurse Practitioner

One of the first roles to emerge in primary care was that of the pediatric nurse practitioner. In settings where overburdened physicians were involved in curative and preventive care of children, the need was acute for a health care worker who could provide primary, family-oriented care. Nurses assumed this role beginning in 1963 and the idea quickly spread. The first formal training program was established in Denver several years later.

Basic to the role of pediatric nurse practitioner (PNP) is the ability to accurately and comprehensively assess the needs of the child, to make sound judgments, and to implement the appropriate action.   In the early seventies, the American Nurses' Association and the American Academy of Pediatrics issued a joint statement called *Guidelines on Short Term Continuing Education Programs for Pediatric Nurse Associates.* The statement contains the functions and responsibilities of the PNP and also goals for educational programs to prepare nurses to work in the role.

THE NURSE PRACTITIONER

There have been few, if any, new positions in nursing that have elicited such a response as that of the nurse practitioner.   Because of that response and the fact that the role has become a prototype, the nurse practitioner merits further discussion.

Roles and Functions

The need for primary care practitioners has been recognized in many settings. Because of the diversification of health care facilities and the trend toward even greater specialization, the nurse practitioner role is hardly uniform. Variety, both in education and practice, is one of the few constants.

The family nurse practitioner is a generalist who combines the basic skills of the pediatric and medical nurse practitioner with the orientation and approach of the public health nurse in order to provide a high level of health care to people of all ages. As a primary care provider in ambulatory settings, she assesses the physical, emotional, and developmental status of individuals and families; analyzes health behavior related to personality, life-style, and culture; makes positive interventions to maintain, restore, or improve health; and critically evaluates the quality and effectiveness of her practice.

By adding medical skills in diagnosis and patient management to her nursing knowledge and skills, she is able to expand her care to include all levels of prevention, that is, health promotion, specific disease protection, early recognition and prompt treatment, and disability limitation and rehabilitation.   Teaching, counseling, and provision of emotional support are important aspects of her practice: she promotes independent positive health behaviors in patients.

The family nurse practitioner is acutely aware of the interrelatedness of community, family, and individual health and approaches her patients using this framework.   She is aware of community needs and resources and collaborates with health and social agencies to meet important community, family, and individual needs.

The family nurse practitioner is able to provide care independently to many patients and works closely with physicians in the joint management of others. She is acutely aware of the limitations of her knowledge and skills, continually seeks to improve her practice, and her primary concern is the health of her patients and the quality of their care.

Fig. 15-3   The Yale University School of Nursing faculty developed this concept of a primary care provider.

The role is frequently referred to as the *expanded* role and *extended* role. Both terms imply that the fundamental aspects of the role are constant, but that new aspects are added. Such is not quite the case. Obsolete or unnecessary aspects of the role are deleted while concurrently new ones are added, changing the dimensions and focus of the role; therefore, *metamorphic* role might really be a more descriptive term. The role of the nurse has changed because the approach and focus of practice has changed, the responsibility has shifted, new tools and skills are used, and the practice is collaborative.

The approach of the nurse practitioner is *holistic,* that is, the emphasis is on the interrelatedness of parts and wholes. The patient is not a fragmented disease entity; he is part of a family and community. The focus of practice is to provide health care to a client rather than to provide nursing service to the employing health care facility. The nurse practitioner must make independent decisions and assume total responsibility for them. When she collaborates with another health professional, the responsibility is shared. If the nurse practitioner is in a setting where physical assessment is necessary, it is essential to learn and use the tools and skills of physical assessment such as the physical examination, health history, and so on. The nurse practitioner has the responsibility and the authority to establish the scope of practice. When the need exists, referrals are made and the nurse collaborates with other health professionals in order to provide the necessary health care services. Trust and interdependence are essential to effective decision making.

Nurse practitioners work in group practice with physicians, in neighborhood and community health care agencies, in nurse clinics, in hospital outpatient and in-service departments, in extended care facilities, in industry, and in schools.

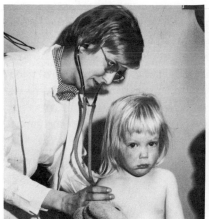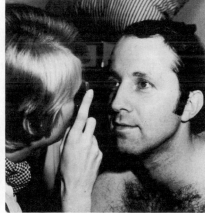

Fig. 15-4 The nurse practitioner who does physical assessment must develop new skills.

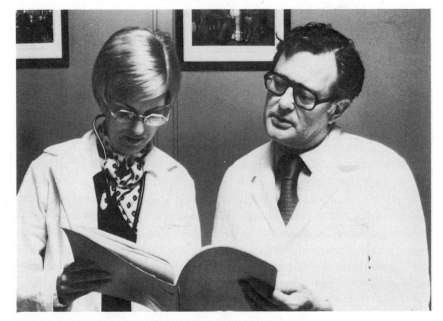

Fig. 15-5   The nurse practitioner collaborates with the physician when the need exists.

Some practitioners are pursuing independent practices in communities or in rural areas where they provide the only health care available. The nurse practitioner can practice in primary, acute, and chronic health care settings.

Preparation of the Nurse Practitioner

Programs which prepare nurse practitioners vary as greatly as the roles which practitioners assume. Short-term programs usually award a certificate for successful completion. Long-term educational programs may lead to baccalaureate or master's degrees. Programs are sponsored by nursing or medical schools of colleges and universities, hospitals, nursing agencies, and private and public community health agencies. Programs vary in length from three weeks to two academic years. Requirements vary from licensure as a registered nurse to a baccalaureate degree in nursing, with up to three years of experience in a specialty. Instruction is provided by collegiate nursing and medical faculty, practicing physicians, other nurse practitioners, and any combination of the aforementioned.

The Issues

Many issues have developed concerning the nurse practitioner. They have been brought about because the role itself is new and not clearly understood.

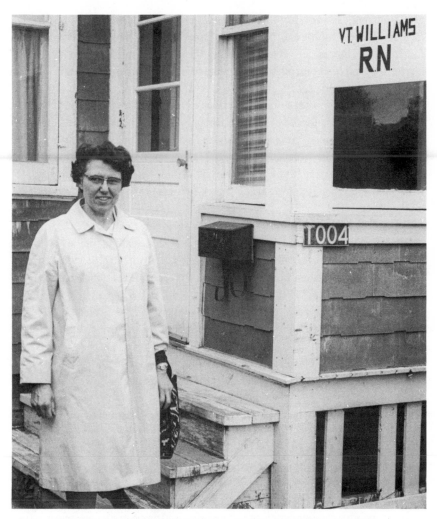

Fig. 15-6 Many nurse practitioners are setting up independent practices.

They have also been brought about because of the suddenness with which the nurse practitioner and practitioner programs emerged. There has not been time or effort made to establish national criteria concerning practitioner programs or what the nurse practitioner can or cannot do. There have been few legislative changes which establish standards or regulations for such practice. However, many of the major professional organizations and official government agencies have made statements on the nurse practitioner.

The ANA supports the concept of the nurse practitioner and has said: "The American Nurses' Association, recognizing the full range of professional services which nursing can provide, firmly believes that no restrictions should be placed on nurses' opportunities to fulfill every aspect of their professional role. The functions of nurses are changing primarily because nurses themselves have recognized and demonstrated their competence to perform a greater variety of services."

It has been stated that nurses in primary care are simply incorporating into their practice, those tools and skills which are not used in the practice of nursing in all settings. Nurses using such tools and skills must be adequately prepared by qualified persons from any number of disciplines. The nurse practitioner and physician will function collaboratively within a mutually designed framework, and thus there is no need for supervision of either group of practitioners by the other.

In the 1971 report *Extending the Scope of Nursing Practice* the Department of Health, Education, and Welfare recommended extending the nurse's role in order to increase the effectiveness and efficiency of health care delivery. In addition, role expansion would provide greater professional opportunity for the nurse to realize the fullest potential.

Dr. Ernest B. Howard, executive vice-president of the American Medical Association, announced implementation of a plan to improve the most urgent problem facing health care: the acute imbalance of supply and demand. It was proposed that with modest training, 100,000 nurses could become associated with physicians in order to expand the physician's ability to serve his patients. The scope of nursing practice would be determined by the physicians serving on various councils of the AMA. The physician would remain the manager of the medical system. Dr. Howard stated that the nurse's professional status would be enhanced by the more responsible nature of her work, and her income would also increase. By using nurse practitioners, home visits would become a reality and would reduce the need for hospitalization. It was implied by Dr. Howard that the nurse would practice medicine under the supervision of a physician. These comments were cited in the American Medical Association News, a weekly publication of the AMA.

It is clear that there is not unanimous agreement on the nurse practitioner's scope of practice and the responsibility for that practice. There have been many conferences, workshops, seminars and discussions held by nurses and interdisciplinary groups to clarify all aspects of the nurse practitioner role and preparation for that role. There have been many issues raised; the major ones focus on: how a nurse practitioner should be prepared, certification, the nature of practice (is it medicine or nursing?), liability, reimbursement for services, and the implications of the practitioner movement for nursing.

NEW NURSING TITLES

COMMUNITY HEALTH
Community Health Nurse
Community Health Nurse Clinician
Community Health Nurse Practitioner
Community Health Specialist
Family and Community Nurse Clinician
Family Health Nurse Clinician
Family Health Specialist
Family Nurse Practitioner
Family Nurse Specialist
Health Nurse Clinician
Primary Care Nurse Practitioner
Public Health Clinical Specialist
Public Health Nurse Clinician
Public Health Nurse
Rural Health Specialist
School Nurse

MATERNAL-CHILD
Ambulatory Child Health Care Nurse
Child Nurse Clinical Specialist
Child Nurse Specialist
Family-Child Nurse Clinician
Family Planning Nurse Practitioner
Maternal Clinical Specialist
Maternal Health Nurse Clinician
Maternal Nurse Clinician
Maternal Nurse Clinical Specialist
Maternal and Newborn Nurse Clinician
Maternal Nurse Practitioner
Maternal Nurse Associate
Maternal-Child Clinical Nurse Specialist
Maternal-Child Nurse Clinician
Maternal-Child Nurse
Maternal-Infant Nurse Clinician
Maternal-Newborn Nurse Clinical Specialist
Maternity Distributive Care Clinical
   Specialist
Maternity Nurse Clinician
Nurse-Midwife
Obstetrical Nurse Clinician
Obstetrical-Gynecological Nurse Practitioner
Parent-Child Nurse Clinician
Pediatric Clinical Specialist
Pediatric Distributive Care Clinical Specialist
Pediatric Nurse Associate
Pediatric Nurse Clinician
Pediatric Nurse Practitioner

MEDICAL-SURGICAL
Adult Health Nurse Clinician
Adult Health Nurse Practitioner
Adult Nurse Practitioner
Adult Nurse Specialist
Aging Specialist
Biophysical-Pathology Nurse Clinician
Cardiac and Respiratory Clinical Specialist
Cardiovascular Nurse Clinical Specialist
Cardiovascular Nurse Clinician
Gerontology Nurse Clinician
Medical Clinical Specialist
Medical Nurse Clinician
Medical Health Evaluation Nurse
Medical Surgical Clinician
Medical Surgical Clinical Nurse Specialist
Medical Surgical Clinical Specialist
Medical Surgical Nurse Clinician
Medical Surgical Nurse Clinical Specialist
Medical Surgical Nurse
Medical Surgical Nurse Practitioner
Ophthalmic Nurse Practitioner
Physiological Nurse Practitioner
Physiological Nurse Clinician

PSYCHIATRIC/MENTAL HEALTH
Adult Psychiatry Clinical Specialist
Adult Psychiatric Nurse Clinician
Child Psychiatric Clinical Specialist
Child Psychiatric Nurse Clinician
Community Mental Health Nurse
Psychiatric-Child Nurse Clinician
Psychiatric Clinician
Psychiatric Clinical Nurse Specialist
Psychiatric Clinical Specialist
Psychiatric-Mental Health Clinical Specialist
Psychiatric-Mental Health Nurse Clinician
Psychiatric Nurse Clinician
Psychiatric Nurse Clinical Specialist
Psychiatric Nurse
Psychosocial Nurse Clinician

REHABILITATION
Chronic Illness and Rehabilitation Clinical
   Specialist
Rehabilitation Nurse Clinician
Rehabilitation Nurse Practitioner

Fig. 15-7 This illustrates the lack of standard titles for nurse practitioners.

Preparation

In reviewing the types of nurse practitioner education programs, there is no general uniformity. Historically in nursing, there has always been an emphasis on developing uniform standards of nurse education in order to guarantee the consumer of the consistency of quality. However, a number of problems prevented the development of such standards in the preparation of the nurse practitioner. The practitioner movement occurred rapidly, before education programs could be established and standardized. There are some nursing leaders who feel that the pluralistic approach to nurse practitioner preparation is healthy, because nurses themselves have not waited to be coerced into developing new roles through formal education and training. They have taken the initiative to assume new roles and to develop programs to train themselves and others.

Another problem which has been cited frequently is that there is no consensus on who should teach in nurse practitioner programs. Some nursing educators feel that nurses should teach all the skills and techniques which the nurse practitioner is required to master. Difficulties have been encountered with this approach because many faculty members are not qualified or prepared to teach these skills. Others feel that physicians should teach these skills because they are qualified to do so. An inherent danger of that approach

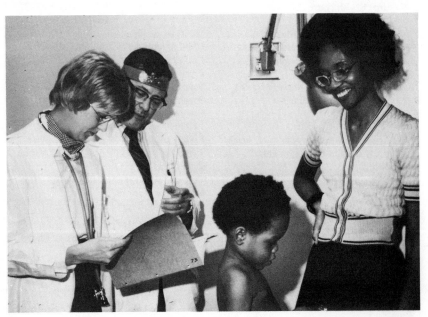

Fig. 15-8 Should the physician be involved in the preparation of the nurse practitioner?

is that once the physician trains nurse practitioners, he feels he must supervise them and be responsible for their practice. On the positive side, involving the physician in the preparation of the nurse practitioner allows him to become acquainted with the capabilities of nurses. This awareness fosters the development of interdependent roles. Some programs have had physicians teach the assessment skills, but only to nursing faculty. This approach is based on the premise that the nursing faculty must know what students are expected to know; also it allows faculty members to serve as role models.

The trend is toward the establishment of broad program objectives and the development of uniform standards concerning entrance requirements, curricula, length of programs, and accreditation of programs. It is generally believed that such standards are necessary to assure the consumer of quality and to prevent further fragmentation of nursing and health care services.

Certification

Certification is the process by which an individual registered nurse is granted recognition for competency by having met certain established criteria or qualifications developed by an ANA Division on Nursing Practice. In some instances certification is required for entrance into the practice of a specialty; for example, nurse-midwife and nurse anesthetist.

The Interdivisional Council on Certification was established in April, 1976 by the Executive Committees of the Divisions on Practice. The Council is composed of chairpersons or designated members of the Executive Committees of the Divisions on Practice, and the Interim Certification Boards of the Divisions on Practice. It is the responsibility of the Council to establish:

1. Definitions related to certification

2. Administrative policies and procedures for certification

3. Guidelines for recognition of specialties for purposes of certification

4. Guidelines for relationships with other organizations in regard to certification

The ANA Certification Program was established in 1973 to provide formal recognition of personal achievement and superior performance in nursing. In July of 1976, a new process was initiated whereby the ANA Divisions on Nursing Practice provided two types of recognition for nurses who demonstrated competency and excellence in practice: *Certification* would attest to professional *competency* in a specialized area. *Diplomate* status would attest to *excellence* in a specialized area. Registered nurses are eligible for certification if they meet the following requirements:

1. Current licensure.

2. Have had a minimum of two years of practice as a registered nurse in a designated nursing practice area; up to one year may have been spent in an organized program in higher education or in a continuing education program.

3. Are currently practicing in the specialty area in which certification is sought.

Consultants, researchers, administrators, supervisors, and educators may seek certification. The certification process involves the following:

- The candidate must meet the established requirements for eligibility.

- The candidate must submit an application to the division of nursing practice in which certification is sought.

- The candidate must take an examination for a certificate of competency in the designated area of practice.

- If the candidate receives a passing score, evidence must be provided of innovativeness and excellence in nursing practice.

- References must be provided by persons familiar with the candidate's nursing practice.

All candidate documents are reviewed and the appropriate ANA Division on Nursing Practice makes the final decision whether to grant certification. The candidate is notified. Certified nurses will use the letters RN, C. or RN, C.S. (Certified Specialist).

Excellence in nursing practice is recognized by membership in the American College of Nursing Practice. Diplomatic status provides prestige for the registered nurse with exceptional expertise. Criteria for membership as a diplomate in the American College of Nursing Practice includes current ANA certification, current practice in the area in which membership is desired, a Master's Degree in Nursing from an accredited institution, and two years of practice following the master's degree. A summary of certification and related information can be found in figure 15-9. To obtain further details and current materials concerning certification, the Certification Unit, Credentialing Department, American Nurses' Association, 2420 Pershing Road, Kansas City, Missouri 64108 should be contacted.

Some states have passed legislation pertaining to the extended role of the nurse. Several states require certification by the Board of Nursing for entry

	CERTIFICATION (for competence)	**AMERICAN COLLEGE OF NURSING PRACTICE** (for excellence)
Definition	Certification is the process by which an ANA Division on Nursing Practice grants recognition to an individual Registered Nurse who has met predetermined qualifications for competency in a designated area of nursing practice, and predetermined qualifications for continuing competency.	Membership as a diplomate is recognition granted to a certified nurse who has met predetermined qualifications for excellence in a designated area of practice and predetermined qualifications for continuing diplomate status. Criteria and qualifications for excellence are determined by the ANA Divisions on Nursing Practice.
Eligibility Requirements	1. Current licensure as a Registered Nurse. 2. Two years of practice as a Registered Nurse in a designated area of nursing practice immediately prior to application, up to one year of which may have been in an organized program of study in an institution of higher learning or in a continuing education program. 3. The applicant must be currently engaged in the practice of nursing in the ANA Division in which certification is sought.	1. Current ANA Certification in the designated area of nursing practice. 2. Current practice in the area in which membership is sought. 3. A Master's Degree in Nursing or a related field from an accredited institution. 4. Two Years of practice in the area of specialization post master's.

For the purposes of recognizing professional achievement and excellence in practice, *practice* is defined as direct involvement in the nursing process in a clinical setting, where the nursing actions and judgments are focused on a particular individual, family, or group of individuals, and where there is professional responsibility and accountability for the outcome of these actions. Consultants, researchers, administrators, supervisors and educators who meet these criteria are eligible to seek certification.

The eligibility requirements listed above are to be common to all Divisions on Practice. Other eligibility requirements may be developed as appropriate by the various Divisions on Practice, which also have the prerogative of certifying nurse specialists.

Within the framework of these basic requirements, the Divisions will develop the qualifications and procedures for certification, including passing a written examination and providing reference vouchers, and for membership in the College, including any documentation or other criteria for demonstrating excellence in their respective areas of practice.

Fig. 15-9 Competence and excellence in nursing practice are recognized. (Adapted from ANA Divisions on Practice, Recognition of Professional Achievement and Excellence in Practice, *Fact Sheet*, dated 5/76)

into practice. Other states are registering nurse practitioner programs and making it mandatory that nurses in extended roles be graduates of these registered programs. Some states permit nurse practitioners to practice if they have certification from any program or agency.

From the consumer point of view, certification may mean anything, everything, or next to nothing. National certification has been proposed as one means of forcing some standardization of practitioner programs and assuring the consumer of the quality of nurse practitioner services.

Medicine or Nursing?

There has been considerable discussion and some disagreement as to whether the nurse practitioner is practicing medicine, nursing, or both. Statements made by the federal government indicate that the nurse practitioner is practicing nursing, but that practice has new dimensions. Professional nursing organizations have repeatedly stated that nurse practitioners are practicing nursing and that they are responsible for their own practice and are accountable to their patients. Generally, most nurses believe that the nurse practitioner practices nursing; she makes traditional nursing judgments and she also makes other decisions about health care in collaboration with the physician and other health

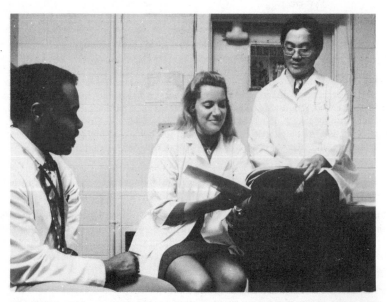

Fig. 15-10 The nurse practitioner (left) makes independent judgments, but can collaborate with the physician (center) and the pharmacist (right) in making some decisions.

professionals. There are some who feel that the nurse practitioner is practicing medicine and, therefore, must be supervised by a physician. The basis for this belief is that in many cases nurses are performing tasks, usually associated with the practice of medicine, which are not nursing responsibilities as defined by many state nurse practice acts. Those who do not understand the role of the nurse practitioner or who feel threatened by it, tend to emphasize the need for legal restrictions of nursing practice or placement of that practice under the direct supervision of the medical profession. This is hardly an unexpected response. Historically, physicians have tried to keep nursing under restraint. An editorial written in 1901 by Lavinia Dock emphasized that nurses needed to define and control their nursing practice, figure 15-11.

Related to this issue is the question of liability and reimbursement for services. It is not yet clear under what circumstances the nurse is exclusively liable and when the nurse and doctor share that liability. It remains to be seen if the increased liability of the nurse practitioner will bring about changes in malpractice insurance plans and premiums. There is also a problem concerning reimbursement for services provided by the nurse practitioner. How the costs and fees will be determined and who will determine them is not yet resolved. The rules and regulations for third-party payment have not been developed to include these new nursing services rendered by an independent practitioner.

"Nothing, I think dear Editor, is more trying to one's toleration than to see men—most of whom never did and never can comprehend what a woman's work really is, what its details are, or how it ought to be done—undertaking to instruct and train women in something so unquestionably her own special field as nursing. I do not limit this statement to men only, but will say that physicians, be they men or women, cannot teach nursing, any more than nurses can teach medicine. Medicine and nursing are not the same; and how-ever much we may learn from the physician about disease and its treatment, the whole field of nursing—as nursing is realized by the *patient* (the centre of the question)—is unknown to him. I agree that he can criticise nursing intelligently, but he cannot show how it ought to be done or do it himself, except in rare instances."

"We need, then, to recognize those qualities and characteristics in our work which are superior to what men can teach us, and to hold firmly to them, refusing to give them up, and most unremittingly should we resist all attempts to take our right of teaching our own work out of our hands, putting nurses out of their true relation to their own calling, and bringing up a set of imperfect imitators of pseudoscientific men, mere satellites of the medical profession, who will be neither doctor nor nurse."

I am, dear Editor, yours sincerely,
L.L. Dock

Fig. 15-11 Lavinia Dock wrote this letter to the American Journal of Nursing Company; it appeared in Volume 2, December 1901 issue of the AJN.

A Pattern for Nursing Education and Practice?

Nursing educators are questioning whether the nurse practitioner movement will bring about new patterns for nursing education and practice, or whether nurses in primary care will constitute a specialty group within the profession. Before these questions can be answered it must be determined whether nurses and the consumer can afford the higher costs of advance preparation; if not, will there be adequate federal funding to support the practitioner programs? Studies must also be done to evaluate and determine the effectiveness of this new role in improving health care.

PROFESSIONAL RELATIONSHIPS

The new roles and responsibilities of nurses have brought about the need for a change in the nurse-doctor relationship. The old traditional relationship of the dominant male physician and the weak, subordinate female nurse is obsolete and must change. Unfortunately, the burden for bringing about that change rests primarily with the nurse. There have been innovations in medical treatment which have facilitated the change in the doctor-nurse relationship. Esther Lucile Brown stated that it is only recently that doctors have had the opportunity to observe the ability of nurses to learn and apply medical theory. The development of intensive care units has forced physicians to relinquish some of their responsibilities to nurses. Initially, physicians taught nurses what they needed to know to assume the responsibility for care of patients in intensive care units. Once the physicians recognized the capability of nurses, they began to realize that nurses could assume greater responsibility.

If nurses are to reach their fullest potential, they must be allowed to make independent decisions. The physician must recognize that the nurse is capable of making sound professional judgments and he must be able to appreciate the contribution of the nurse in providing comprehensive health care. It is at this point that the nurse-doctor relationship becomes an interdependent, collaborative, peer relationship.

Practicing nurses involved in primary care have stressed the need for nurses to develop an interdependent working relationship with the physician. The nurse must be self-confident and must be able to demonstrate her competence to the physician. The nurse must guard against falling into the subservient role, which is easy to do because both doctors and nurses have been comfortable with such a role for so many years. At this point, nurses and doctors are developing a colleague relationship on a one-to-one basis. In professional education, there is a need to include a philosophical orientation which recognizes the practice of doctors and nurses as different, but equal. There must be a sharing of power and the elimination of unilateral decision making by physicians.

SUMMARY

The role of the nurse is changing and individual responsibility for nursing practice is growing. Nursing practice is much more sophisticated. Nurses are incorporating new theory, techniques, skills, and tools into that practice so that they can provide health care services to meet the needs of the health care consumer. It is unanimously agreed that the growth or expansion of the nurse's role is both necessary and desirable. However, there is disagreement as to whether some aspects of that role are nursing practice or medical practice. The changing role of the nurse has led to the development of many new programs designed to prepare the nurse to use new skills and to assume new responsibilities. There is no standardization of such programs; therefore, there are no fixed standards of quality. As in the past, nurses themselves must define nursing practice and assume the accountability for the quality of nursing practice. If they do not, other health care professionals will be more than happy to do it for them. It is to the credit of nursing that the need for new roles has been recognized and that nurses are moving into these roles. However, nurses must not be so shortsighted as to leave it at that.

SUGGESTED ACTIVITIES

- Contact a local independent nurse practitioner and request to spend a few hours with her to observe the overall routine and scope of her practice. Report to the class what you have witnessed.

- Interview three physicians on the staff of your local hospital and elicit their personal feeling about the expanded roles of the registered nurse. Decide whether these persons are progressive in their thinking or bound to tradition.

- Obtain information regarding admission requirements and the program design of local nurse practitioner programs. Compare the programs and note the differences.

REVIEW

A. Multiple Choice. Select the best answer.

1. The American Nurses' Association recognizes excellence in clinical practice
   a. by admitting those qualified to the Academy of Nursing.
   b. through the process of certification.
   c. through the process of accreditation.
   d. through the presentation of yearly awards.

2. The major focus of episodic care is
   a. curative care in a hospital setting.   c. maintenance of health.
   b. prevention of illness.   d. all of these.

3. The current trend in nursing is a renewed interest in
   a. health education.   c. clinical practice.
   b. nursing administration.   d. team management.

4. A health care facility where nurses are the primary therapeutic agents is
   a. City of Hope Medical Center.
   b. Loeb Center for Nursing and Rehabilitation.
   c. called an extended care facility.
   d. recommended by DHEW.

5. The focus of distributive care is
   a. maintenance of health.
   b. curative care in a hospital setting.
   c. the development of intensive care facilities.
   d. all the above.

6. The maintenance of health and prevention of illness can best be achieved by a health care professional who has a one-to-one relationship with the patient; this concept is called
   a. prepaid group practice.   c. primary care.
   b. episodic care.   d. the ANA.

7. A professional organization which feels that nurse practitioners are practicing medicine is
   a. DHEW.   c. AMA.
   b. ANA.   d. JCAH.

8. The consumer of health care may consider certification of nurse practitioners a meaningless process because
   a. certification requirements vary considerably.
   b. there are many types of certification.
   c. certification does not guarantee standards or quality.
   d. all the above.

9. The nurse-physician relationship is
   a. an interdependent relationship.   c. a dependent relationship.
   b. a collaborative relationship.   d. a and b.

10. The clinical specialist, usually prepared at the graduate level, is an expert
    a. in nursing education or administration.
    b. in clinical practice.
    c. in primary care.
    d. diagnostician.

B. Briefly answer the following questions.

1. List the common characteristics of the nurse practitioner role.

2. What does certification mean?

3. In what ways do nurse practitioners differ?

chapter 16
THE HEALTH
CARE TEAM

STUDENT OBJECTIVES

- List the occupations which provide health care services in community health facilities.

- Explain the major roles and functions of each member of the health care team.

- Discuss two alternative approaches available to the nursing team in providing patient care.

The health care industry is the most rapidly growing industry today. There are at least 125 major health occupations, with about 300 job classifications. However, the doctor, dentist, and nurse are generally considered the major health care providers. New scientific and technological developments and major socioeconomic changes have created a demand for new health occupations and more highly skilled health workers.

HEALTH CARE TEAM

All of the individuals who provide health care services to the patient and family are collectively called the *health care team.* Theoretically, the goals of the individual members of the team are similar, if not identical. However, the functions and roles of each member of the team are very different because each member has a different perspective and, therefore, identifies different problems. It is easy to visualize this team in an organized health care facility like the hospital. However, the members of the health care team do not have

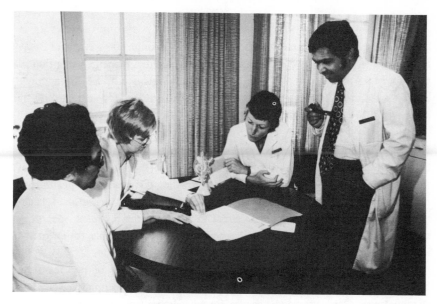

Fig. 16-1 The health care team

to be employed in the same facility or by the same employer. A health care team could include a family physician (self-employed), a school nurse (employed by a school district), a public health nurse (employed by the county), a pharmacist (self-employed), and a physical therapist (employed by a hospital). The team becomes effective when all team members have an understanding of and appreciation for the contribution of each member. It would be impossible to discuss all the health occupations in a single chapter. Therefore, the health occupations which will be discussed are those generally associated with a large, organized, community health facility.

ADMINISTRATION/ BUSINESS	THERAPY	LABORATORY	CORE GROUP

Hospital Administrator
Personnel Director
Public Relations
  Director
Purchasing Agent
Controller
Admitting Officer
Medical
  Transcriptionist
	Electroencephalograph
	Electrocardiograph
	Inhalation Therapy
	Operating Room
	  Technician
	Radiology Technologist
	Rehabilitation Therapist
	Speech Therapist
	Social Services
		Pathologist
		Medical Lab
		  Technologist
		Microbiologist
		Blood Bank
		  Technologist
		Histologic
		  Technician
		Cytotechnologist
			Doctor
			Nurses
			Pharmacist
			Dietitian

Fig. 16-2 Some major health careers

Administration

Hospitals and other large health care facilities require the services of many individuals with training in business and management. With the exception of the admitting officer or clerk, the patient will probably not see the administrative personnel. However, without these individuals, quality care would be an impossibility.

Hospital Administrator. Hospitals are a big business and need a chief executive officer who possesses a keen sense of business operation and knowledge of finance; this officer is the administrator. Providing comprehensive health care at the lowest possible cost is the major concern of the administrator. Leadership and organization skills are essential in directing the complex operations of a large institution. The hospital administrator is responsible for enforcing the decisions of the policy-making board.

Formerly, nurses, doctors, members of religious orders, or persons from business positions, were placed in the role of the hospital administrator. On-the-job training was provided because formal educational preparation was not available. Today, persons employed as hospital administrators are usually required to have an undergraduate degree in business or psychology and a master's degree in hospital administration; this includes a residency period in an accredited hospital.

Personnel Director. The personnel director plays a vital role in the health care industry because he has the responsibility to recruit and interview applicants who wish to fill the many positions in the institution. Generally the basic requirement is a bachelor's degree, with a major in personnel administration, and knowledge of staffing needs and selection criteria. The personnel director is mainly concerned with interviewing the job applicant, and reviewing past work experiences and educational background. Determination of salary and final job placement is done in collaboration with the appropriate department head.

Public Relations Director. It is important that the community is made aware of the available health care facilities and the services provided by them. The purchase of new equipment, such as the kidney dialysis machine, or the appointment of a highly specialized medical staff member, is not only news but also important information to the people in the community. The public relations director issues news releases, makes public appearances to promote the institution, and prepares internal news bulletins, brochures, and publicity articles.

The public relations director is also expected to be able to identify the needs and feelings of the members of the community and brief the hospital on a continual basis. A baccalaureate degree in public relations or journalism is often required by the employing institution.

Purchasing Agent. A good background in business and a degree in economics is helpful to the purchasing agent, who is responsible for the ordering and maintenance of the supply of all equipment and materials used by members of the health care team. He must keep abreast of current prices, economic trends, and product quality. Ordering equipment and supplies to correspond with the need is a vital skill.

Controller. The hospital controller is the business manager. He is supervisor of the business office and is responsible for the hospital finances. A college degree in accounting and finance is essential to understand correct procedures for the disbursement of monies, and for budget planning. Also necessary is the ability to interpret the accounts to the policy-making board, and in some cases, the community. In very large institutions, this position requires the competence of a certified public accountant (CPA).

Admitting Officer. The admitting officer and clerks are responsible for the assignment of patients to rooms. The placing of patients in an efficient, safe, and congenial manner requires planning. Patients are generally assigned to beds on the basis of sex, age, disease, socioeconomic background, common interests, and even smoking habits. The educational requirements for admitting personnel vary; however, a sociology and psychology background are highly recommended.

Medical Transcriptionist. The role of the medical transcriptionist is vital to the health team and requires highly skilled training. The position entails typing the medical dictations of the physician at high speed and with accuracy. Knowledge of medical terminology, names of medications and procedures, and the ability to remain discreet in highly confidential matters are requisites for this position. These records are often utilized by attorneys, insurance companies, and medical specialists.

Therapy

Therapists and trained technicians have an extremely noteworthy place on the health team. They are directly concerned with the diagnostic evaluation and treatment procedures of the patient. Their roles are interrelated with those of the core group of health professionals in providing total patient care.

EEG and EKG Technicians.   The *electroencephalograph* (EEG) technician is trained to operate the machine used to record brain waves. Physicians, usually neurologists, interpret the tracings in order to diagnose organic brain disease. The technician prepares the patient for the procedure, observes symptoms and behavior of the patient during the procedure, and is responsible for the complex equipment.

The *electrocardiograph* (EKG) technician is trained to operate the equipment used to record heart rhythmicity. Physicians, especially cardiologists, use the EKG reading for the purpose of detecting heart abnormalities and to follow up patients with known cardiac problems. A total understanding of the equipment is essential to ensure accurate readings.

EEG and EKG technicians have been prepared through on-the-job training. However, the trend is toward the development of highly specialized programs in large hospitals and junior colleges. To become a registered EEG technician it is necessary to pass the registry examinations given by the American Board of Registration of EEG Technologists.

Inhalation Therapist.   Oxygen therapy, until recently, was administered by the nurse or physician and required only very basic equipment. Now, procedures

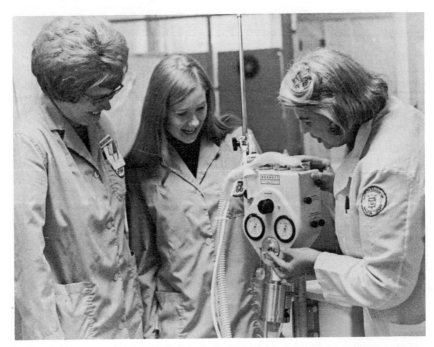

Fig. 16-3 Inhalation therapists

and equipment are very complex and the services of highly skilled therapists are necessary to help the patient maintain adequate gas exchange. The inhalation therapist has an important role on the emergency team in cardiopulmonary resuscitation. Also, the incidence of lung and heart diseases is on the rise, requiring increased special respiratory care. The inhalation therapist supervises the respiratory therapy and maintains the equipment. The inhalation therapist must have a thorough knowledge of the complex equipment and the physiology of respiration. A good math and science background are essential. It is necessary to pass the examinations given by the American Registry of Inhalation Therapists to become a registered therapist.

Operating Room Technician. Until recently, registered nurses were employed to prepare the operative area for surgery, to assist the surgeon by handing instruments, to apply postoperative dressings, and to care for surgical supplies. Now these functions have been delegated to the operating room technician (surgical technician). Military service personnel may be given specialized training in this field and practical nurses are being given on-the-job training in hospitals.

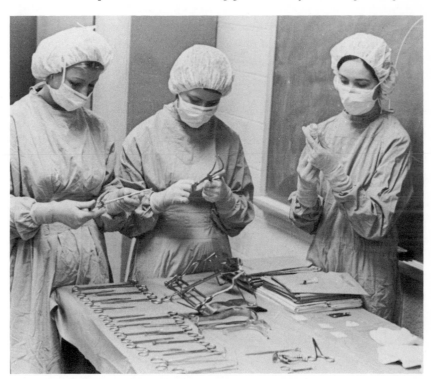

Fig. 16-4 Operating room technicians

Aptitudes necessary for this position include neatness, accuracy, alertness, precision, and a team spirit. To become certified, one must take the national certification examination through the Association of Operating Room Technicians, Inc.

Radiologic Technologist. The radiologic technologist works under the supervision of a radiologist, who is a licensed physician. However, the duties of the technologist have expanded markedly and today the technologist performs complex procedures. Technologists may specialize in special procedures, radiation therapy, and nuclear medicine. Knowledge of mathematics and physics is necessary as well as knowledge of anatomy in order to position patients for proper exposure to the X ray. Two and four-year college courses are offered. Preparation requirements vary with the specialty area and the degree of responsibility. Good manual dexterity and physical strength are needed in the handling of heavy equipment and the lifting of patients. To become certified, one must pass the examinations given by the American Registry of Radiologic Technologists.

Rehabilitation Therapy. Professionally trained therapists work as members of the health care team. The goal is to assist the patient to return to maximum physical and mental health. Occupational therapists help the patient, incapacitated

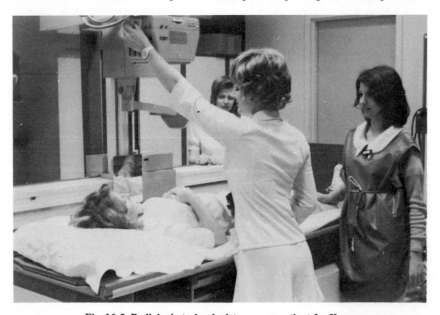

Fig. 16-5 Radiologic technologists prepare patient for X rays

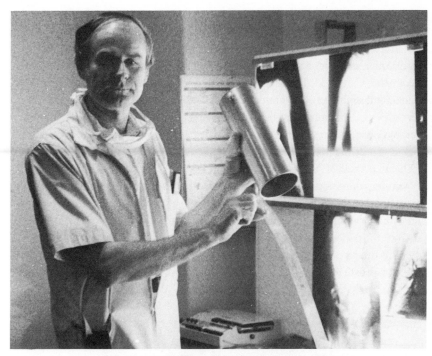

Fig. 16-6 A certified radiologic technologist at work

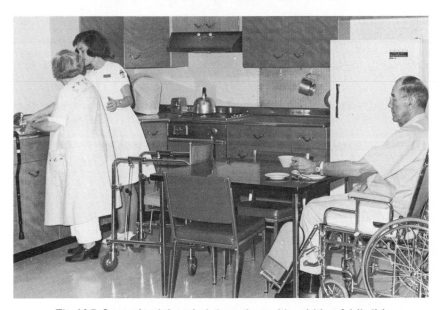

Fig. 16-7 Occupational therapist helps patients with activities of daily living

by emotional, physical, or other functional disturbance, to cope with the problems of daily living. The therapist works in collaboration with the physician and nurse, and plans experiences to meet individual needs. Activities of a recreational, creative, and educational nature are utilized. Occupational therapy encompasses areas of disease prevention and health maintenance, occupational adjustment, and medically prescribed treatment programs. Educational requirements for the therapist may be bachelor or master's degrees. The occupational therapy assistant may earn an associate degree. For professional registration, one must pass the national examination conducted by the American Occupational Therapy Association.

Another important member of the rehabilitation team is the physical therapist who also works in collaboration with the physician and nurse. Accident and stroke victims, and persons born with crippling defects, comprise a large portion of patients assisted by the rehabilitation therapist. In addition to teaching the patient to regain use of a paralyzed limb, crutchwalking, or how to use a prosthetic device, the physical therapist provides massages, whirlpool

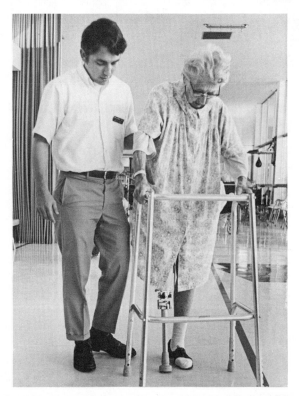

Fig. 16-8 The physical therapist assists with ambulation activities.

treatments, and electrical stimulation. Patient and family teaching is done frequently. Good manual dexterity, coordination, and strength are needed. There are three types of educational programs, granting a baccalaureate degree, associate degree, or a certificate. A master's degree in physical therapy may also be earned. Graduates of approved schools may apply for licensure by examination.

Speech Therapist. Speech therapists are specialists in verbal communication. Speech and hearing sciences are taught in colleges and universities at the undergraduate, graduate, and doctoral level. Certification from the American Speech and Hearing Association (ASHA) is based upon demonstration of clinical competence and the ability to meet the standards and qualifications established by ASHA. Speech therapists work with hospitalized patients and outpatients. Victims of stroke, patients recovering from laryngectomies, and persons with speech impediments and hearing losses are referred to the speech therapist by members of the health care team.

Social Services. In the hospital, social workers and case aides are usually assigned to specialty areas. The case aide is an individual with a baccalaureate degree,

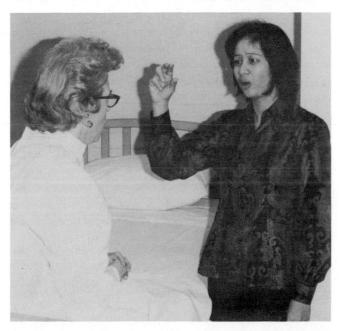

Fig. 16-9 The speech therapist assists a patient with a communication problem.

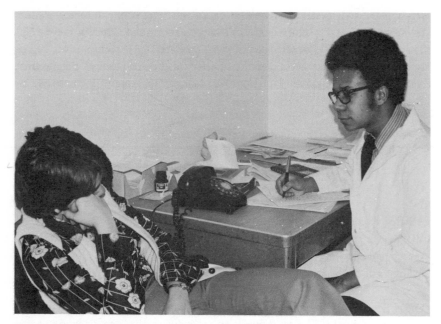

Fig. 16-10 A case aide helps a family member plan for a relative's return to the home.

usually in sociology or psychology, who is primarily concerned with discharge planning for hospitalized patients. The clinical social worker has a master's degree in social work and is involved in counseling activities. Patients are referred by all members of the health care team. Discharge planning includes nursing home placement, planning for home care, transportation, referrals to community resources, and follow-up. Counseling is done on a one-to-one basis, or it may involve the family or large groups. The social worker might, for example, counsel a patient who is recovering from a heart attack and who is having difficulty coping with restricted activity. In order to be effective, the social worker may have to work with the patient's spouse or family. It is possible that the social worker might work with a group of recovering cardiac patients if that approach seems appropriate.

Laboratory

Medical laboratory careers are greatly diversified and specialized. Diagnosis and treatment rely heavily on the functions of the laboratory technicians and technologists. Opportunities are available to persons with or without a college degree.

Pathologist. The pathologist is a physician who completes a three to four year residency, in addition to the regular medical training, and is certified by the American Board of Pathology in clincial or anatomical pathology, or both. He performs postmortem examinations (autopsies), examines tissues excised during surgical procedures, and often teaches nursing and medical students.

Medical Technologist. The medical technologist works under the direction of the pathologist. The work in the clinical laboratory includes analyzing blood samples to detect the cause of disease. The technologist may draw blood samples from the patient, count blood cells, and do blood groupings. The technologist prepares tissue specimens and identifies microorganisms, in addition to doing chemical tests of body fluids. Equipment is complex and is continually being updated. Medical technologists must possess a minimum of a bachelor's degree. Some go on to teach and must earn a master's degree. To become certified, it is necessary to take the national examination of the Board of Registry of the American Society of Clinical Pathologists.

Other Laboratory Personnel. Certification and/or registration is awarded specialists in nuclear medicine technology, chemistry, microbiology, blood bank

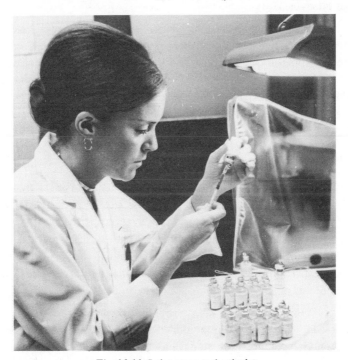

Fig. 16-11 Laboratory technologist

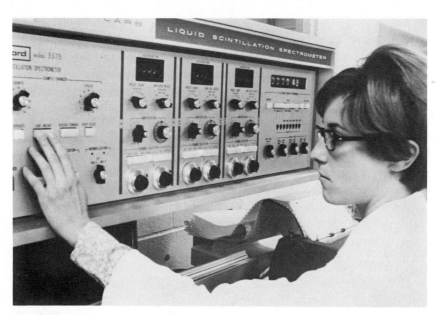

Fig. 16-12 A medical technologist measures amount of radioactivity in blood sample (Courtesy Pfizer, Inc.)

technology, cytotechnology and histology. One of the newer categories in laboratory careers is the medical laboratory technician. Programs for medical laboratory technicians are being offered mainly through the junior/community colleges. The technicians work in the areas of radioactive isotopes, immunology, detection of body cell changes, the preparation of body tissues for malignancy diagnoses, and the collection, classification, processing and storing of blood.

Core Group

Persons involved with the daily care of the hospitalized patient are the nurse, physician, dietitian, and pharmacist. The nurse has the most contact with the patient and therefore is able to make observations as to how the patient is responding to the illness and the treatment. The physician makes a diagnosis and treats the pathology. Since food is an essential part of daily living, the dietitian is actively involved in health care. Most ill persons require medication dispensed by the pharmacist.

The Physician. The doctor is responsible for diagnosing and treating pathology. Approximately nine years of study and the successful completion of state licensure examination are required before a doctor can practice. Traditionally, the physician has been self-employed and collects a fee for services. However, there is a trend towards more physicians becoming salaried employees. The physician has had the most difficulty in understanding the team concept. Unfortunately, most doctors see themselves working independently of others. If the doctor works with other health professionals, the tendency is to direct the work of others rather than share responsibility. However, in the rapidly developing specialty care units, the doctor is learning to work as part of a team. It is the patient who ultimately benefits when all the members of the health care team contribute to their fullest potential.

The Dietitian. An essential member of the health team is the dietitian. Throughout history, the importance of good diet habits has been stressed. In many cases health maintenance depends upon proper diet intake. Therapeutic dietitians teach patients how to maintain health by proper diet control. A bachelor's degree is required, with a major in foods and nutrition, or biochemistry. To become registered, one most pass the test of the American Dietetic Association and participate in continuing education activities.

The Pharmacist. It is the role of the pharmacist to prepare and dispense medications prescribed by the physician. Precision and accuracy are imperative. Whether employed in the hospital or local drugstore, this member of the health team has a direct relationship and responsibility to the patient and family. Pharmacy programs grant a bachelor's degree in five years and a doctorate degree in six years. To become licensed, one must pass the examination given by the Board of Pharmacy.

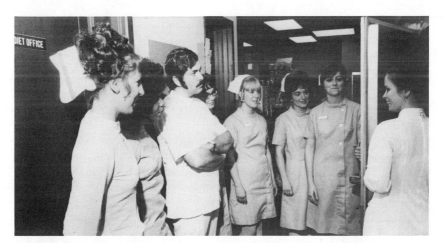

Fig. 16-13 The dietitian explains her role to other members of the health team.

THE NURSING TEAM

The nursing team is made up of all the individuals who are involved in rendering nursing care to the patient. Composition of the nursing team varies according to available personnel, patient census, type of unit, and affiliated nursing education programs. Each member of the team makes a unique contribution and has an important part in the total health care team. It is necessary to keep

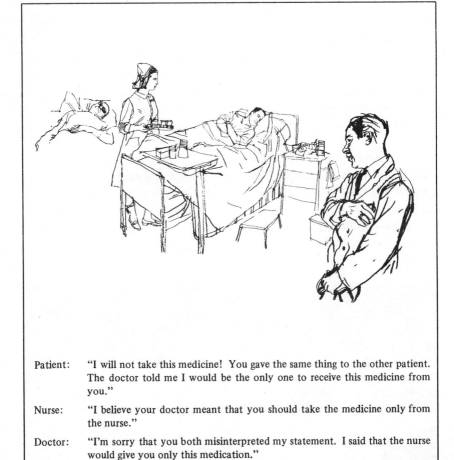

Patient: "I will not take this medicine! You gave the same thing to the other patient. The doctor told me I would be the only one to receive this medicine from you."

Nurse: "I believe your doctor meant that you should take the medicine only from the nurse."

Doctor: "I'm sorry that you both misinterpreted my statement. I said that the nurse would give you only this medication."

Fig. 16-14 Example of a communication error, centered around a misunderstanding of only

in mind that the patient is the focal point of all team effort. This necessitates cooperative planning, good communication and good interpersonal relationships. Being part of a well-organized functioning team provides a sense of security for all members and promotes job satisfaction.

All members of the nursing team must have the ability to communicate effectively. Many errors are made because someone did not clearly state what was meant, or understand what was read or heard. The meaning of a sentence may be changed when the modifier is placed incorrectly, figure 16-14. It is essential to develop the skills necessary to give and to correctly interpret both verbal and written communication pertaining to nursing care and medical treatment. When people work in large institutions, their work is constantly interrelated to the work of others. The quality of patient care is in direct ratio to the quality of the communication that takes place.

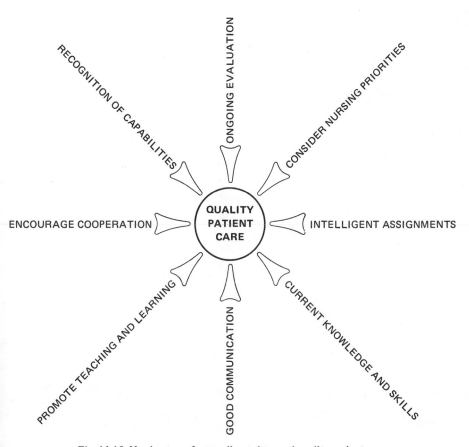

Fig. 16-15 Nursing team factors directed toward quality patient care

Recognition of the need for varying levels of expertise will foster good relationships. Each member of the team must understand his role, his co-worker's role, and how each member relates to the other. An understanding of the educational preparation of all members of the nursing team is also most helpful.

The nursing team can be organized and function in a variety of ways. Two approaches are in vogue at present. They are team nursing and primary care nursing. Both approaches can be modified to meet the particular needs of the health care facility or unit. A third approach, which is often seen but seldom encouraged, is functional nursing. In this approach one nurse changes beds, one passes medications, another takes blood pressures and so on. The ultimate result is fragmentation of care and poor quality nursing.

Primary Nursing

The University of Minnesota Hospital originated the concept of primary care in 1958. Primary care is a new term for total patient care which many nurses have long desired. It permits a one-to-one relationship between the nurse and patient. The primary nurse is given complete responsibility for several patients, generally four or five. She develops the admission-to-discharge treatments and nursing care plans. While the primary nurse is in charge of the nursing care of the patient, she may delegate certain tasks to other nursing personnel. Writing the progress record, making necessary referrals, and initiating

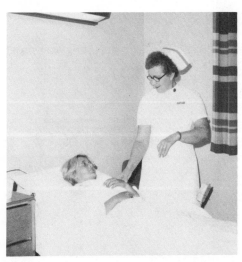

discharge or transfer plans are responsibilities of the primary nurse. The major focus of primary care is the patient. It is not task oriented or functional nursing.

The primary nurse is responsible for total patient care around the clock. This is unlike the team leader in team nursing who plans for patient care on an eight-hour shift. Some hospitals have developed plans to implement primary nursing care. Most of the proposed plans utilize an all professional nurse staff. The major difficulties are

Fig. 16-16 The nurse doing primary nursing has total responsibility for the nursing care of her patient.

to convince the employing agency administration that it is not more costly than team nursing or functional nursing, and to reassure the staff affected by the change to primary nursing care.

Team Nursing

A team is generally composed of a team leader, registered nurses, licensed practical nurses, nursing assistants, and orderlies. The team leader, in collaboration with her immediate supervisor, assigns specific work to each team member and supervises the work of each member. Work assignments are based upon nursing diagnoses and an understanding of the ability and potential of each team member. The team leader is responsible for the coordination and quality of nursing care provided by members of the team. Careful planning is absolutely essential if team nursing is to be effective. The team

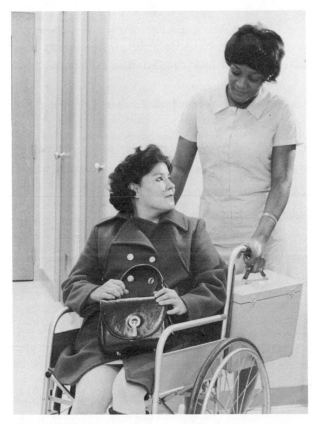

Fig. 16-17 The nursing assistant is a member of the nursing team.

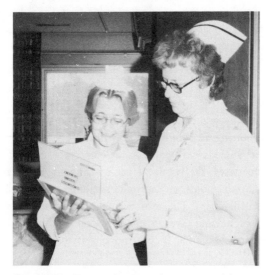

Fig. 16-18 The nursing supervisor acts as advisor to the staff nurse who is team leader.

leader should consider the following factors in making assignments for team members:

1. Know the patients and their individual needs.

2. Write assignments clearly.

3. Distribute work load in accord with ability of team members.

4. Consider priorities of patient care.

5. Revise assignments as emergencies arise.

6. Use sound suggestions offered by team members.

7. Promote growth and optimal functioning of each team member.

8. Evaluate the effectiveness of patient care.

9. Provide atmosphere for job satisfaction.

10. Be a teacher as well as a leader.

One of the most important aspects of team nursing is utilization of the team conference. There is no set number of people required to be present in order for a conference to be held. It is essential, however, that the conference be well planned, brief but comprehensive, and interesting. The team leader is the chairman of the conference, which should be held in a quiet room conducive to listening and discussion. The purpose of the conference is to gather pertinent information about patients assigned to the team in order to plan the nursing

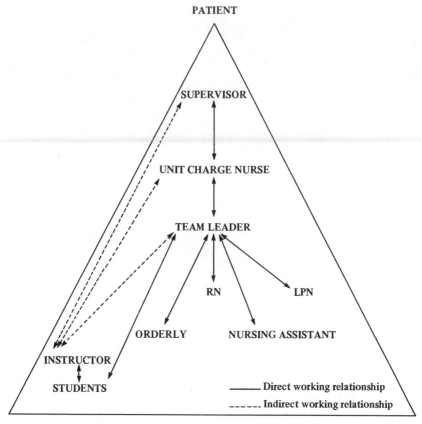

Fig. 16-19 Lines of communication in team nursing

care for new patients and update, evaluate, and/or revise care of the others. Team nursing cannot function properly without team conferences. They afford the opportunity for all personnel to evaluate patient care as a cooperative effort. Patients frequently have problems which can be solved through team discussion. Specific, sometimes crucial, needs of the individual patients may be brought to light through the conference. By active participation in group discussion, each team member has an opportunity to learn, and the team leader is able to evaluate both the nursing care plans and the practice of the individual team member.

SUMMARY

Health care is extremely complex and requires the skills of a wide variety of health care personnel, professionals, and occupational groups. Nursing,

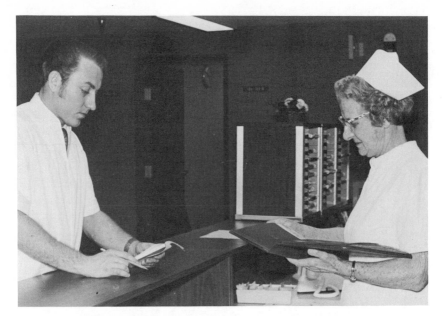

Fig. 16-20 The team leader gives report to the charge nurse

like other health occupations, has varying levels of preparation and expertise. The skills and contributions of all levels of health workers must be utilized and understood.   In order to provide the highest quality health care, each health worker must be allowed and encouraged to contribute to his greatest potential.   The team concept effectively coordinates the efforts of all in order to reach that goal.

SUGGESTED ACTIVITIES

- Role play a team conference which is to last for about fifteen minutes.   The student playing the role of team leader should prepare a mock assignment sheet and nursing care plans for six patients.   Evaluate the outcome.

- Panel Presentation.   The roles of six members of the health team should be explained by a student representing each health occupation.   Show relationships among health team members.

- Conduct a survey in your college or school. How many programs prepare persons in health occupations?   How do the programs differ in content and length?

REVIEW

A. Multiple Choice. Select the best answer.

1. The major members of the health care team are the
   a. nurse, dietitian, and therapist.
   b. physician, dentist, and nurse.
   c. radiologist, physician, and nurse.
   d. physician, microbiologist, and nurse.

2. The efforts of the health care team are directed toward the
   a. hospital.   c. patient.
   b. physician.   d. nurse.

3. The functions of a nursing team leader include
   a. coordination of team activities.
   b. guidance of team members.
   c. planning and organizing assignments.
   d. all of the above.

4. The person on the health care team who analyzes blood to determine the cause of disease is the
   a. medical technologist.   c. pathologist.
   b. blood bank technologist.   d. none of these.

5. When a nurse is assigned around-the-clock total care of several patients from admission of the patient to discharge, it is called
   a. special duty nursing.   c. special care nursing.
   b. team nursing.   d. primary nursing.

B. Briefly answer the following questions.

1. Name the four health care occupations that are always involved with daily care of hospitalized patients.

2. What is the purpose of the nursing team conference?

3. Name five members of the nursing team.

4. Explain why each member of the nursing team is important in order to provide total nursing care.

5. State the educational preparation required for the following health care positions:

Registered Nurse	Pharmacist
Licensed Practical Nurse	Physician
EKG Technician	

C.   Match the following health team members in Column II to the duties they perform in Column I.

<table>
<tr><td colspan="2" align="center">Column I</td><td align="center">Column II</td></tr>
<tr><td>1.</td><td>Has the most contact with patients and is able to make observations of symptoms and behavior.</td><td>a. Admitting Officer</td></tr>
<tr><td></td><td></td><td>b. Hospital Administrator</td></tr>
<tr><td></td><td></td><td>c. Nurse</td></tr>
<tr><td>2.</td><td>Responsible for assigning rooms to incoming patients.</td><td>d. Operating Room Technician</td></tr>
<tr><td>3.</td><td>Prepares the operative area for surgery, hands instruments to the surgeon, applies postoperative dressings and cares for surgical supplies.</td><td>e. Pathologist
f. Pharmacist
g. Public Relations Director</td></tr>
<tr><td>4.</td><td>Responsible for compounding and dispensing drugs ordered by physicians.</td><td>h. Rehabilitation Therapist</td></tr>
<tr><td>5.</td><td>Professionally trained individual who assists patients with physical handicaps or emotional problems to live to their fullest potential.</td><td></td></tr>
<tr><td>6.</td><td>Responsible for the management of the hospital in accordance with established policy.</td><td></td></tr>
<tr><td>7.</td><td>Specially trained to supervise all medical laboratory activities and performs postmortem examinations.</td><td></td></tr>
<tr><td>8.</td><td>Responsible for the release of news concerning the hospital and patients.</td><td></td></tr>
</table>

SECTION 5
THE NURSING COMMUNITY AND THE LAW

chapter 17
PROFESSIONAL
ORGANIZATIONS

STUDENT OBJECTIVES

- List the functions and goals of the major national nursing organizations.
- Identify the official publications of the national nursing organizations.
- Explain the value of being a member of a nursing organization.

Man has long recognized the value of belonging to a group and the advantages of cooperative endeavor. Throughout the history of nursing there is evidence of achievement through group effort and unselfish cooperation. Much can be accomplished when individuals direct their efforts toward a common goal. Graduate nurses have the opportunity to contribute to the progress of nursing as members of national nursing organizations. The organizations are the official spokesmen of individual nurses at the local, state, national, and international level. These organizations can be no better than the members which constitute them. Therefore, all nurses should join and participate in one or more organizations. To facilitate participation, most national associations have state and local levels.

AMERICAN NURSES' ASSOCIATION

The American Nurses' Association (ANA) was founded in 1896 as the Nurses Associated Alumnae of the United States and Canada. In 1911 the Association adopted its present name. The ANA is the national professional organization of registered nurses in the fifty states, the District of Columbia, Guam, Panama Canal Zone, Puerto Rico, and Virgin Islands. The ultimate purpose of the ANA is the provision of quality nursing care through the promotion of professional and educational standards.

Membership is open to all persons licensed to practice as a registered nurse in one or more states. Membership within the United States involves the district, state, and national levels. Nurses who reside outside of the country may have direct membership on the national level only. Associated members pay one-half the dues but share the privileges of full membership. Unemployed registered nurses, full-time students, new graduates, or those eligible for social security may qualify for associate membership. National dues are uniform but state and district dues are established at the local level. The American Nurses' Association headquarters are located at 2420 Pershing Road, Kansas City, Missouri 64108.

Through membership in ANA, dental, hospital supplemental, disability, life and malpractice insurance is available at group rates.

At the request of an individual nurse, the ANA will compile a cumulative record of professional education and experience. This record is kept on file at ANA headquarters and is sent, at the nurse's written request, to potential employers, colleges, or universities. Employment references and verification of basic nursing education is kept on file; however, academic transcripts must be obtained from the schools attended. This service is referred to as the American Nurses' Association Professional Credential and Personnel Service and is provided for all ANA members at a nominal charge.

ANA publishes *The Nation's Nurses: 1972 Inventory of Registered Nurses* which is an inventory of registered nurses and a summary of data related to nurses in the United States since 1949. Another widely used publication is *Facts About Nursing,* a reference book concerning data from the latest studies on registered nurses, salary information, nurse supply, nursing school admissions, enrollments, graduates, and licensure information. Information on fellowships and grants is also provided. Membership in the association offers a reduced subscription rate to the official publication, the *American Journal of Nursing.* *The American Nurse,* a newspaper which provides the latest news on issues affecting nursing is sent without additional cost to members.

The ANA staff represents registered nurses in the nation's capital by reviewing, and then supporting or lobbying against, legislative action which affects nursing and health care. ANA also assists state associations with legislative issues affecting the profession, the individual nurse, and the patient. The Washington ANA office at 1030 15th Street, N.W., Washington, D.C. 20005, publishes the *Capital Commentary* for the purpose of keeping nurses updated on issues which concern them. The ANA is comprised of five divisions on practice: community health, geriatric, maternal and child health, medical-surgical,

AMERICAN NURSES' ASSOCIATION

1976-1978 ASSOCIATION PRIORITIES

STRENGTHEN THE AMERICAN NURSES' ASSOCIATION BY:

- Improving the abilities of the organization to respond to the multipurpose interests and needs of the members
- Increasing membership at least 20% in the biennium
- Improving opportunities for participation in guiding the directions of the association
- Responding to representation of nurses in gaining authority for practice and for determination of employment conditions
- Implementing Affirmative Action throughout organization

STRENGTHEN THE CAPACITY OF THE ORGANIZATION TO PARTICIPATE IN THE DETERMINATION AND EXECUTION OF PUBLIC POLICY RELATED TO HEALTH BY:

- Participating and contributing to health planning (to include attention to all segments of the population, i.e., the poor, the aged, the disadvantaged, the minorities)
- Implementing a coherent manpower policy for nursing resources
- Evolving a coherent system of credentialing including accreditation of educational programs and service agencies, certification and licensure
- Developing systems to assure the profession's accountability for practice, for delivery of services, for education, and for the economic and general welfare of nurses
- Expanding public relations endeavors within and without the profession

STRENGTHEN THE PROFESSION OF NURSING BY:

- Fostering organizational arrangements to protect rights of all members of profession
- Unifying the occupation of nursing
- Improving relationships with other organizations, professional, consumer, government
- Providing the consultation and information system necessary to assist SNAs in collective action (including collective bargaining)

STRENGTHEN RESEARCH AND DATA-GATHERING SYSTEMS FOR THE PROFESSION BY:

- Improving and maintaining information base about the profession
- Studying and evaluating economics of health care
- Expanding knowledge base for practice of nursing
- Promoting a stable financial base for the conduct of research

Adopted by the Board of Directors, May 2, 1976
Endorsed by the House of Delegates, June 11, 1976

The ANA 1976 Platform (Courtesy ANA, Kansas City, Mo.)

psychiatric and mental health nursing. These divisions establish standards of practice and encourage research to advance nursing practice.

Biennial national conventions are held in the even numbered years in various cities throughout the country. The main purpose of these meetings is to exchange ideas and information of interest to nurses in all positions. Clinical conferences and forums promote professional growth.

NATIONAL STUDENT NURSES' ASSOCIATION

The National Student Nurses' Association (NSNA), which maintains a close relationship with the ANA, is a separate legal corporation. It is recognized as the preprofessional organization for nursing students. Through committee and board interrelationships, registered nurses and students work together in promoting excellence in nursing. The Committee on Common Interests and Goals, which is comprised of ANA and NSNA members, identified the following common goals: to further the aims of nursing; to encourage membership in the ANA; and to provide guidance to state and district associations.

The national student organization was formed in Cleveland in 1953 by students from forty-three states and the District of Columbia. The Coordinating Council of the ANA and NLN assumed sponsorship for the student association. Prior to this time schools were united at the local level through district and state associations. Active participation in the school organization prepares

---

1. Don't attend meetings; but if you do, come late.
2. Always leave before adjournment.
3. Never speak up at any meeting. Wait till you get outside.
4. Sit in the back of the room where you can chat freely with other members.
5. Vote in favor of every action. Then go home and do nothing.
6. Find fault with the officers and other leaders every chance you get. It keeps them on their toes and enables you to say, "I told you so," if something does not go well.
7. Take all you can get in the way of benefits and services. Give as little as possible in return.
8. Keep your ideas to yourself. But be a good listener and pick up all the tips you can from others.
9. Never ask anyone to join. Only fall guys serve on a committee.
10. Only serve on a committee if they make you chairman. Do as little as possible and try not to call a meeting. You can always report progress.

Fig. 17-1 Ten ways to sink an organization

the nurse for membership in district, state, and national levels of the professional association.

The NSNA sends delegates to the ANA and NLN biennial conventions in order to foster a close relationship between student nurses and the professional nursing organizations. One member from the ANA Board and one from the NLN Board serve on the Advisory Council. Attendance and student involvement at the NSNA conventions indicate the deep sense of responsibility felt by the majority of students toward professional development.

NATIONAL LEAGUE FOR NURSING

The National League for Nursing (NLN) is committed to maintaining and improving standards of nursing education. The NLN has both individual and agency members. Over 20,000 individuals from all the allied health professions, in addition to nursing and medicine, hold memberships. Over 1,800 schools, colleges, and universities offering nursing programs, and institutions providing nursing services, hold agency memberships in the NLN.

The NLN conducts one of the largest professional testing services in the country. Pre-entrance testing to assist schools in the selection of potentially successful students, and achievement testing to measure student progress, is done on a wide scale. The National League for Nursing, Division of Measurement, is the test service agency for the State Board Test Pool Examinations for registered nurse and practical nurse licensure. NLN publications include *NEWS,* the monthly news communication sent to the membership, and *Nursing Outlook,* the NLN official magazine. Two annual research reports are the directories *State-Approved Schools of Nursing for Registered Nurses* and *State-Approved Schools of Nursing for Practical Nurses.*

The NLN offers continuing education programs in the form of workshops, seminars, and conferences to inform practicing nurses of new developments in nursing practice. The NLN staff possess expertise in their specialty areas of nursing and provide consultation on the initial planning and development of new programs; the organizational and administrative problems of programs already in operation; and curriculum revision. NLN headquarters are located at 10 Columbus Circle, New York, N.Y. 10019.

The National League for Nursing was formed in 1952 as a result of the merger of seven national nursing groups: the National League of Nursing Education, the American Nurses' Association, the National Association of Colored Graduate Nurses, the National Organization of Public Health Nursing, the American Association of Nurse Anesthetists, the Association of Collegiate Schools of Nursing, and the American Association of Industrial Nurses, Inc.

After numerous studies were conducted to determine the best organizational structure, the two major organizations were formed: The American Nurses' Association, with membership open to nurses only, and the National League for Nursing, open to nurses and lay persons. A coordinating council assures coordination between the two organizations. The NLN and the ANA sponsor a nursing careers program as a joint effort to assist individuals in the selection of schools and to provide scholarship information.

The NLN has been recognized by the U.S. Office of Education as the official accrediting agency for master's, baccalaureate, associate degree, diploma, and practical nursing programs. The NLN has been designated by the National Commission on Accreditation as the accrediting agency for schools of nursing in colleges and universities. The National Federation of Licensed Practical Nurses recognizes NLN accreditation of practical nursing programs. The NLN, along with the American Public Health Association, accredits home health agencies and community nursing services.

NATIONAL ASSOCIATION FOR PRACTICAL NURSE EDUCATION AND SERVICE, INC.

National Association for Practical Nurse Education and Service, Inc. is the oldest nursing organization dedicated exclusively to practical nursing. The organization provides both service and education for licensed practical nurses (or licensed vocational nurses, as they are called in Texas and California). Although NAPNES is interested in raising public consciousness with respect to the role and function of licensed practical nurses, it is not a major aim. The major goals are to establish, develop, and maintain high educational standards for practical nursing preparation, to provide opportunities for voluntary continuing education, and to encourage licensed practical nurses to take advantage of the opportunities available to them. Its efforts are also directed toward meeting consumer health needs and improving delivery of all health care services.

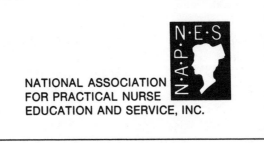

Fig. 17-2 NAPNES emblem

To create visibility and to bolster recruitment, NAPNES makes use of all the communications media and distributes educational literature. NAPNES also supplies speakers for schools, clubs, service organizations, and other interested groups.

Registered nurses, educators, health care agency administrators, physicians, and lay persons are members of NAPNES. Practical nursing students may become student members of NAPNES. The fee for student membership is a reduced rate. Membership entitles the licensed practical nurse to attend educational seminars, apply for malpractice insurance at group rates, attend the annual national convention, wear the NAPNES membership pin, and receive a monthly copy of the *Journal of Practical Nursing,* the official publication.

NAPNES was the first agency recognized by the United States Office of Education to accredit schools of practical nursing. NAPNES has also developed and published guidelines for continuing education. The organization approves continuing education programs for credit, and also sponsors workshops and continuing education programs for licensed practical nurses.

NATIONAL FEDERATION OF LICENSED PRACTICAL NURSES

The National Federation of Licensed Practical Nurses was founded in 1949 as a national organization for licensed practical nurses. The membership is open to licensed practical nurses and includes district, state, and national levels. Upon the payment of state dues, membership in the national organization is automatic.

The NFLPN has adopted a code of ethics for the licensed practical nurse which serves as a guide for the practicing nurse. The organization is dedicated to promoting high standards of nursing education for practical nurses. The NFLPN was instrumental in changing the composition of the State Boards of Nursing Examiners to include a licensed practical nurse. NFLPN also has been involved in obtaining the right for licensed practical nurses to

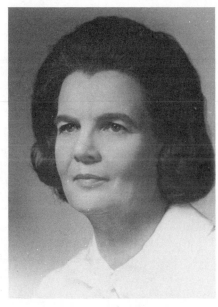

Fig. 17-3 Muriel R. Smith, Executive Director of NFLPN, 1977

constitute an appropriate unit for the purposes of collective bargaining. The organization also sponsors workshops and seminars which carry continuing education credits. The official publication of NFLPN is *Nursing Care.*

SIGMA THETA TAU

Six students enrolled in the Indiana University Training School for Nurses in 1922 conceived the idea of an honor society in nursing. Sigma Theta Tau was granted its charter and Articles of Association from the State of Indiana in October of the same year. In 1959 Sigma Theta Tau was admitted to the Association of College Honor Societies, which has established the criteria for identification of an honor society. The society has grown tremendously since 1959 and many chapters have been established in colleges and universities having accredited baccalaureate or higher degree programs in nursing.

The purposes of the honor society include the recognition of superior achievement and leadership qualities; the fostering of high professional standards; the encouragement of creative work; and the strengthening of commitment to the

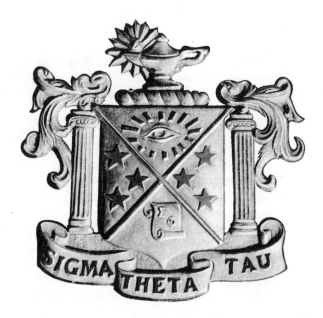

Fig. 17-4   Emblem of the Honor Society in Nursing. (Reprinted with permission from *Nursing Outlook.* ©1972, The American Journal of Nursing Company and Sigma Theta Tau)

ideals and purposes of the nursing profession. The name, Sigma Theta Tau, stands for the Greek words, *storgs, tharos,* and *tima,* which mean love, courage, and honor.

Five elected national officers comprise the National Council which meets several times a year. To help the council in organizational business matters, each chapter elects two delegates, forming the House of Delegates, which meets biennially. The society elects national honorary members who have achieved national recognition in nursing or a related field. The society conducts workshops and sponsors research projects. Local chapters also conduct programs, workshops, and seminars which generally focus on excellence in nursing practice, education, and current research findings and applications. The official publication *Image* is sent to members three times a year. Membership in Sigma Theta Tau is approved by the local chapter on the basis of the demonstration of superior scholastic achievement and professional leadership.

INTERNATIONAL COUNCIL OF NURSES

The International Council of Nurses (ICN) was the first international organization of professional women. The organization represents over half a million nurses and in many countries it is the only professional nursing organization. The idea of an international organization for nurses was discussed in 1893 at the Columbia Exposition in Chicago. A provisional committee representing nine countries laid the groundwork. In 1899 ICN was founded during the meeting of the International Council of Women in London. In 1900 the constitution of the ICN was adopted. The organization is committed to the maintenance of high standards of nursing service and education and the promotion of professional ethics. Membership is open to national nursing associations and not to individuals. The ANA holds the membership for nurses in the United States.

WORLD HEALTH ORGANIZATION

It was at the United Nations founding meeting, held in San Francisco in 1945, that delegates from Brazil and China suggested that the United Nations might set up an international health program. The aftermath of World War II revealed vast medical and social problems. The World Health Organization (WHO) was dedicated to promoting health as a state of physical, mental, and social well-being. The official publication of WHO is the *Guide for National Studies of Nursing Resources.* Other publications are the *Chronicle of the World Health Organization* and *World Health,* published in English at Palais des Nations, Geneva, Switzerland.

The World Health Organization has assigned a nurse to four regional offices based in Alexandria, Egypt; New Dehli, India; Bangkok, Thailand; and Washington, D.C. Each WHO team, composed of a doctor, a nurse, and a sanitary engineer, functions to meet the needs of the people by providing assistance in nursing care, preventive medicine, and sanitation. Since the founding of WHO, almost 150 American nurses have gone to twenty-one countries to teach midwifery, nutrition, and dispensary work. One hundred thirty-four nurses are employed by WHO and are involved in nursing activities in twenty-nine countries. The ICN standards are the basis for the nursing activities throughout the world.

Type 1.   *"Wishbones"* who spend their time wishing someone would do the work.

Type 2.   *"Jawbones"* who do all the talking, but very little else.

Type 3.   *"Knucklebones"* who knock everything that anyone tries to do.

Type 4.   *"Backbones"* who get under the load and do the work.

Make no "Bones" about it . . . . A successful association takes a lot of Backbone . . . . it needs yours.

Fig. 17-5 Four types of organizational members

SUMMARY

Progress in nursing comes as a result of the efforts of the dedicated members of nursing organizations. The individual nurse gains from the united efforts of members striving to promote the interests of organized nursing. Because these nursing organizations are dedicated to high standards of nursing education and practice, the consumer of nursing services also benefits. Nursing's real power and potential lies with individual nurses who can unite and work together for common purposes. The individual alone has little power, but many nurses working together can accomplish much. The nursing organizations need the input and efforts of every individual nurse in order to truly represent the interests of the profession and to have the benefit of a united front. Therefore, each nurse should support and participate in a professional organization at the local, state, and national level. Note the directory of international and national nursing organizations.

DIRECTORY OF MAJOR NURSING RELATED ORGANIZATIONS		
INTERNATIONAL		
International Council of Nurses	Box 42, 12111	Geneva 20, Switzerland
International Committee of Catholic Nurses	Square Vergota, 43, B-1040	Brussels, Belgium
Pan American Health Organization	525 23rd St., N.W. WHO Regional Office for the Americas	Washington, DC 20037
World Health Organization	Avenue Appia	Geneva, Switzerland
NATIONAL		
American Nurses' Association	2420 Pershing Road	Kansas City, MO 64108
American Nurses' Foundation	2420 Pershing Road	Kansas City, MO 64108
American Association of Critical-Care Nurses	631 E. Chapman Ave.	Orange, CA 92667
American Association of Industrial Nurses	79 Madison Ave.	New York, NY 10016
American Association of Nephrology Nurses and Technicians	Middle City Station P.O. Box 2368	Philadelphia, PA 19103
American Association of Neuro-surgical Nurses	51813 Westhaven Dr.	Indianapolis, IN 46254
American Association of Nurse Anesthetists	Suite 929 111 E. Wacker Dr.	Chicago, IL 60601
American Cancer Society	219 E. 42nd St.	New York, NY 10017
American College of Nurse Midwives	50 E. 92nd St.	New York, NY 10028
American Heart Association	44 E. 23rd. St.	New York, NY 10010
American Hospital Association	840 N. Lake Shore Dr.	Chicago, IL 60611
American Indian Nurses Association	Griffin Memorial Hospital	Norman, OK 73069
American Medical Association	535 N. Dearborn St.	Chicago, IL 60610
American Public Health Association	1015 18th St., N.W.	Washington, DC 20037
American Red Cross Nursing Programs	National Hq. 17th & D Sts., N.W.	Washington, DC 20006

DIRECTORY OF MAJOR NURSING RELATED ORGANIZATIONS (Continued)		
NATIONAL (Continued)		
Association of Operating Room Nurses	10170 E. Mississippi Ave.	Denver, CO 80231
Emergency Dept. Nurses Association	P.O. Box 1566	East Lansing, MI 48823
Gay Nurses' Alliance	Box 5687	Philadelphia, PA 19129
National Association for Practical Nurse Education and Service	122 E. 42nd St. Suite 800	New York, NY 10017
National Black Nurses Association, Inc.	P.O. Box 8295	Canton, OH 44711
National Federation of Licensed Practical Nurses	Rm. 323-25 250 W. 57th St.	New York, NY 10019
National Joint Practice Commission	875 N. Michigan Ave.	Chicago, IL 60611
National League for Nursing	10 Columbus Circle	New York, NY 10019

SUGGESTED ACTIVITIES

- Interview an officer of the district association of one of the nursing organizations and report to the class on information relative to what territory the district covers, types of programs offered, meeting dates and places, membership, and student involvement.

- Attend the Student Day activities at the annual State Nurses Association convention and report on the event as a learning experience.

- Review the constitutions of the district associations and make a comparison chart of the standing committees of each.

REVIEW

A. Multiple Choice. Select the best answer.

1. A record of nursing education and experience may be compiled through the Professional Credential and Personnel Service of
    a. Sigma Theta Tau.   c. ANA.
    b. NLN.   d. NAPNES.

2. The nursing organization which conducts a testing service and is the test service agency for the State Board Test Pool is
   a. ANA.
   c. ICN.
   b. all the state nursing associations.
   d. NLN.

3. Two international nursing associations are
   a. ICN and WHO.
   c. ANA and WHO.
   b. ICN and ANA.
   d. NLN and WHO.

4. The NLN is recognized by the U.S. Office of Education as
   a. the official nursing organization in the United States.
   b. the ultimate authority on nursing practice.
   c. the profession's lobby organization.
   d. the official accrediting agency for nursing programs.

5. The nursing organization which has the purpose of recognition of superior achievement and leadership in nursing is
   a. NLN.
   c. Sigma Theta Tau.
   b. ANA.
   d. a and b.

B. Match the organization in Column II with the appropriate statement in Column I.

Column I	Column II
1. An organization proposed at the 1945 meeting of the United Nations.	a. ANA
	b. NLN
2. The oldest nursing organization dedicated to practical nursing exclusively.	c. NSNA
	d. NAPNES
3. Formerly the Nurses Associated Alumnae of the United States and Canada, the organization is promoting professional nursing practice standards.	e. NFLPN
	f. Sigma Theta Tau
4. A three-level national organization which has as its official publication, *Nursing Care.*	g. WHO
5. An organization designed to familiarize student nurses with the professional organizations.	h. ICN
6. A professional nursing organization which has individual and agency membership and permits nonnurses to join.	
7. A nursing organization with members being national nursing associations rather than individuals.	
8. The national honor society in nursing.	

C.   Briefly answer the following questions.

      1.   Why should nurses join a professional nursing organization?

      2.   List the official publication of

         a. ANA   d. NAPNES

         b. NLN   e. NFLPN

         c. Sigma Theta Tau   f. WHO

chapter 18
NURSING PRACTICE
ACTS AND LICENSURE

STUDENT OBJECTIVES

- Explain the process of individual licensure.
- Explain the concept of institutional licensure.
- Explain government regulation of nursing practice.

In the United States, each state has the right to control occupations or professions which are related to the health, safety, or welfare of its citizens. Therefore, every state has its own definition of professional and practical nursing practice and regulations governing that practice. Such regulations are meant to protect the public and do so by restricting practice to only those individuals who have demonstrated that they possess the qualifications determined by the state. The actual regulation of nursing and the definition of nursing practice varies from state to state. However, there are similarities in terms of nurse practice acts, licensure, and registration.

NURSE PRACTICE ACTS

In each state the legislative bodies establish the definition of nursing, the qualifications to practice nursing, the mechanics of licensure and registration, the definition of misconduct and unlawful acts, disciplinary actions, the state agency which shall administer the laws and how that agency will function. The legislation or laws (nursing practice acts) regulating nursing practice vary considerably from state to state. Therefore, it is possible for a nurse to practice independently in one state; yet she must work under the supervision of a licensed physician or dentist in another. In one state licensure may be required for practice; in another, licensure may be voluntary.

The Legal Definition of Nursing

The nurse must practice nursing within the legal scope of the definition of nursing in the state in which she practices. There has been considerable dialogue for many years about what nursing really is. Regardless of the academic definition developed by nurses, nursing practice must be within the scope of the legal definition. For this reason, nurses and nursing organizations in many states have attempted to change the legal definition of nursing so that it is in keeping with the current concepts of nursing practice. Changing state law is no small task, because many other groups, particularly hospitals and physicians, have an interest in how nurses practice. State hospital associations and medical societies can provide a very strong opposition to nurses who seek to change the legal scope of nursing. However, it is possible when nurses work together. If all the nurses in a state will unite and push legislative reform, they become more powerful because they constitute a large group of registered voters. The trend is to revise obsolete definitions of nursing, and the state nurses associations are the vanguards in that movement.

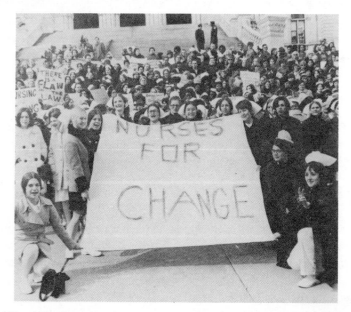

Fig. 18-1   Nurses working together to change an obsolete nurse practice act.

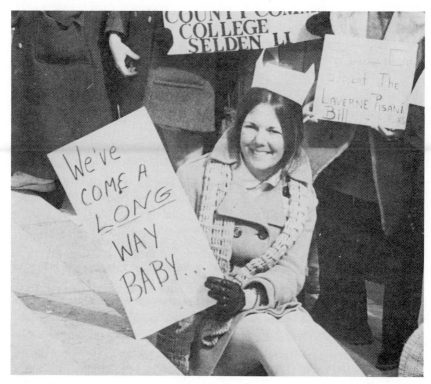

Fig. 18-2 Nurses meet strong opposition when they attempt to make changes, but with a united front it can be done.

Qualifications for the Practice of Nursing

Each state establishes the qualifications which must be met before an individual can practice nursing. Most states require proof that the applicant has satisfactorily completed a course of study in nursing at a school approved or accredited by the state agency or a recognized, similar agency in another state (for example, the National League for Nursing). Most states require the payment of a fee; this nominal charge accompanies the returned application form. Some states have minimal age requirements, and others may also require that the applicant be of good moral character. Citizenship is no longer a requisite for licensure. A decision of the United States Supreme Court declared it unconstitutional to require United States citizenship, or the filing of a declaration of intent to become a citizen, prior to the taking of a licensing examination. The states also require that the applicant pass an examination satisfactorily and in accordance with the regulations developed by the agency. A *license* (permission to practice) is granted when an applicant meets the requirements established by the state law and the administering agency. That license is valid during the life of the holder, unless it is revoked or suspended for some reason. *Registration* is the listing of the license with the state, for a fee. This requirement, of registration, must be met before the nurse can legally practice in that state. The duration of the registration varies from state to state but it is generally two to three years. The license must be registered with each state in which the nurse practices. It must be renewed in accordance with the regulations of each state.

Reciprocity or *endorsement* refers to the mutual acceptance of previously issued state licenses, without additional requirements. States vary in the rules and regulations governing licensure by reciprocity. In order to alleviate many reciprocity problems, the Council of State Boards of Nursing recommended single dates for nationwide testing. This was established in May, 1975 and the identical examination is given by each participating board.

Application for licensure begins with writing to the state nursing board for the proper form. The form is completed by the applicant and the administrator of the school or department from which the nurse graduated. The school seal is affixed by the academic institution, and the applicant verifies the information by signing the form in the presence of a notary public. Most forms require notarization and attachment of a passport-sized photo. A nominal fee is submitted with the application. It is essential to specify whether the application is for licensure by examination or endorsement, and for professional or practical nursing. The name of the applicant must be entered exactly as it appears on the school certificate or degree. Documentary proof must be submitted for a change of name. This process is fairly standard in all states; however, requirements for licensure as a registered nurse and practical nurse are different and vary from one state to another.

STATE BOARDS OF NURSING

Each nurse practice act specifies the agency which will administer the licensure laws. In most states a nursing board, which is usually an arm of a larger agency (such as the state health department or state education department), is given the responsibility for carrying out the procedures designated by the act. The board of nursing is also responsible for the rules and regulations for administering the act. Its members are usually appointed by the governor and represent the nursing profession. The board reviews all applications for licensure, and issues licenses to qualified applicants. The board has the responsibility to establish educational standards for nursing programs and must register or approve nursing programs in the state on the basis of those standards. Most

The registered nurse practitioner shall:

1. be familiar with the Illinois Nursing Act, Code of Ethics for Nurses and ANA Functions and Standards.

2. plan, implement and evaluate nursing care needs of patients.

3. supervise all nursing activities relating directly and indirectly to patient care.

4. promote the improvement of patient care.

5. coordinate the nursing care plan with the medical plan.

6. make appropriate observations, report and record accurately.

7. act to safeguard the patient when his care and safety are affected by incompetent, unethical or illegal conduct of any person.

8. promote and participate in patient education and rehabilitation.

9. collaborate with members of related health disciplines in implementing care.

10. utilize community resources for continuity of care.

11. work with other members of health professions and citizens in promoting efforts to meet health needs of the public.

12. maintain ability to function in an emergency and disaster.

13. accept responsibility for new and expanded functions only after assurance that:

    a. the group delegating the functions is ready to do so.

    b. the individual assesses own readiness to accept responsibility.

    c. adequate instruction and practice to assume responsibility to administer the new function safely has been provided.

14. assume responsibility for own standard of care, own acts, and judgments.

15. assume responsibility for individual professional and personal growth and education.

16. participate in professional organizations that contribute to own area of practice.

17. participate in studies and research.

Fig. 18-3 Standards of practice for the registered nurse, State of Illinois

schools of nursing easily meet the standards of the state board, and many meet the higher standards which are required for accreditation by the NLN. The board is also responsible for the reregistration of licenses. The board Standards are enforced and the board takes the necessary disciplinary action when indicated.

The state board of nursing is also responsible for determining the standards relating to the licensing examination. Licensing examinations are developed and distributed to each state by the National League for Nursing. The completed tests are returned to the NLN for grading and evaluation. The State Board Test Pool is under the jurisdiction of the Council of State Boards of the American Nurses' Association. Examinations are given in specifically designated testing centers on prescheduled dates two or more times annually, and are carefully monitored by the board of nurse examiners to insure test item secrecy.

Composition of a committee of nurse examiners may vary among states but generally there are representatives from the different professional educational programs in nursing, nursing service, and practical nursing programs. Standardized tests are used. Test items are evaluated and kept current and consistent with nursing trends. The National League for Nursing Division of Measurement provides test booklets, answer sheets, and grading service for the State Board Test Pool examinations for licensure of registered and practical nurses.

The state board reviews all charges of misconduct and usually makes recommendations to the larger agency (e.g., the state education department) concerning disciplinary steps. The state law defines professional misconduct but the administrative agency has the authority to interpret the law. Obtaining licensure fraudulently, practicing with gross incompetence or negligence, practicing while impared by alcohol or drugs, and conviction of crime are examples of conduct which would usually lead to revocation or suspension of the license to practice.

INSTITUTIONAL LICENSURE

Licensure as it has been discussed previously in this chapter refers to individual licensure. *Institutional licensure* is terminology which has been used by the health care industry for several different plans for licensure. In some cases, it refers to the proposal that the state should not license individual health workers, but should license health care institutions instead. In other proposals, institutional licensure refers to licensing of individuals by health care institutions. Both definitions advocate the abolishment of individual licensure.

Advocates of institutional licensure contend that individual licensure facilitates professional obsolescence because there is no requirement for the individual to update knowledge or to demonstrate continued proficiency. They also claim that the state licensure boards are composed of the same professionals that are being licensed, and this has led to self-serving policies and practices. Proponents of institutional licensure also state that the laws requiring strict conformance to educational preparation designated by the board, prevent experimentation and change in academic programs. Likewise, the laws allow the health worker to practice only within the rigid scope of the definition of the practice, again preventing experimentation and stifling individual growth.

In 1976, there were over 250 different health care occupations. Many of these new occupations are licensed under voluntary or mandatory state systems. At least twenty-five health occupations are subject to mandatory licensure. Simultaneously, the need for health care workers has increased. By enforcing mandatory licensure, the number of individuals allowed to practice is restricted to those who meet established requirements.

With institutional licensure, the institution would determine that individuals meet certain standards and qualifications for work in that institution. Hospital administrators claim that continuing education could easily be built into the system of establishing and maintaining the appropriate credentials: (a) evaluation of individual performance is much easier to do on the job, (b) the institution would have the flexibility to experiment and test new programs of instruction or new types of personnel, and (c) career mobility would be facilitated because the worker would continue to advance to his fullest potential.

In 1970, the American Hospital Association (AHA) proposed that health care institutions should be given complete responsibility for the quality of health care provided by all of the health workers who were employed by the institution or who had contractual relationships with the institution. The American Medical Association (AMA), in that same year, suggested that institutional licensure might be appropriate for dependent practitioners such as nurses, but that independent practitioners (doctors) should maintain individual licenses. In 1973, AMA's House of Delegates opposed institutional licensure for doctors and nurses. In the early 1970s, the Department of Health, Education, and Welfare (DHEW) proposed that pilot projects in institutional licensure be initiated. Illinois and Pennsylvania have been the two states to participate in these studies, which are still going on.

Essentially, institutional licensure is a management rights concept. It would give the health care facility the legal right and responsibility for selecting, training, evaluating, supervising, and establishing standards for all who provided health care within the institution. Advocates of institutional licensure assume that such an approach will promote efficiency and cut costs. There is little mention of improved quality of health care. Many nurses feel that the training and evaluating of health workers would increase costs rather than reduce them. Individuals assume the cost of *individual* licensure, but it seems likely that the public will have to pay the bill for *institutional* licensure. Nurses claim the institution might exclude qualified personnel and, instead, hire or train others who will work for a lower salary. It is conceivable that the numbers of nurses would be reduced and nursing functions delegated to nonnurses. Nurses would not determine the scope of their practice; the institution would develop the job descriptions for all health workers.

For nurses one of the more serious drawbacks of institutional licensure is that mobility would be severely thwarted. If each institution developed its own training and positions, it is not likely that an individual could move to another institution and be found qualified to hold the same or similar position. Furthermore, there would be little need for professional or technical nursing education unless the institution decided formal nursing education should be a qualification.   There is no guarantee that such standards would be established.

Inherent in the proposals for institutional licensure is the belief that licensure boards are self-serving.   In a health care institution, the ultimate authority rests with the board of directors or a similar body.   Members of the board are usually selected because of their business, financial, or social background, and not because of their training in health care.   Their concern is the business of health care rather than the quality of services.   It is possible, nurses contend, for such a board to be as self-serving as the licensure board.

The American Nurses' Association (ANA) has long promoted individual licensure because individuals should be held accountable for the quality of services rendered.   The House of Delegates approved a resolution in 1972, which reinforced the importance of: individual accountability; career and geographic mobility; and the profession's right and responsibility for establishing the scope and standards of practice. The National League for Nursing (NLN) also has publicly opposed shifting the accountability from the individual to the institution.   Generally, the nursing community has opposed the concept of institutional licensure because the quality of health service is directly related to individual responsibility.   By abolishing or reducing individual responsibility, the safety of the health care consumer will be seriously jeopardized.   Individual licensure does provide for standardized levels of competence and education, giving the public some measure of protection.   Institutional licensure gives no guarantee of consistency or quality.   The consumer would place his safety and health in the hands of a business, the health industry, rather than in the hands of licensed professional health workers who are legally responsible for the services provided.

SUMMARY

The legal regulation of nursing practice is a prerogative of state government. The state board of nursing, or a similar group, administers the state nurse practice act.   The actual content of the practice act and the policies and procedures set by the board of nursing vary from state to state.   In the past, differences in qualifications from state to state led to difficulties.   However, those problems have been resolved in part by the establishment of the State Board Test Pool and single dates for nationwide testing.   In the early seventies, institutional licensure was proposed as an alternative to individual licensure.   Nurses have strongly opposed the concept because it necessitates shifting the accountability for practice from the individual to the institution.   This would tend to foster lower standards and poor quality of care.

DIRECTORY OF STATE BOARDS OF NURSING

ALABAMA State Administration Bldg., Room 153 Montgomery 36104	**INDIANA** 100 N. Senate Avenue, Room 1018 Indianapolis 46204
ALASKA 2702 Denoli Street, Room 206 Anchorage 99503	**IOWA** 300 - 4th Street Des Moines 50309
ARIZONA 1645 W. Jefferson, Suite 254 Phoenix 85007	**KANSAS** 701 Jackson Street, Room 314 Topeka 66603
ARKANSAS 9107 Rodney Parham Road Little Rock 72205	**KENTUCKY** 6100 Dutchmans Lane Louisville 40205
CALIFORNIA 1020 N Street Sacramento 95814	**LOUISIANA** 150 Baronne Street, Room 907 New Orleans 70112
COLORADO 1525 Sherman Street Denver 80203	**MAINE** 295 Water Street Augusta 04330
CONNECTICUT 79 Elm Street, Room 101 Hartford 06115	**MARYLAND** 201 W. Preston Street Baltimore 21201
DELAWARE Cooper Bldg., Room 234 Dover 19901	**MASSACHUSETTS** 1509 Leverett Saltonstall Bldg. Boston 02202
FLORIDA 6501 Arlington Expressway, Bldg. B Jacksonville 32211	**MICHIGAN** 1033 S. Washington Avenue Lansing 48926
GEORGIA 166 Pryor Street, S.W. Atlanta 30303	**MINNESOTA** 717 Delaware Street, S.E. Minneapolis 55414
HAWAII P.O. Box 3469 Honolulu 96801	**MISSISSIPPI** 135 Bounds Street, Suite 101 Jackson 39206
IDAHO 481 N. Curtis Boise 83704	**MISSOURI** 3523 N. Ten Mile Dr., Box 656 Jefferson City 65101
ILLINOIS 628 East Adams Springfield 62786	**MONTANA** 601 N. Davis Helena 59601

DIRECTORY OF STATE BOARDS OF NURSING (Continued)	
NEBRASKA P.O. Box 94703 Lincoln 68509	SOUTH DAKOTA 132 S. Dakota, Suite 200 Sioux Falls 57102
NEVADA 100 Vassar Street, Room 202 Reno 89502	TENNESSEE 217 Capitol Towers Nashville 37219
NEW HAMPSHIRE 105 Loudon Road Concord 03301	TEXAS 7600 Chevy Chase, Suite 502 Austin 78752
NEW JERSEY 1100 Raymond Blvd., Room 319 Newark 07102	UTAH 330 E. 4th S. Street Salt Lake City 84111
NEW MEXICO 505 Marquette, N.W. Albuquerque 87101	VERMONT 126 State Street Montpelier 05602
NEW YORK 99 Washington Avenue Albany 12210	VIRGINIA 6 N. 6th Street, Room 404 Richmond 23219
NORTH CAROLINA P.O. Box 2129 Raleigh 27602	WASHINGTON P.O. Box 649 Olympia 98504
NORTH DAKOTA 219 N. 7th Street, Upper Suite 5 Bismarck 58501	WASHINGTON, D.C. 614 H Street, N.W., Room 112 Washington, DC 20001
OHIO 180 E. Broad Street, Suite 1130 Columbus 43215	WEST VIRGINIA 1800 Washington Street, E., Room 416 Charleston 25301
OKLAHOMA 4545 Lincoln Blvd., Suite 76 Oklahoma City 73105	WISCONSIN 201 East Washington Avenue Madison 53702
OREGON 1400 S.W. 5th Avenue Portland 97201	WYOMING 1902 Thomas Avenue Cheyenne 82001
PENNSYLVANIA Box 2649 Harrisburg 17120	GUAM P.O. Box 2816 Agana 96910
RHODE ISLAND Health Bldg., Davis Street Providence 02908	PUERTO RICO P.O. Box 3271 San Juan 00904
SOUTH CAROLINA 1777 St. Julian's Place Columbia 29204	

SUGGESTED ACTIVITIES

- Write to the state board of nursing for information concerning licensure of registered nurses. List the requirements for licensure.

- Review the nursing practice act of the state in which you plan to practice and that of another state, and compare them.

- Take a stand on either institutional or individual licensure and write a position paper for class presentation.

REVIEW

A. Multiple Choice. Select the best answer.

1. State board examinations in nursing are prepared by the
    a. committee of nurse examiners. c. National League for Nursing.
    b. state board of nursing. d. State Board Test Pool.

2. The examinations are graded by the
    a. committee of nurse examiners.
    b. members of the state board.
    c. members of the ANA.
    d. Division of Measurement of the NLN.

3. Legal regulation of nursing practice is a prerogative of the
    a. nursing profession. c. federal government.
    b. employers of nurses. d. state government.

4. The rules and regulations concerning licensure of nurses are developed by the
    a. legislative body. c. state board of nursing.
    b. state health department. d. none of these.

5. The legal scope of practice of any licensed health care worker is determined by the
    a. state practice act for each licensed health occupation.
    b. employing agency.
    c. members of the profession.
    d. licensing board.

6. When a state agrees to accept the license issued by another state, it is called.
    a. certification. c. reciprocity.
    b. endorsement. d. b and c.

7. The usual requirements for licensure as a registered nurse are
   a. United States citizenship.
   b. references which vouch for the applicant's moral character.
   c. a baccalaureate degree in nursing.
   d. a passing score on the state board examination.

8. The license of a registered nurse is usually
   a. good for two to three years.
   b. registered, for a fee, with the state.
   c. noncertified if there is conviction of a serious crime.
   d. b and c.

9. Institutional licensure refers to a concept which advocates
   a. abolishing individual licensure.
   b. licensure by institutions.
   c. that institutions be licensed.
   d. all the above.

10. Restricting the number of individuals who can practice in a given profession to those who meet established requirements,
    a. limits the number of individuals in the profession.
    b. is typical of institutional licensure.
    c. does not guarantee even minimal standards.
    d. is not the wish of most professional health workers.

B. Briefly answer the following questions.

1. What is the difference between registration and licensure?

2. Why do nurses oppose institutional licensure?

chapter 19
LEGAL RIGHTS
AND RESPONSIBILITIES

STUDENT OBJECTIVES

- Name at least four rights of nurses.
- Identify the responsibilities of nurses.
- Define the terms: *malpractice, collective bargaining, bargaining agent, liability, torts,* and *contract.*
- Identify the advantages of the collective bargaining process for the employee.

Historically, nurses have had a tendency to confuse the terms *right* and *responsibility.* Nurses have long been aware of their responsibilities but they are just beginning to identify their rights. Professional nursing organizations have developed and passed resolutions pertaining to the rights of nurses. However, the resolutions seldom state rights which are independent of responsibility. There is no question that the nurse assumes responsibility when she practices nursing. The nurse is legally responsible to practice as defined by the state law. Many aspects of her practice carry legal liability. In order for the nurse to claim what is rightfully hers and to avoid legal suit for abrogation of responsibility, it is vital that she be aware of and understand the rights and responsibilities of nurses.

NURSES' RIGHTS

According to Webster's dictionary one of the definitions of *right* is: *the power or privilege to which one is justly entitled.* To have a right implies the

> *RESOLVED, That the nurse practitioner has the responsibility to inform employers, present and prospective, of her educational preparation, experience, clinical competencies and those ethical beliefs which would affect her practice, and be it,*
> *RESOLVED, That the nurse practitioner has the responsibility to alter, adjust to or withdraw from situations which are in conflict with her preparation, competencies and beliefs, and be it,*
> *RESOLVED, That the employer shall provide the resources through which health services are made available to the recipient, and be it,*
> *RESOLVED, That the nurse practitioner has the right and responsibility to collaborate with her/his employer to create an environment which promotes and assures the delivery of optimal health services, and be it further,*
> *RESOLVED, That the nurse has the right to expect that her/his employer will respect her/his competencies values and individual differences as they relate to her/his practice.*

Fig. 19-1   Resolution of the Michigan Nurses' Association on nurses rights

ability to demand, with justification, that which is moral and legal. Nurses began to claim rights when participation in procedures and modes of treatment, which contradicted basic beliefs and philosophy, was expected and required. Nurses recognized they had the right not to participate. This awareness led the International Council of Nurses and state nurses' associations to develop statements about the rights of nurses. Some of these statements failed to list rights of nurses, but instead tended to emphasize the responsibilities of the nurse. However, as nurses look more closely at their responsibilities, roles, and relationships with other health professionals, they are beginning to identify their rights as well.

Rights of Nurses

The nurse has the right to *economic reward* which is commensurate with responsibility and qualifications. These rewards refer to salary, paid vacation, paid sick days, paid holidays, insurance, pension plans, and so forth. Nurses, like all other individuals, cannot live on the good will earned for dedication and service. Living requires money. To practice nursing, an education is required, which also costs money. Therefore, the nurse has the right to demand salary and benefits which reflect her value and responsibility.

The nurse has the right to *working conditions* which do not jeopardize her physical or mental health or well-being. The nurse should neither be expected to work in an environment which is not safe, nor should she be expected to work an excessive number of hours or days without adequate time off duty. The nurse has the right to a work environment which has all the resources necessary to provide safe, quality care.

The nurse has the right to *pursue activities which would lead to professional development.* Such activities include educational meetings, workshops, conferences, and formal, structured, academic courses offered by colleges or universities. Continuing education is essential if the nurse is to maintain and develop higher levels of competency. The employer must not restrict or prevent participation in such activities by demanding that the nurse work tours of duty which would preclude such activity.

The nurse has the right to *control professional practice as defined by state law.* Too often, the control over nursing practice is assumed by the employer, other health professionals, and large agencies or organizations. Closely related to the right to control, is the right to participate in decision making which affects nursing. Nurses should be involved in decision making in the local health facility and in all other agencies and levels of government, including Congressional action. Nurses have the right to be informed and involved in any decisions made about any aspect of nursing, because nurses have been

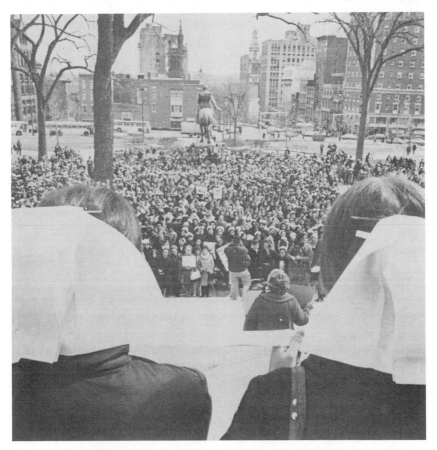

Fig. 19-2 Nurses have the right to take collective action

legally mandated to assume responsibility for nursing. It is impossible to assume responsibility for practice without having the right to control and participate in decisions made about that practice.

Nurses have the right to *collective action* in order to preserve these rights. Not only do nurses have the right to join nursing organizations but they also have the right to take political action in behalf of nursing and the health care consumer.

Nurses have the right to *set standards for nursing practice and education.* They also have the right to enforce such standards, to promote optimal health care services and delivery, and to support or draft and introduce legislation which enables nursing and the health care industry to meet these standards.

Rights of Women

In 1976, only 1.3 percent of registered nurses in the United States were males; the other 98.7 percent females. Thus, most nurses are faced with the problems all women face in terms of equal rights, privileges, and opportunities. Women, as human beings, have the right to dignity and the freedom to pursue a career which permits the utilization of individual talent and formal education. Women have the right to participate in the decision-making processes of every aspect of economic, political, and social life, and share with men the responsibility for the welfare of the nation. Men, by assuming total responsibility and control, have shortchanged themselves as well as women. Complete equality for men and women, nurses and doctors, cannot help but lead to a society which draws upon all resources and potential to improve the well-being of every individual.

Rights of Employees

Many nurses are employees; as such, they have employee rights which are provided by federal, state, and local labor laws. Under the National Labor Relations Act, employees have the right to self-organization; to join labor organizations; and to select a labor organization to represent them for the purpose of collective bargaining. Nurses and other employees in proprietary institutions have had the right to bargain under the auspices of the National Labor Relations Act (NLRA) since 1964. The NLRA was amended in 1974 (Taft-Hartley Amendment) to include employees of voluntary hospitals. One of the difficulties encountered under the NLRA was that employees who are considered supervisors (as defined by the Act) are excluded from the *bargaining unit* (a group of employees recognized as appropriate under the NLRA, to bargain collectively with the employer). ANA and state nurses associations are seeking to clarify that definition, which was developed for the industrial setting and is not appropriate in describing professional authority. Employees in Veterans Administration hospitals have the right to collectively bargain under an Executive Order. Nurses employed by counties, cities, and states do not all have such rights; however, Public Employee Relation Acts have been passed in many states, and some of these acts do give nurses the right to bargain collectively.

Collective bargaining is a process which introduces the concept of democracy in the establishment of employment conditions within the work setting. Through collective bargaining, individual employees have the right to participate in the establishment of their conditions of employment and thereby exercise a measure of control over such conditions. *Collective bargaining* is the bilateral determination of conditions of employment and the administration of the agreement reached through the bargaining process. The process consists of two parts: the development of a contract (negotiation of a new contract or changes in an existing contract) and administration of the contract (processing of problems which arise according to the provisions of the contract).

Through the process of collective bargaining, the individual has a voice and is not subject to arbitrary decisions made by the employer. The individual participates in the decisions made concerning salaries, wages, working conditions, and standards. Before, it was stated that nurses had the right to set standards, control practice, to work in a safe environment, and fair compensation. These rights are not guaranteed by law, but are rights which are morally justified. They can become guaranteed by law (relating to contractual agreements) which is one of the benefits of collective bargaining.

The *bargaining agent* is an organization certified by a government agency to represent a group of employees for the purpose of collective bargaining; it can be selected from any number of labor organizations. Most labor organizations or unions have a single purpose, that of representing employees for the purpose of collective bargaining. Most nurses have turned to their professional organizations for such services, because they require services which can only be provided by those who are familiar with nursing. The state nurses associations have developed programs which are totally responsible for promoting the economic and general welfare of registered nurses. Each program has a professional staff prepared to assist practitioners: the achievement of employment standards consistent with those of the profession and in the development of employment conditions essential to the practice of nursing. The primary purpose of such programs is the improvement and correction of those conditions which impede the practice of nursing. Nurse educators may elect the National Education

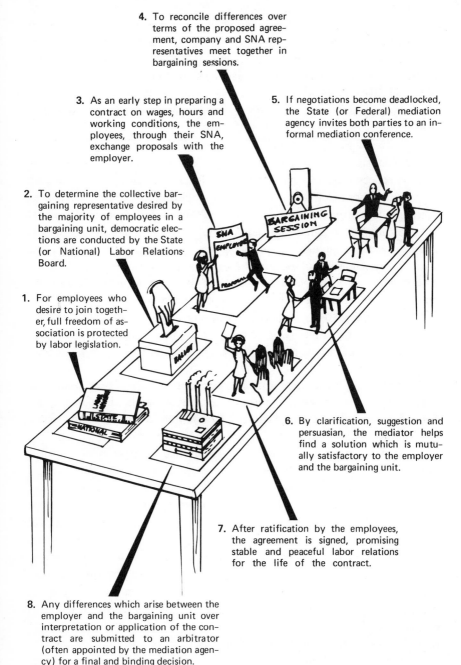

4. To reconcile differences over terms of the proposed agreement, company and SNA representatives meet together in bargaining sessions.

3. As an early step in preparing a contract on wages, hours and working conditions, the employees, through their SNA, exchange proposals with the employer.

5. If negotiations become deadlocked, the State (or Federal) mediation agency invites both parties to an informal mediation conference.

2. To determine the collective bargaining representative desired by the majority of employees in a bargaining unit, democratic elections are conducted by the State (or National) Labor Relations Board.

1. For employees who desire to join together, full freedom of association is protected by labor legislation.

6. By clarification, suggestion and persuasion, the mediator helps find a solution which is mutually satisfactory to the employer and the bargaining unit.

7. After ratification by the employees, the agreement is signed, promising stable and peaceful labor relations for the life of the contract.

8. Any differences which arise between the employer and the bargaining unit over interpretation or application of the contract are submitted to an arbitrator (often appointed by the mediation agency) for a final and binding decision.

Fig. 19-3 Setting the table for collective bargaining

Association, American Association of University Professors, or the American Federation of Teachers as their bargaining agent.

CONTRACTS

A *contract* is a legally binding agreement between two or more parties. A group contract is a written agreement between the employees and the employer, which contains the conditions of employment applicable to each position. An individual contract is a written or unwritten agreement between an individual and an employer, containing the terms of employment of the individual. A contract is not legal unless it is mutually understood. Generally, a contract requires the signature of both parties; however, some merely imply an agreement or understanding between two parties. The contract may be dissolved by mutual agreement. There is a legal and moral obligation to fulfill the terms of a contract. If one of the parties to a contract does not fulfill all of the terms as promised, it is called a *breach of contract* and the law provides remedies for breach.

NURSES' RESPONSIBILITIES

A contract can guarantee rights but it also usually implies legal responsibility. *Responsibility* is the state of being held to blame or accountable. To be responsible, it is assumed that there is a capacity for rational thought, decision, and action. Like rights, responsibility can be morally justified or legally mandated.

The responsibility of the nurse is found in the state nurse practice act. A licensed registered nurse is totally responsible for practicing nursing as it is legally defined. If the nurse fails to do so, she is *liable* (obligated by law) for all acts of omission and commission. She is further responsible for changing or withdrawing from conditions or situations which are in conflict with existing individual, professional, or legal standards.

The nurse is responsible to the health care consumer for quality nursing services and the promotion of health care services and delivery which meet the needs of the consumer. The nurse is responsible for maintaining and promoting the highest standards of practice for herself and the nursing community. The nurse has the responsibility for ethical conduct and should take appropriate action if another nurse is failing to assume that responsibility. The ANA has a code of ethics which provides broad guidelines for the registered nurse. NAPNES has a similar code for the licensed practical nurse.

As an employee, the nurse has the responsibility to accept and work in accordance with the rules and regulations established by the employer, provided

THE NURSE'S PLEDGE

solemnly pledge myself before God and in the presence of this assembly, to faithfully practice my profession of nursing.   I will do all in my power to make and maintain the highest standards and practices of my profession.   I will hold in confidence all personal matters committed to my keeping in the practice of my calling.   I will loyally assist the physician in his work and will devote myself to the welfare of my patients, my families and my community.   I will endeavor to fulfill my rights and privileges as a good citizen and to take my share of responsibility in promoting the health and welfare of my community.   I will constantly endeavor to increase my knowledge and skills in nursing and to use them wisely.   I will zealously seek to nurse those who are ill wherever they may be and whenever they are in need.   I will be active in assisting others in safeguarding and promoting the health and happiness of mankind.

Squibb Nurses Notes, 1964

Marion G. Howell, R.N., Dean Emeritus
Frances Payne Bolton School of Nursing
Western Reserve University, Cleveland, Ohio

Fig. 19-4 The Nurse's Pledge

they do not conflict with established professional responsibilities and ethics. If there is a contract, the nurse has the responsibility to fulfill the responsibilities as defined in the agreement.

The nurse is often involved in a number of situations which involve legal responsibility. The nurse should be particularly aware of legal responsibilities as ignorance is no protection.

Signing of Legal Papers

Ocassionally, a nurse may be asked to witness the signing of a will. The nurse should not become unnecessarily involved in legal situations and should make no statements which might be interpreted as "exerting influence." Usually, there is no reason why a nurse cannot witness a will; however, it is advisable to investigate the policy of the hospital or employer in this matter.

Consent Forms

There are various consent forms used in health care facilities. The most frequently used consent form is the one granting permission to the patient's doctor to perform a specific procedure. The physician or a designated surgeon is responsible for explaining the nature of the operation to the patient. The role of the nurse is generally to witness the signature of the consenting patient. This type of consent is called an *informed consent,* which simply means the patient agrees to have certain procedures performed on his body, *after having had the procedure explained to him.* The nurse should not witness such a consent unless she is positive that the patient has been informed, either by the doctor or nurse. Other forms which usually require the signature of a witness include a permission for autopsy (figure 19-6, page 325) and a release against medical advice. If a patient is a minor, the signature of the parent or guardian is required. In most states a minor can sign a legal document only if married.

Incident Report

Whenever a patient is injured or has a potential injury, there exists the possibility of a lawsuit. Such incidents must be immediately and accurately recorded. Incident reports should be completed when a patient slips on a wet floor, falls from a chair or bed, faints in the bathroom, cuts a finger on hospital equipment, and so forth. An incident report may be written for situations involving a patient, visitor, or employee. Incident report forms should be made out in duplicate by the person who was present at the time the incident occurred.

CONSENT TO OPERATION

PATIENT _____ DATE _____ TIME _____

1. I HEREBY AUTHORIZE THE PERFORMANCE UPON _____
   (myself or name of patient)
   OF THE FOLLOWING OPERATION _____
   (state nature and extent of operation)
   TO BE PERFORMED UNDER THE DIRECTION OF DOCTOR _____.

2. I recognize that, during the course of the operation, unforeseen conditions may necessitate additional or different procedures than those set forth in Paragraph 1. I, therefore, further authorize and request that the above named surgeon, his assistants, or his designees perform such procedures as are, in his professional judgment, necessary and desirable, including, but not limited to, procedures involving pathology and radiology. The authority granted under this Paragraph 2 shall extend to remedying conditions that are not known to Doctor _____ at the time the operation is commenced.

3. I consent to the administration of such anesthetics as may be considered necessary or advisable by the physician responsible for this service with the exception of
   _____ .
   (State: "None", "Spinal", etc.)

4. I consent to the administration of Blood Transfusions and/or Blood Derivatives if such is deemed necessary, and will not hold the hospital responsible if an unforeseen blood borne infection results from its administration.

5. I am aware that the practice of medicine and surgery is not an exact science, and I acknowledge that no guarantees have been made to me as to the results of the operation or procedure.

6. Check one:
   A. _____ I hereby authorize St. Therese Hospital to preserve for scientific or teaching purposes or for the use in grafts upon living persons, or to otherwise dispose of the dismembered tissue, parts, or organs resulting from the procedures authorized above.
   B. _____ I will be fully responsible for making disposition arrangement of amputated limbs. Removal of said limbs will be accomplished within ten (10) days after surgery; failure to remove before ten (10) days have passed will constitute approval of disposition by St. Therese Hospital.

7. I am aware that sterility may result from this operation. I know that a sterile person is incapable of becoming a parent.

8. The undersigned hereby agrees to indemnify St. Therese Hospital, Inc., from all costs, judgments, attorneys' fees and any other expenses which may be incurred by the said St. Therese Hospital, Inc., as a result of any claims or litigation arising out of the furnishing of blood or blood derivatives on the above named patient.

I CERTIFY THAT I FULLY UNDERSTAND THE ABOVE CONSENT TO OPERATION, THAT THE EXPLANATIONS THERE-IN REFERRED TO WERE MADE, AND THAT ALL BLANKS OR STATEMENTS REQUIRING INSERTION OR COMPLETION WERE FILLED IN, AND INAPPLICABLE PARAGRAPHS, IF ANY, WERE STRICKEN BEFORE I SIGNED.

SIGNED _____
(Patient or person authorized to consent for patient)

WITNESS _____

WITNESS _____

Fig. 19-5 Consent to operation form. (Courtesy of St. Therese Hospital)

AUTHORIZATION FOR AUTOPSY

Date _____ 19 _____

1. I hereby authorize Dr. _____, and such persons as he may designate, to perform and attend an autopsy on the remains of _____ for the purpose of determining the cause of death. Authority is also granted for the preservation and study of any and all tissues or parts which may be removed.

   SPECIFIC DESIGNATIONS, IF ANY: _____.

2. It is understood that due care will be taken for avoiding disfigurement of the body.

3. This authorization is given with the understanding that no charge will be made.

   Signature of Next of Kin _____

   Relationship _____

   Address _____

   _____

Witness _____

Address _____

_____

Witness _____

Address _____

_____

Fig. 19-6 Autopsy Permit. (Courtesy of St. Therese Hospital)

Everything pertinent to the incident must be written in that person's own words and penmanship. The physician must be notified immediately and the exact time of that notification, as well as the time of the physician's examination must be noted (and charted). It is the physician's responsibility to state the nature of the injury. The signatures of all persons present at the time of the incident and the physician must be entered on the incident report.

Administration of the wrong medication or dosage is an incident which could lead to a lawsuit against the nurse. Injecting a contaminated needle into a patient could cause an infection; striking a nerve or artery, or giving medication via the wrong route are all serious malpractice situations. Also, the nurse must be careful never to give a medication without proper identification of the patient. The nurse must always inquire as to whether the patient has known allergies. For some drugs, a sensitivity test is advisable if there is any doubt at all. If the patient has an allergy, every precaution must be taken to assure that the patient does not receive the *allergen* (substance that causes the allergy).

MEDICATION INCIDENT REPORT

PATIENT _____ ROOM _____ DOCTOR _____
        Last   First

HOSPITAL # _____ AGE _____ SEX _____

DRUG ORDERED _____ DATE _____

    STRENGTH _____ ROUTE _____ SCHEDULE _____

DRUG REQUISITIONED _____ BY _____

    STRENGTH _____ ROUTE _____ SCHEDULE _____

DRUG DISPENSED _____ BY _____

    STRENGTH _____ ROUTE _____ SCHEDULE _____

    HOW LABELED _____

DRUG GIVEN _____ # OF DOSES _____

    DATES & TIMES _____ BY _____

    STRENGTH _____ ROUTE _____ SCHEDULE _____

HOW ERROR DISCOVERED _____

_____

    DATE _____ BY _____

REMARKS _____

_____

_____

CORRECTED BY _____ DATE _____ HOW _____

REPORT FILLED OUT BY _____ DATE _____

NURSE'S SIGNATURE _____ DATE _____

PHYSICIAN'S SIGNATURE _____ DATE _____

PHARMACIST'S SIGNATURE _____ DATE _____

NURSING SUPERVISOR _____ DATE _____

Fig. 19-7 Medication incident report. (Courtesy of St. Therese Hospital)

Immediately upon recognizing a medication error, the nurse should notify the physician and complete an incident report or similar form.

Charting

Charting should always be done immediately after a procedure is performed, an observation is made, or noteworthy statements are made by either the nurse or patient. The nurse is liable for what she says or does in the performance of her duties. Very often the chart is the sole record of a nurse's action. Recording on the chart after the patient has left the institution is highly improper and may be questioned if the chart is taken to the courtroom. Black ink is preferred because it gives a clear reproduction. If penmanship is not legible, the nurse should print the entries. Charting that cannot be read is worthless. All data entered on the patient's chart should be pertinent and accurate. Only standard abbreviations are to be used. When making an entry on the chart, always note the time of day or night the incident occurred, the procedure was done, the medication was given, the observation was made, the patient left for other departments and returned to the nursing unit, and so forth. It is advisable to record the exact time the physician responded to a call or visited the patient. Comments should be comprehensive yet concise. Never erase or skip a line. The nurse must sign her name to the entries made by her and should be prepared to defend them in the event the record goes to court.

Emergency Care

In some states, a licensed professional nurse who provides emergency care without remuneration and in good faith, to a victim at the scene of an accident or in the event of nuclear attack, is exempt from civil liability. Legally, a nurse is not obligated to provide emergency assistance, although she may be ethically responsible to provide such care. Good Samaritan Laws have been passed in many states to encourage nurses and physicians to give emergency care to accident victims: the nurse will not be held liable for malpractice if she performs within the limitations of the nursing practice act of the state. A nurse is held responsible for the quality of care given. The nurse should avoid providing services if she does not have the necessary background, knowledge, and skills to provide safe care.

Negligence

Negligence is the failure to do something that an equally qualified person would do in a similar circumstance. Negligence is one of the most common

Type of Tort	Definition	Example
Assault and	Threat or attempt to touch another person.	Nurse who forces a treatment upon patient against his will and in absence of consent can be charged with assault and battery.
Battery	Carrying out the threat.	
False Imprisonment	Unwarranted restriction of the freedom of an individual.	Nurse who uses restraints on a patient who is of sound mind and not in danger of injuring himself may be charged with false imprisonment.
Invasion of Privacy	All individuals have the right to privacy and may bring charges against any person who violates this right.	A nurse who discloses information about a patient which is considered private knowledge, or photographs a patient without consent, can be charged with invasion of privacy.
Defamation (libel and slander)	Verbal (slander) or written (libel) remarks which may cause an individual to lose his good reputation.	A nurse who makes a statement about a patient which could cause him a ruined reputation or loss of employment, can be charged with defamation.
Negligence	Failure to do something that an equally qualified person would do in a similar circumstance.	Loss of patient property. Medication error. Burns from improperly used equipment. Failure to observe and/or report a change in the patient. Inaccurate sponge count in operating room.
Malpractice	Any professional act that causes injury, damage or loss to the patient.	Euthanasia. Nurse who makes an inaccurate medical diagnosis and prescribes the wrong treatment. Nurse who does not follow doctor's orders.

Fig. 19-8 A tort is a legally wrongful act, intentional or unintentional, against another individual. The chart lists some torts which allow patients to take civil action against nurses.

legal problems in nursing and is often brought about by the simple failure to use good judgment. Negligence is an unintentional *tort* (legally wrongful act) and may occur due to failure to properly apply knowledge to practice. The employer does not have to take the responsibility for acts of negligence; the nurse can be held legally responsible for an act of negligence, and charged with malpractice. A nurse charged with negligence may be required to pay money damages to the person harmed by the negligent act. If the act is serious enough, it may be considered a crime and the consequences may be severe.

Malpractice

Malpractice is any professional practice that results in damage, injury, or loss to a client. Negligent acts of persons rendering services of a skilled, professional, or highly technical nature are classified as malpractice. Rarely is an act of malpractice willfully done, If it were, the offender could be convicted

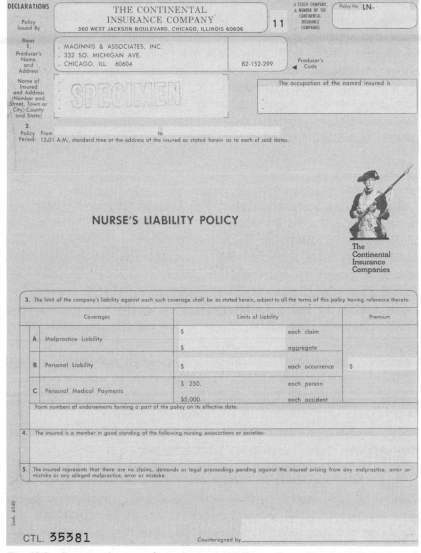

Fig. 19-9 Sample of a nurse's professional liability policy. (Courtesy, Maginnis and Associates)

of a criminal offense and punished by law. Failure to carry out a specific function normally associated with the performance of safe nursing care would be considered malpractice.

Malpractice Insurance

The incidence of malpractice suits filed in the courts is steadily increasing. Because the public is aware that most physicians and nurses are covered by malpractice insurance, there is little hesitancy to sue. The cost of such insurance for nurses is relatively small, especially if it is obtained through the professional nursing organization. The nurse must not assume coverage by the employer; the nurse must assume responsibility for professional liability insurance. In many cases, employer malpractice insurance will be inadequate for the nurse. The individual may determine the amount of coverage, commensurate with the type of nursing duties performed.

STUDENT RIGHTS

Student nurses have a right to learn. This places responsibility on the faculty to provide experiences which will facilitate the highest level of learning. The student, like the patient, has the right to be treated as an individual. Each student has different potentials, abilities, aptitudes, and interests. Students adjust and learn at different rates. The student nurse has the right to be informed about what is expected of her. Students have the right to a complete bibliography of all pertinent reference materials appropriate to each course. They should be notified well in advance of due dates for assignments and of examination schedules. Penalties for past due assignments and makeup exams should be clearly explained to the student. The student should be well informed of all the evaluation tools utilized. Test papers should be returned as soon as possible. All tests and assignments should be learning experiences and treated as such.

SUMMARY

Nurses have rights as human beings, women, and health care professionals. These rights have often been abrogated by employers of nurses, other health professionals, local, state, and federal governments, and by nurses themselves. Nurses are becoming aware of and demanding their rights. Nurses must act together to protect their rights, for as a unified force they have influence and power. If nurses remain divided and/or disinterested, they will never have control over their own practice nor will they be included in major decision making on issues involving nursing and health care.

The nurse also has both legal and ethical responsibility. If the nurse does not practice as defined by law or if a patient suffers damage or injuries because of the acts of a nurse, she is liable and may be sued. The nurse must be constantly aware of the legal consequences of nursing practice.

SUGGESTED ACTIVITIES

- Procure a copy of the job description for the staff nurse position in three local health care facilities and make a comparison.

- Interview a member of the faculty council or association charged with collective bargaining in your institution. Find out what the objectives of the local group are.

- Watch newspapers and magazines for news items pertaining to malpractice, liability suits, and other legal actions involving hospitals, and medical and nursing personnel. Bring clippings to class for discussion or a bulletin board display.

REVIEW

A. Multiple Choice. Select the best answer.

1. The National Labor Relations Act, amended in 1974, gives the right to bargain collectively to
   a. nurses in federal hospitals.
   b. nonsupervisory nurses in voluntary hospitals.
   c. all nonsupervisory employees in state health facilities.
   d. all the above.

2. If the terms of a contract are not met by one of the parties, it
   a. is called a breach of contract.
   b. is a nullification of the contract.
   c. gives the other party the right to ignore the terms of the agreement.
   d. none of the above.

3. If the patient agrees to have a certain procedure performed on him after having had the procedure explained to him, it is called
   a. a consent.   c. an informed consent.
   b. a consent for surgical procedure.   d. a verbal or written consent.

4. If a nurse is asked to witness a will, she should
   a. remember that nurses should avoid signing legal statements unnecessarily.
   b. check the hospital policies.
   c. avoid trying to influence anyone concerned with signing the will.
   d. all the above.

5. Some states have laws which protect a health care professional who gives emergency care at the scene of an accident or injury called
   a. medical and nurse practice acts.   c. right to work laws.
   b. State Labor Relations Act.   d. Good Samaritan Laws.

6. Which of the following is not a moral or legal right of a nurse?
   a. Economic reward for services rendered.
   b. A safe environment in which to practice.
   c. The right to refuse to participate in a procedure which conflicts with individual beliefs.
   d. The right to wear street clothes rather than uniform, regardless of hospital policy.

7. Collective bargaining is defined as
   a. a process which allows laborers to control management.
   b. a process which facilitates making arbitrary decisions.
   c. the bilateral determination of conditions of employment.
   d. all the above.

8. If the nurse discovers she has made a medication error, the first thing she should do is
   a. check to see if the patient is allergic to the drug.
   b. file an incident report, describing the error.
   c. tell the patient what has happened.
   d. call the doctor.

9. The nurse who comes upon an accident on the highway should remember that she
   a. has a legal responsibility to offer assistance.
   b. has a moral responsibility to offer assistance.
   c. may be sued for offering assistance in most states.
   d. all the above.

10. Malpractice can be best defined as
    a. an act of negligence.
    b. a criminal act.
    c. an intentional professional act of negligence.
    d. any professional act which leads to injury, damage, or loss.

B. Briefly answer the following questions.

1. List four rights to which nurses are justly entitled.

2. Explain why a nurse should have individual malpractice insurance.

3. In your own words, explain the following terms:

malpractice

contract

collective bargaining

bargaining agent

liability

torts

SECTION 6
OPPORTUNITIES
TO
GROW

chapter 20
EMPLOYING AGENCIES AND JOB OPPORTUNITIES

STUDENT OBJECTIVES

- Identify some major employment opportunities for nurses.
- List factors to be considered in selecting a nursing position.
- List the steps involved in seeking employment as a staff nurse.

The greatest number of nursing opportunities are available in the community setting, although nurses are usually able to find positions in all parts of the United States in a variety of agencies and facilities. Nursing positions are usually available in the community for the graduate of a community school. In an attempt to recruit personnel, the employing health care facilities may even contact students prior to graduation. However, employment opportunities for nurses do become more scarce during national employment crises and inflationary periods. The new graduate should be aware of what job opportunities are available. It is necessary that she re-examine her educational background, skills, interests, and professional goals in order to find a position which will be enjoyable and challenging. There is a direct relationship between the nurse who is happily employed and the quality of nursing care she gives. The new graduate also should know how to apply for a job and the proper conduct during an interview. A rational, mature approach to job selection will be more likely to result in a wise choice.

A SURVEY OF NURSING OPPORTUNITIES

It would be impossible to discuss every type of employment available to nurses in this chapter. It is possible to give an overview of such opportunities.

It is necessary to keep in mind that there are many kinds of jobs available in each area discussed. Some positions have education and experience requirements. If the nurse needs further information, she should contact an appropriate employer or health care agency.

Private Duty Nursing

The most outstanding appeal of private duty nursing is the direct patient contact and the close nurse-patient relationships. The private duty nurse remains at the bedside of the patient and gives the individualized care required by the patient. She is able to identify the physical, mental, spiritual, and socio-economic needs of the patient. The work of the private duty nurse is varied, as she is called upon to care for patients with various medical diagnoses. Private duty nurses are often able to choose the shift, type of clinical cases, and place of practice (hospital, extended care facility, or private home). Private duty is the oldest form of nursing. Prior to World War II, about 80 percent of the registered nurses did private duty. Today, over half of the calls for private duty nurses go unanswered because enough nurses are not available.

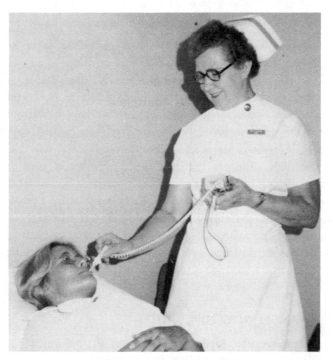

Fig. 20-1 A private duty nurse

Camp Nursing

In addition to a basic nursing education, camp nurses need a good understanding of food preparation, food handling, and an understanding of psychological problems, such as homesickness, enuresis, and sleeping disorders. Injuries which require first aid and orthopedic problems are most frequently encountered. Camp nursing often appeals to the nurse, enrolled in an academic program, who has the summer months free of other commitments. Employment dates extend from the end of June to the end of August. The camp nurse must have a love of the outdoors, travel, and enjoy children of all ages. Salary and living accomodations are generally good.

Occupational Health Nursing

An occupational health nurse practices in industry, commercial or government agencies; she provides health care for the employees. A synonymous term for occupational health nurse is industrial nurse. Positions are open to both licensed practical and registered nurses. Generally, the industrial nurse works the day shift but a few of the larger companies work evening and night shifts. Direct nursing care is not always required. An extensive amount of paper work is necessary, such as completing insurance forms of various kinds. Typing ability, knowledge of office management procedures, and emergency room experience are desirable prerequisites. Job duties include administering first aid to employees, maintaining records, performing or assisting with physical examinations, issuing safety glasses, operating the plant blood bank, disseminating preventive medicine information, and counseling employees with family or mental health problems. Frequently, the industrial nurse serves on a safety committee and is responsible for detecting safety hazards which may prove a threat to the welfare of the employee.

Public Health Nursing

The public health nurse serves the citizens of a geographically distinct area. Providing nursing services in the home on a scheduled assignment basis, planning the continuity of care for the patient discharged from the hospital, and collaborating with physicians, psychologists, and educators in meeting health needs are the main functions of the public health nurse. This is usually a day shift job, with opportunities for advancement; a baccalaureate degree is usually required.

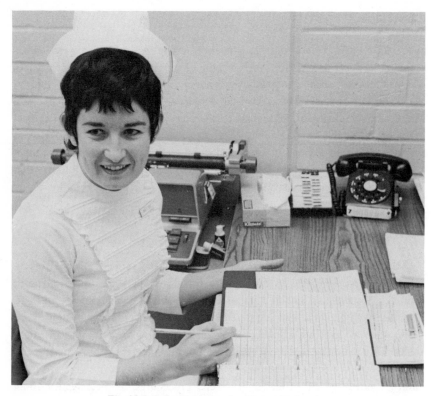

Fig. 20-2 Industrial nurse checking patient roster

School-Health Nursing

One of the most important public health positions is school nursing. Miss Lillian Wald returned from England in 1902, inspired to institute a comparable school-nursing service in New York. She placed nurses in four schools which had the highest absentee rate. The nurse was responsible for ascertaining the reason for the absence and for providing medical care.

In 1904, the city of Los Angeles placed nurses in the school system. Today, the role of the school nurse is accepted universally. The nurse provides health services at all levels of educational institutions: elementary, secondary, colleges, and universities. The major function of the school-health nurse is the prevention of disease through health education.

Hospital Nursing

General staff nursing opportunities are usually available in a wide range of clinical settings. Areas include the burn unit, medicine, surgery, obstetrics,

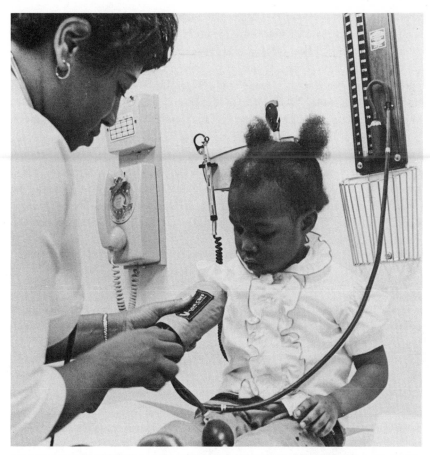

Fig. 20-3 The staff nurse in a hospital outpatient department

psychiatry, operating room, pediatrics, rehabilitation, orthopedics, neurosurgery, intensive and coronary care units as well as outpatient services. There are nursing positions in diagnostic areas (X ray, cardiopulmonary), renal units, drug abuse and treatment centers, and many subspecialty areas such as premature intensive care units and pediatric cardiology. Administrators are needed in the nursing service office to guide, direct, and coordinate nursing practice and to determine and maintain standards of nursing practice. There are also positions available for clinical specialists with graduate education.

The Veterans Administration Nursing Service

Based on *Facts On Nursing,* there are about 171 VA hospitals, 200 outpatient clinics, and over 80 nursing home care units located in rural, urban, and suburban areas throughout the country. Bed capacity ranges from 150 to 2000. Approximately 20,000 registered nurses are presently employed in the VA system. In addition, over 5,000 licensed practical nurses and over 25,000 nursing assistants play a large part in the nursing care of the nation's veterans. Positions in nursing education, administration, research, nurse practitioner roles and general staff nursing are available. Nearly half of the hospitals are affiliated with medical and nursing schools. Licensure in any state qualifies the applicant to obtain placement in a VA hospital located elsewhere in the country. No civil service examination is required. The primary function of the Veterans Administration Nursing Service is the rendering of nursing care to veterans, male and female; a variety of medical diagnoses is present. The VA hospitals provide continuing education programs for staff development and tuition reimbursement for academic courses. The Veterans Administration is the nation's largest hospital system.

Military Nursing

As a Navy nurse, it is possible to practice in pediatrics, obstetrics, or gynecology. Opportunities are available for advanced educational preparation which

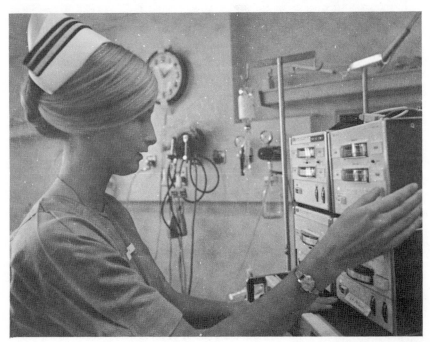

Fig. 20-4 Navy nurse monitoring care

may lead to teaching positions in the Corps School or administrative positions in nursing service. The full-time Navy nurse is an officer with all the privileges and status; this includes a thirty-day paid vacation per year and an opportunity for world travel. For more detailed information the Navy Nurse Corps Nursing Division of the Bureau of Medicine and Surgery, Navy Department, Washington, D.C. 20390 should be contacted.

As an Army nurse, full commissioned officer's rank and privileges are enjoyed. The registered nurse with a Bachelor of Science degree in nursing may be placed in a head nurse, teaching, or staff position. Many Army nurses continue advanced study. Licensed practical nurses may enlist as clinical specialists with the Army Medical Service. For information, the Army Nurse Corps, Office of the Surgeon General, U.S. Army, Washington, D.C. 20314 should be contacted.

Air Force nursing may be a full-time career; in the Reserves it may be a part-time career. The scope of positions covers public health, obstetrics, medical-surgical, coronary care, psychiatry, orthopedics, anesthesia, operating room, midwifery, and pediatric practitioner. Educational opportunities are available for many with steady promotions. Full-time nurses live in modern facilities and have a thirty-day annual paid vacation. Part-time reservists spend one weekend per month plus fifteen days per year on active duty. As an Air Force officer, duty assignments include world travel. For information, the Air Force Nurse Corps, Office of the Surgeon General, Headquarters USAF/SGN, Washington, D.C. 20314 should be contacted.

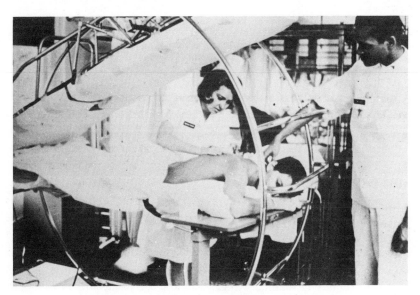

Fig. 20-5 An Army nurse operating a CircOlectric bed

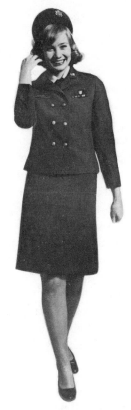

Fig. 20-6 The Air Force nurse in dress uniform

Aerospace Opportunities

Aerospace research has openings for nurses interested in research. An understanding of the physiological and psychological responses in extraterrestial environments is a necessity. Advanced preparation in the behavioral sciences is desirable. Nursing techniques must be adapted to changes brought about by changes in the environment. Adventurous nurses would find this field most interesting and challenging.

Peace Corps/VISTA (ACTION)

A variety of nursing functions are routinely performed by the nurses serving as Peace Corps volunteers in remote areas of the world. In the sparsely populated bush country in southern Africa, the nurse spends much time visiting the patients in their own homes. A primary task is the innoculation of children.

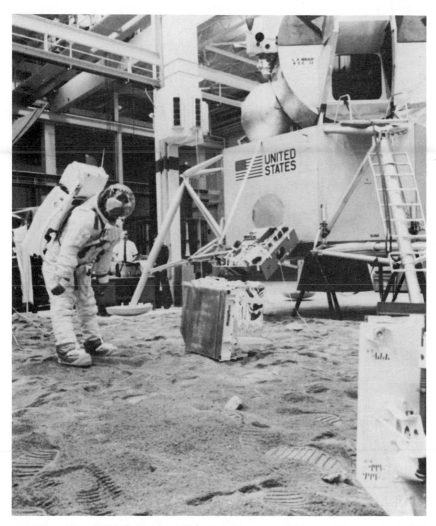

Fig. 20-7 Nursing positions are available in aerospace research to follow up physiological and psychological responses.

Teaching hygiene and nutrition to the villagers is a vital part of the daily routine. Maternal and child health clinics are often staffed by nonnursing personnel, with a nurse in charge. In areas where nursing education programs have been developed, there are teaching positions available. Many diseases rarely seen in the United States are frequent causes of death and disability in other countries. Malaria, tuberculosis, leprosy, malnutrition, and parasitic diseases require skilled care. Over fifty countries seek nurses through the Peace Corps. Graduate experience in a specialty area is highly desirable. The ability to organize working

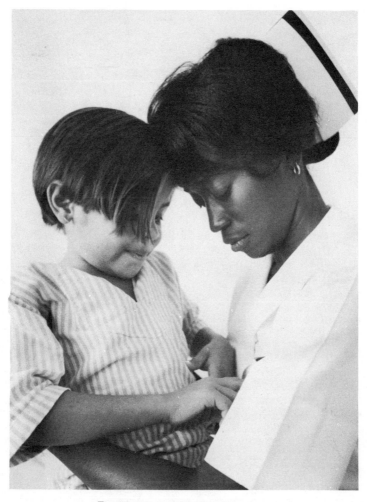

Fig. 20-8 Peace Corps Volunteer nurse

areas, supervise health care workers, and teach hygiene and health standards are requisites.

VISTA nurses serve the poor in the United States, Puerto Rico, and the Virgin Islands, They work and live in ghettos, rural communities, migrant labor camps, and on Indian reservations. In many areas, the people have never before visited a physician or dentist. The work is hard and challenging. The nurse must be able to cope with frustrations, work under adverse conditions, and adapt to different cultures and life-styles. For more information contact ACTION/Peace Corps, Office of Citizen Placement, 806 Connecticut Ave., N.W., Washington, D.C. 20525.

Independent Nurse Practitioners

More and more nurses across the country are opening private offices to begin independent practice in the delivery of primary health care. The independent nurse practitioner takes health histories, does physicial examinations, conducts screening tests, gives nursing care to patients in their homes, and assists the patient in the prevention of illness. The nurse who contemplates opening a private practice must be aware of the expenses involved in renting office space, purchasing equipment, and the sometimes slow process of acquiring clients. Unlike the physician, the nurse practitioner is willing to make home

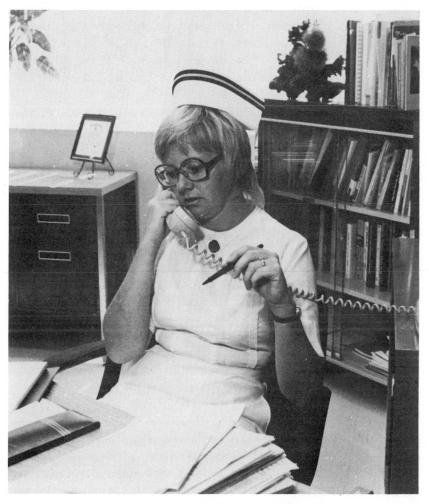

Fig. 20-9 A psychiatric nurse practitioner

visits. Often, the physician will refer patients to the nurse practitioner for follow-up visits or follow-up care at home.

THE APPLICATION PROCEDURE

The problem confronting the majority of graduate nurses is making the decision where to work. Occasionally, a student whose clinical performance has been observed in a cooperating agency, will be contacted and offered employment upon graduation. In this instance, references and the letter of inquiry are often waived. The interview then consists of discussion of salary, personnel policies, and shift assignment. The graduate nurse often accepts the first offer made and fails to thoroughly assess the job. Thoughts of the future are neglected and the gratification of immediate job security suffices. All too frequently, first jobs are unpleasant experiences due to the lack of foresight.

The Resume

Every professional person should prepare a *resume* which clearly states the data which may be of interest to a potential employer. The resume, once started and progressively added to or revised, is a permanent record of education and experience. It should be typewritten on standard white typing bond. Name, current address, phone number, license number, and the state which issued the license must be included. List educational background in reverse chronological order. Give specific dates of attendance and the degree conferred, or courses completed, including the number of credits earned. Working experience is of prime concern as it indicates the specific skills and experiences which were probably acquired. List positions previously held, again in reverse chronological order; list the most recently held position first. Generally, only experiences related to nursing are of interest to employing agencies, although it is appropriate to list community activities. List professional memberships and committee memberships or offices held in professional organizations. Indicate all published articles or unpublished studies or projects. If the nurse has a file with the American Nurses' Association Professional Credential and Personnel Service, it should be indicated under a section on references. Persons in responsible positions willing to attest to the professional abilities and character.of the applicant, are listed as references. Be sure to include addresses of references. The resume will be a valuable tool in attaining a desirable position if it is well written and complete. The resume should accompany the application letter.

The Application Letter

The letter of application is extremely important as it represents the applicant to the employer. The letter should be typewritten on standard white bond. It is advantageous to learn the name and accurate title of the person to whom the letter will be directed. The letter should be brief, in business form, and be void of mistakes (spelling, grammar, or typographical). The purpose for writing should be clear, the position desired should be mentioned, and any restrictions to employment should be given; for example, being unable to rotate shifts or work weekends. Briefly state any previous working experiences, and education. Identify the school from which you graduated, when you graduated, and the name of the director of the nursing program. Suggest two or three references and offer a time when you could be reached by phone to schedule an appointment for an interview.

Generally, an application form will be given or sent to you prior to the interview. This will become part of your permanent file if you are hired. Read questions carefully and answer them thoughtfully and neatly, using black ink whenever possible. Be able to supply the social security and nursing registration numbers.

The Interview

The interview should be structured so as to provide an opportunity for both the prospective employee and employer to adequately evaluate the potential

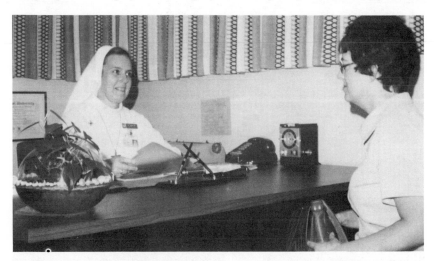

Fig. 20-10 The director of nursing interviews a nurse applying for a beginning staff nurse position.

assets of each. The beginning nurse is understandably insecure, and sometimes frightened, during the first interview.

It is important that the job aspirant honestly appraise both shortcomings and assets. Demanding and expecting too much from an employer is unfair to the employing agency. On the other hand, it is unfair to the individual to underrate capabilities and accept employment conditions not in line with education, experience, and skills. Self-evaluation pertaining to career goals, abilities, interests, temperament, physical endurance, and even religious beliefs concerning moral issues should be conscientiously scrutinized. The nurse who has completed this self-appraisal will be able to communicate her expectations to the interviewer. If the position being sought is not available, the duty hours do not conform to the applicant's preference, or the salary range is not satisfactory, there is no need to pursue an interview.

Once an appointment has been made, the applicant should carefully plan for the meeting. Good grooming is essential. It is advantageous to arrive on time, looking well rested and mentally alert. Clothing should be appropriate for the occasion. The interviewer should be addressed by name. The applicant should offer a handshake and not sit until asked to do so. The interviewer should start the conversation. The applicant should respond briefly, honestly, and with an enthusiastic manner. It is wise to avoid unnecessary and irrelevant

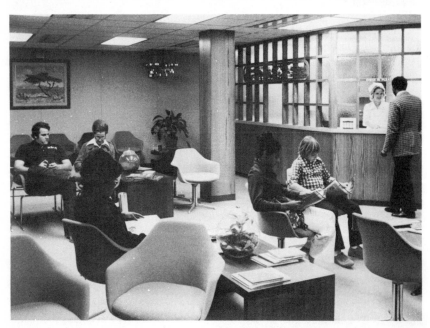

Fig. 20-11 Nursing in a group medical practice

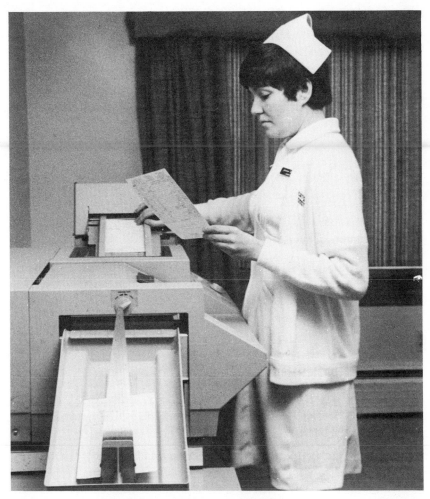

Fig. 20-12 The nurse in data processing

chatter. It is appropriate to request to visit the working area to which you expect to be assigned simply to make an appraisal of the physical environment.

SUMMARY

There are challenging positions available in nursing for new graduates of all nursing programs. The graduate should seek employment which will allow her to achieve her fullest potential, thereby providing job satisfaction. The purpose, philosophy, and goals of the employer must be completely understood and compatible with those of the nurse. Therefore, the graduate nurse must establish goals, assess her interests and aptitudes, and also be aware of any personal responsibilities or conditions which must be considered in selecting a job.

SUGGESTED ACTIVITIES

- Ask the instructor to allot class time for nurse recruiters from several facilities to present current employment opportunities and benefits.

- Role play a job interview session between a personnel director or director of nursing service and a recently graduated nurse.

- Prepare a resume and start a professional file which will be kept updated throughout your nursing career.

- Have nurses from a variety of employment settings present a panel discussion of their roles, experiences, and so forth.

REVIEW

A. Multiple Choice. Select the best answer.

1. The largest employer of nurses is
    a. the Veterans Administration.   c. the military.
    b. community health facilities.   d. cities and states.

2. A summary of professional education and experience is referred to as
    a. a professional portfolio.   c. a letter of application.
    b. a resume.   d. all of these.

3. Officer's rank is given to the registered nurse in
    a. the Navy Nurse Corps.   c. the Air Force Nurse Corps.
    b. the Army Nurse Corps.   d. all of these.

4. The American Nurses' Association service which may be of value to the nurse in procuring employment is
    a. continuing education.
    b. certification.
    c. Department of Special Services.
    d. Professional Credential and Personnel Service.

B. Match the statement in Column II with the job in Column I.

Column I	Column II
1. Private Duty Nursing	a. An opportunity for world travel and health teaching.
2. Camp Nursing	
3. Military Nursing	b. The oldest nursing position.
4. Peace Corps Nursing	c. Officer's rank and privileges.
5. Public Health Nursing	d. A nice summer job.
6. Veterans Administration	e. The largest employer of nurses.
7. School-Health Nurse	f. Health education is the major focus.
8. Industrial Nursing	g. Usually requires a baccalaureate degree.
	h. The opportunity to practice nursing in a large pharmaceutical plant.
	i. Innoculating children in a small Caribbean village.

C. Briefly answer the following questions.

1. List the items that should be included on the resume.

2. List three things you would do in seeking employment in a community health facility.

chapter 21
NEW DIMENSIONS
IN NURSING
EDUCATION

STUDENT OBJECTIVES

- Identify factors which contributed to the new interest in career mobility.
- Explain the concept of open curriculum.
- List the major approaches to an open curriculum system.

In recent years, educators have begun to seriously study curriculum design and content of nursing education. Researchers have found that the most difficult problem facing nursing education and nursing students is the absence of *articulation* (a common or shared bond, interest, or body of knowledge) between the various levels of preparation. This deficiency tends to minimize opportunities for licensed practical and registered nurses who wish to continue their education and advance their career opportunities without great expense and repetition. A number of factors have contributed to a growing pressure on nursing educators and educational facilities to develop programs which facilitate *upward mobility* (increased status and earning power, due to higher educational preparation and credentials). A number of approaches have been developed and the trend is toward nontraditional programs of study.

THE OPEN CURRICULUM

The *open curriculum* is a system which encompasses programs and practices designed to meet the needs and goals of the student. Such designs provide the student with opportunities to enter and leave the system at various levels and also to utilize all past education and experience. Actually, the term *open curriculum* is used by educators synonymously with many new educational approaches such as the career ladder, university without walls, multiple entry and exit, and so forth. The open curriculum is an alternative to the traditional, rigid, nursing education system.

The Manpower Development Training Act provided funding for the establishment and operation of vocational health training programs. The programs were developed to provide opportunities for members of minority groups to develop skills which would upgrade their earning power. These newly trained individuals soon found that it was almost impossible to move on to more highly skilled and better paying jobs, because to do so meant expensive, full-time academic study; also required was the meeting of rigid entrance requirements. Previous experience and training was not recognized. If she desired to enter a basic nursing program, a licensed practical nurse received no credit for her educational program. However, a student in the basic program, after one year of study, could take the state examination for PNs and be licensed as a practical nurse. Highly trained military medics, who returned home after active duty discovered that their education and experience were disregarded by employers and educational facilities. The nurse who graduated from a diploma school found that when application was made to a collegiate nursing program, little or no credit was given for the basic nursing school education. Nurses who graduated from associate degree programs found that all their credits would not transfer to a baccalaureate nursing program. Many people felt thwarted by the inflexibility of the educational system, and pressure began to build. Legislators, who were sensitive to the dissatisfaction of their constituents, brought about passage of legislation which encouraged greater flexibility. Some legislation proved effective while other laws merely added confusion to the inflexibility. Nevertheless, it is obvious that if the educational system does not change, the legislative bodies will change it, for better or for worse.

There is also a trend for increasing enrollment in community colleges and a drop or leveling off in the enrollment of senior colleges and universities. It was found that students preferred the community college because it was close, offered evening and weekend courses, and was less expensive. Therefore, senior colleges and universities have been forced to experiment with new educational approaches in order to attract students.

The National Commission for the Study of Nursing and Nursing Education in its report, *An Abstract for Action* (published in 1970) stated that planning was necessary in order to eliminate obstacles that prevented "the orderly transfer and acceptance of qualified individuals who wish to pursue higher career goals." The report gave recommendations which were synonymous with the open curriculum concept.

Upward mobility was supported by the NLN Board of Directors in 1970. An Open Curriculum Pilot Project Planning Committee was formed in May, 1972. This committee selected fifty-one schools to participate in a pilot project. In 1973 and 1974, the NLN conducted forums on the open curriculum.

THE OPEN CURRICULUM IN NURSING EDUCATION

A Statement Approved by the Board of Directors,
National League for Nursing, February 1976

An open curriculum is one educational approach designed to accommodate the changing career goals and learning needs of students. It facilitates entry into and exit from educational programs by capitalizing on the student's relevant education and experience. The open curriculum in nursing recognizes areas of achievement common to the graduates of various types of educational programs, as well as the value of learning that takes place outside the academic setting. This is one of nursing's responses to the needs of students for more flexibility in entering the nursing education system.

The National League for Nursing supports the open curriculum in nursing education. NLN believes that:

- Individuals who wish to change career goals in nursing or enter nursing from other fields should have the opportunity to do so without unnecessary repetition of course content or clinical experience. In any type of nursing program, opportunity should be provided to students to validate previous learning and to facilitate advanced placement.

- Prospective students should be provided with effective guidance to select the nursing education program best suited to their career goals and to assist them in all stages of their nursing education.

- Schools of nursing should be supported in their efforts to experiment with innovative patterns in nursing education, including open curriculum concepts. All phases of an open curriculum program must be carefully planned with continual and follow-up evaluation as an integral part of the program's accountability to society. Open curriculum programs also need assurance of continuing financial support and of academic and community resources.

- Faculty in open curriculum programs are encouraged to carefully develop curriculum designs that meet NLN's criteria for accreditation. League accreditation is based on a nursing program's meeting the specified criteria of an appropriate NLN education council, on the "general excellence" of the program, and on the program's ". . . achievement with regard to its stated objectives."[1]

NLN will continue to provide a forum for nursing schools interested in the development of educational innovations, including the open curriculum concept. This policy reflects the League's continuing commitment to assist nursing education in meeting society's needs.

[1] *Policies and Procedures of Accreditation for Programs in Nursing Education*, New York: National League for Nursing, 1976, p.2.

Fig. 21-1 NLN Statement (Courtesy National League for Nursing, 10 Columbus Circle, NY, NY.)

Representatives of the fifty-one schools met to discuss progress and problems in implementing innovative approaches to nursing education. The Division of Research conducted extensive surveys and published the *Directory of Career Mobility Opportunities in Nursing Education.* The Directory includes the NLN position statement on the open curriculum in nursing, the list of schools with career mobility opportunities, and a directory of Boards of Nursing. A brief description of career mobility patterns is given and examinations and other methods of evaluation are explained.

Most state boards of nursing encourage the open curriculum and are available for guidance. Actual program development is the responsibility of the individual program. Experimental programs which were given full approval by the state boards of nursing are in operation; an important factor in the evaluation of such programs is the satisfactory performance of the graduates on the State Board Test Pool Examination for licensure.

In spite of wide support, the open curriculum concept is not without controversy. Many educators charge that articulation is not possible because basic nursing education is not based upon the same body of knowledge acquired by students in a practical nurse program. Others contend that individuals feel pressured to continue their education when they are really not qualified to do so. Many also feel that practices associated with the open curriculum are educationally unsound and that standards of nursing education are being lowered.

---

1. *It's* been done this way for 15 years, why change now!

2. We don't have enough time for *it.*

3. *It's* too different.

4. We don't do *it* that way.

5. *It's* never been done before.

6. *It's* too late now to make changes.

7. *It's* too soon to make changes.

8. We can't stop for *it* now.

9. Let someone else try *it* first.

10. We'll get back to *it* later.

11. They won't like *it.*

12. *It's* impossible.

Fortunately, there are plenty of us who ignore these poor excuses and go ahead and get the job done!

Fig. 21-2 Twelve reasons why "it can't be done"

CAREER MOBILITY PATTERNS IN NURSING EDUCATION

There are several basic patterns or approaches to achieve upward mobility in nursing and there are many variations on each pattern. Advanced placement, independent study, the career ladder, and the external degree are the most talked-about approaches.

Advanced Placement

Advanced placement means that courses generally required by a collegiate program are waived and the student receives credit for them. Generally, advanced placement is done by testing. Examinations are used to assess levels of knowledge in order to grant credit and advanced placement; these are called *challenging examinations.* Standardized tests are most often used, but teacher-made tests are used to cover nursing subjects and reflect the emphasis of an individual program. Some programs evaluate clinical performance in the clinical agency or campus nursing laboratory.

NLN Examinations. Standardized tests from the National League for Nursing cover nursing content. The basic achievement tests from the NLN Evaluation Service for basic medical-surgical nursing, obstetric nursing, nursing of children, basic nutrition, basic pharmacology, anatomy, and physiology are often used. Each faculty must decide the amount of credit to be given for tests passed. Other NLN achievement tests might be used for the admission of aides or orderlies to practical nursing programs, and registered nurses to baccalaureate programs.

College Proficiency Examination Program. The New York State Education Department initiated the College Proficiency Examination Program (CPEP) in 1960. New York recognized the need for licensed practical nurses and registered nurses to apply credit, for previous education and experience, toward an associate or baccalaureate degree. Committees were formed to represent the baccalaureate, associate and diploma nursing programs in New York. Five proficiency examinations in nursing were developed. Each test covers a nursing major and is three hours in length. Each test includes 150 questions. The licensed practical nurse wishing to enroll in an associate degree program may take the Fundamentals of Nursing and Maternal and Child Nursing written examinations. The three baccalaureate level tests are: Medical-Surgical Nursing, Psychiatric-Mental Health Nursing, and Maternal-Child Nursing.

Standards for granting credit for CPE scores vary within institutions. Registered nurses or licensed practical nurses considering advanced placement should check with the university or college of their choice regarding proficiency examination policies. Interest has grown at a rapid rate, indicated by the rapid increase in registration for the examinations. This program greatly facilitates career mobility for nurses.

Pre-Tests. Highly qualified nursing educators from the Yale School of Nursing, Cornell School of Nursing, and the Waterbury Medical Center have written, reviewed, and edited a series of test items comprising Pre-Tests for the National Standardized State Nursing Boards and Practical Nurse Licensure examinations. The Pre-Test packages have been published by Pre-Test Service, Inc., in Hamden, Connecticut for group testing programs or individual self-help study. Many schools utilize the materials as challenge exams for advanced placement purposes.

Independent Study

Independent study refers to an approach which permits each student to learn and progress at his own rate. It also gives the student the opportunity to study or take courses particularly needed to continue in a program or to move into another program. The approach allows for rapid movement; the student can quickly complete individual courses. It also allows the slow learner, or student with language handicaps, to work at a slower pace. Such a program requires facilities and faculty which can help students to work at their own pace. Some course work may be structured; at other times it might be independent study or a student-teacher discussion. Therefore, great flexibility is necessary on the part of both student and teachers, if the program is to be a success.

Hospitals and schools, such as the Michael Reese Hospital School of Nursing in Chicago, Illinois, have developed a special program to prepare applicants who are seeking admission to a professional school of nursing. This type of program, called an *enrichment studies* program, attempts to meet the needs of persons who are academically competent but are deficient in some of the admission criteria. Each participant must have fulfilled the general admission requirements of the particular school sponsoring the enrichment studies program. The emphasis of this type of program is on individualized instruction, which is planned to assist the student in developing study skills necessary for success in the nursing program. Curriculum content includes classes in language arts, mathematics, scientific concepts, speech, and communication skills. The courses are usually eight-week summer sessions. Financial assistance is available.

The Career Ladder

Career ladder is an approach which focuses on the articulation of educational programs. This permits advancement without repetition or loss of credit.

There are many variations currently in existence. It is the approach most often used in the open curriculum system.

Multiple Entry and Exit Pattern. Multiple-exit programs provide opportunities for students to leave at designated points in the program. They have the opportunity to receive a certificate as a nursing assistant or orderly, prepared for local employment; or a practical nursing certificate with eligibility to write the state licensure examination for practical nurses. Variations in this system exist within schools. For example, a program may offer any one of the following, with termination at the completion of the program.

- Aide to practical nurse to registered nurse model.

- Licensed practical nurse to registered nurse at the associate degree level.

- Licensed practical nurse to registered nurse at the associate, baccalaureate, master, or doctoral levels.

This is referred to as core curriculum, or a spin-off system at the basic nursing education level. There is an articulated curriculum from the lower division levels to the senior or upper division levels and on through graduate programs if desired.

Core Curriculum. Many professional schools have attempted to define a core curriculum for the health sciences; it is based on the assumption that there is knowledge basic to all health education programs, as well as alternatives or specialties specific to one profession. This concept is applicable to the nursing profession, with its varying levels of education and variety of practitioner roles. It is the hope of progressive educators that effective articulation will result from the studies and research on new approaches to nursing education.

The core curriculum approach seems the most logical in institutions which offer basic nursing education programs for practical nurses and registered nurses. Most nursing tasks are performed by both groups and there is knowledge common to both programs. Common learning needs can be identified and incorporated in broad subject areas. Surveys show, however, that few programs utilize a core curricular approach.

Some community colleges offer a core of educational experiences for related health occupational programs. The first semester is a comprehensive core program which meets the basic educational requirements of all students. Nursing programs in the community colleges could benefit both the institution and the student by instituting a core curriculum. Educational costs could be lowered, faculty assignment could be improved, and indecisive or inadequately screened students could be counseled into the career best suited for them.

Programs leading to state licensure may have problems due to the rigid rules and regulations of accrediting bodies.

Core Courses. Nursing core courses should be developed to provide vertical and horizontal career mobility. There should be progressive and increasing depth and breadth of content and learning. The beginning or basic nursing knowledge, processes, and skills are offered to all nursing levels: the nursing assistant or orderly, the practical nurse, and the registered nurse. The second core area includes theories, research, and application of principles for patient care through a problem-solving approach. In the third core area, emphasis is placed on the community health care needs in relation to socioeconomic and political influences. The fourth core area provides opportunities for intensive clinical experiences, in which students may: (1) develop nursing care plans, (2) practice leadership skills, and (3) apply theory and research in the assessment of current issues and problems.

Community College Articulation. The number of basic nursing education programs within the setting of community colleges is rapidly increasing. Although the setting is ideal for the implementation of the core curriculum, it is unrealistic to presume that all colleges will eventually adopt a common core program. The ideal community college program would provide common core courses with termination options at three career levels: nurse assistant, licensed practical nurse, and registered nurse. Some experimental programs provide easy transfer into the third year of the baccalaureate program at a senior college. Students terminating at the end of the first year qualify for the practical nurse licensing examination, and students completing two years of the program qualify for the registered nurse licensing examinations. In such programs, identifiable components are transferable and the first year forms the base upon which the second year is further developed. Competencies are defined clearly for each level and expected skill achievement for the licensed practical nurse and associate degree graduates are clearly delineated.

External Degrees

The *external degree program* is one which gives credit for an individual's knowledge, regardless of when or how that knowledge was acquired. To be eligible for a degree, the individual only has to meet the requirements of the program. The external degree program is a means by which a degree-granting institution enables students to learn without the rigid rules and regulations of traditional academia. During the decade of the sixties, many college students protested against traditional requirements which seemed to lack relevancy to the social problems of the time. Some college campuses experienced the burning of buildings; administrators were held as hostages; severe property destruction took place; and even human deaths resulted. Because of these protests, some required courses were either dropped or changed; new courses were added to the curriculum. New areas of interest emerged in courses such as black studies, urban studies, and the psychology of women. Such changes laid the groundwork for the development of the external degree program.

Some of the major advantages of external degree programs are:

- The student assists in the development and planning of a personalized learning experience.
- Community resources are better utilized.
- Tuition rates are lower.

Credits are granted for work experience and knowledge gained outside the degree-granting institution. This is done in a variety of ways: (1) credit is allotted for personal life experiences, (2) transfer credit is given for courses taken and completed satisfactorily at another college, (3) credit is granted based on various testing programs such as passing proficiency examinations to the satisfaction of the specific institution.

The University of the State of New York presented the Regents External Degree Program for nurses at a meeting of the Council of Associate Degree Programs in 1973. It was established under the leadership of Dr. Dolores Wozniak, consultant for the Regents External Degrees in Nursing program. The New York State Commissioner, Dr. Ewald B. Nyquist, presented the plan to grant a Regents Associate in Applied Science Degree in Nursing. All candidates must pass specific college-level tests and performance examinations in two components: general education and nursing. Upon receipt of the degree, the individual is entitled to take New York's registered nurse licensing examination; namely, the same State Board examinations.

This external degree program eliminates unnecessary repetition of courses. Time and expenses incurred in moving upward in nursing can be kept to a minimum. The estimated cost of obtaining the degree was approximately $700.00. A faculty committee composed of eighteen members representing all levels of nursing education programs developed the guidelines of the program; no one particular curricular design was followed. Each participant is expected to maintain the competency of a graduate from an associate degree program in New York State. A copy of the nursing degree requirements may be obtained by writing to Regents External Degree, 99 Washington Avenue, Albany, N.Y. 12210.

In 1975, Carrie B. Lenburg, coordinator of the program, announced that the first two groups of Regents External Degree nursing graduates who took the State Board Test Pool Examination for licensure as registered nurses achieved significantly higher scores than graduates of traditional nursing programs. The scores demonstrated that individuals can learn in many ways and that quality education can be provided with such a nontraditional approach. Follow-up studies are being conducted to evaluate the work performance of the graduates. Preliminary findings indicated that the graduates performed as well as or better than graduates of traditional associate degree programs.

University Without Walls

The *university without walls* approach is a baccalaureate nursing program which permits a registered nurse to take courses in a local college in lieu of taking the course on the campus of the university conferring the degree. Most baccalaureate programs are geared for the basic nursing student and do not meet the specific needs of a diploma school graduate. In this type of program, courses are offered which allow a greater degree of flexibility. Past educational and work experiences form the basis for an individualized program. Generally, a student is assigned to an on-campus adviser and an off-campus adviser; both guide the learning activities. Learning opportunities are provided by community agencies in areas of specific interest to the student. Participation in institutes in other cities may be accepted. The traditional grading system and recording of credit hours is not utilized. A file is kept by the individual participant on all activities and is received and reviewed by an advisory board at regular intervals. When the program is satisfactorily completed, a bachelor of arts degree is awarded.

University without walls (UWW) programs are accredited by regional accreditation associations or the accrediting agency for the Union for Experimenting Colleges and Universities. If the program meets accreditation standards, it is supported by a grant from the U.S. Office of Education and the Ford Foundation. Advantages to this type of program are the flexibility of the curriculum; less time usually required to obtain the baccalaureate degree; ability to remain employed full-time while working on the degree; opportunity to apply newly acquired knowledge to specific employment; and the elimination of regular travel to and from a campus. Michigan State University School of Nursing is a pioneer in the establishment of an extension program which enables registered nurses to complete the baccalaureate degree requirements without the traditional residency requirement. Skidmore College in Saratoga Springs, New York also has a popular UWW program.

INNOVATIONS IN TEACHING TOOLS AND METHODS

Many of the nontraditional approaches to nursing education require the development of tools and methods which facilitate learning in the very flexible open curriculum programs. Learning laboratories, clinical laboratories, audiovisual materials, and printed supplemental materials may be necessary to provide individualized programs of study. Many new materials have been developed specifically for use in open curriculum programs.

Learning Experience Guides

Learning Experience Guides (LEGS) for nursing students, is a multimedia system designed by nursing instructors with expertise as nurse educators and consultants. The codevelopers of the LEGS Self-Instructional Package are Anne Roe and Mary Sherwood. The flexible curriculum is designed to assist the student in the attainment of specific behavioral objectives. Self-tests enable the student to conduct self-evaluation.

Learning Experience Guides provides for individualized nursing instruction and effective utilization of time and effort for faculty and students. The learning modules are kept in loose-leaf volumes which are updated as necessary. Faculty may adapt LEGS to meet specific program needs by simply adding supplemental materials of their own design. Slides, cassettes, films and games are available to students in all types of nursing education programs. LEGS is presented in four volumes and covers all areas of an associate degree nursing program curricula.

Multimedia Materials

Innovative teaching techniques include wise selection and utilization of multimedia materials in the curriculum. The faculty is responsible for insuring the use of quality materials to enhance learning. Often, the operational budget hampers the selection process. Not only should faculty preview, review, and evaluate materials but students should also be represented on the team.

The audio-cassette is the most commonly used audio medium. Audio-cassettes may be used as lectures for enrichment purposes; tutorial exercises to clarify faculty presentations; and as self-instructional study aids. Documentary films are useful during regularly scheduled class periods when laboratory practice is limited or nonexistent; or they may be used for a dramatic presentation of content material. Film loops provide simulation of basic conceptual materials and are often useful in independent study. The use of mass media such as television, radio, and the newspaper will enrich the educational experience.

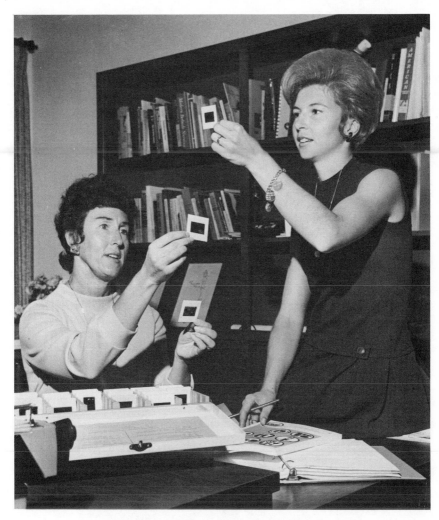

Fig. 21-3 Nursing educators review a multimedia system, LEGS.

Tests can be very useful as study tools. Some faculty members have constructed series of tests which are corrected by a computer, thereby providing results almost immediately. This type of learning activity is termed Computer-Managed Instruction (CMI). Some computers are programmed to suggest remedial references, learning activities to correct wrong answers, and also to maintain progress records of individual student achievement. Computer-Assisted Instruction (CAI) is a process by which interaction takes place between the student and the computer and the information is relative to specific content areas.

SUMMARY

In the past, nursing students have been the victims of a poorly articulated system of education. Opportunities for career advancement were limited. To be truly effective, the educational process should be flexible and responsive to individual needs of students, no matter what the terminal goal might be. The educational system should be designed so that educational standards are not compromised. Students should be able to move through the system without repetition or loss of credit. Changing career goals should be accommodated by the system. The material presented in this unit is not all-inclusive and is no doubt being continually expanded and improved upon as more current social and economic pressures influence community planning and educational needs. These educational concepts merely offer some insight into a few of the innovative, progressive, and nontraditional approaches to nursing education.

SUGGESTED ACTIVITIES

- Have members of the class with prior educational preparation in military corps schools or other allied health fields discuss similarities in course content and clinical experiences.

- Organize a panel with a moderator to discuss the open curriculum patterns presented in this chapter. After researching relevant current literature, each panel participant should discuss a pattern and why it is educationally sound.

- Survey six schools offering a core curriculum in basic nursing education and compare core courses.

REVIEW

A. Multiple Choice. Select the best answer.

1. The enrollment in higher education programs continues to increase except in
    a. the western part of the United States.
    b. associate degree programs.
    c. senior colleges and universities.
    d. open curriculum programs.

2. The amount of credit to be given for successful completion of standardized tests for advanced placement is
    a. the same in all accredited schools of nursing.
    b. determined by the National League for Nursing.
    c. determined by the state board of nursing.
    d. determined by the faculty of each school.

3. Ideally, community college nursing programs would provide common core courses with options for termination at
   a. three levels.
   b. nursing assistant, licensed practical nurse, and registered nurse levels.
   c. levels which offer three career opportunities.
   d. all the above.

4. Open curriculum programs are approved by the state board for nursing on the basis of
   a. the grants received for support of the program.
   b. the performance of graduates on State Board Test Pool Examination.
   c. accreditation visits twice a year.
   d. reports made by the institution sponsoring the program.

5. The most common method of obtaining credit for advanced placement is by
   a. challenging exams.
   b. tests from NLN Evaluation Service.
   c. College Proficiency Examinations.
   d. all the above.

6. The multimedia four-volume system of learning modules with self-evaluation tests is called
   a. Computer-Managed Instruction.   c. LEGS.
   b. Computer-Assisted Instruction.   d. enrichment studies.

7. Interest in a more flexible educational system developed because
   a. many health care workers did not have upward career mobility.
   b. legislation was passed, forcing schools to give credit for all previous education.
   c. institutions of higher learning found experimental programs very successful.
   d. all the above.

8. The career ladder approach provides for
   a. credit given for all previous education, regardless of where or when it was acquired.
   b. single entry and exit.
   c. articulation between components.
   d. independent study and paced learning.

9. The core curriculum approach is most appropriate
   a. in institutions with both practical nursing and associate degree programs in nursing.
   b. in baccalaureate nursing programs.
   c. for diploma school graduates.
   d. b and c.

10. University Without Walls programs are
    a. accredited by the NLN.
    b. funded by a grant, if accredited.
    c. conferring only associate degree in nursing.
    d. designed particularly for licensed practical nurses.

B.   Briefly answer the following questions.

1. Define open curriculum.

2. List five major approaches to the open curriculum system.

chapter 22
SCHOLARSHIPS,
FELLOWSHIPS,
GRANTS AND LOANS

STUDENT OBJECTIVES

- Identify financial resources available for students who wish to pursue basic and graduate nursing education.
- Describe the various kinds of financial assistance available.
- Identify sources for information regarding financial assistance.

Nursing students and potential students of nursing should be aware of possible sources of financial assistance. Occasionally, financial problems arise after the student has begun a program of studies. The faculty has an obligation to inform students of local, state, and federal resources available. Students should be aware of the various kinds of assistance available and generally where monies are available. No qualified candidate for a career in nursing should be kept from seeking such a goal due to lack of money. Nurses wishing to continue their education or to carry out research also have available to them a number of sources of financial aid.

TYPES OF FINANCIAL ASSISTANCE

In addition to many sources of financial assistance for nursing education, there are several types of assistance available. In order to find financial assistance, the individual must know his particular need and the type of financial aid which would be most appropriate. Basically, assistance falls into three categories: loans, scholarships, and grants. Students obtaining professional education may also obtain fellowships and traineeships.

Loans

A *loan* usually refers to money provided temporarily for the borrower's use. In other words, the money which is borrowed must be paid back to the lender. In most cases, the borrower pays a fee (in the form of interest) to the lender for the opportunity to borrow the money. In some cases, an educational loan may be interest free; generally there is an interest, but at a reduced rate. Oftentimes, the loan does not have to be repaid until the education is obtained and the graduate has started to work. Educational loans can be obtained from banks, businesses (credit unions, insurance companies, educational associations), schools, alumnae associations, and state and federal agencies.

Scholarships

A *scholarship* is usually a gift of money. A scholarship is often a recognition of academic excellence although some scholarships are given on the basis of demonstrated need. Many associations, organizations, and foundations provide scholarships to high school graduates, nursing students, and practicing nurses. The size of the scholarship may vary from a twenty-dollar book scholarship to one which will pay all expenses for the entire education. Scholarships are also available to veterans and their dependents. State and federal agencies also award individual scholarships. Most nursing schools have some kind of scholarship award for students in financial need.

Grants

A *grant* may be a gift, or it may be money given with certain conditions. Grants are awarded to individuals and institutions. Generally, a grant is given to fund a particular project. The individuals receiving the grant money have the responsibility to fulfill the conditions under which the grant was awarded. Students may receive state or federal grants to allow them to complete their nursing education. Associations, foundations, and industries award grants for research.

Fellowships

A *fellowship* usually refers to the appointment of an individual to a position which grants a *stipend* (fixed sum paid at regular intervals). A fellowship is usually associated with graduate, doctoral, or postdoctoral study or research. Fellowships may also be given to cover the expenses of advanced study which may be pursued abroad.

Traineeships

Traineeships usually are monies given to cover the cost of the specific training or education of individuals. Sometimes stipends are provided to cover living expenses. Traineeships are often awarded to universities or colleges. They have the authority to establish the requirements which must be met by individuals who wish to receive a traineeship.

PROFESSIONAL NURSING ORGANIZATIONS

A major goal of professional nursing associations is the promotion of quality nursing care. The establishment of funds in the form of grants, scholarships, or loans to enable capable nurses to gain competency in a special field of nursing helps to assure well-educated nurses who can provide leadership and quality patient care.

Nurses' Educational Funds, Inc.

Nurses' Educational Funds, Inc. (NEF) began with the establishment of two memorial funds in honor of early nursing leaders. The two memorial funds starting the concept of NEF were in honor of Isabel Hampton Robb in 1910 and Isabel McIsaac in 1914. Later, alumni from Teachers College, Columbia University nursing education program became the third group to provide financial aid to nurses through NEF. These three funds became known as Nurses' Educational Funds, Inc. in 1954. That same year, the National League for Nursing offered clerical assistance and administrative consultation to the board members of NEF. The American Journal of Nursing Company assumed the administrative responsibilities for NEF in 1973. However, since the NEF board establishes its own policy and criteria for the granting of awards and fund handling, it remains a separate entity. Since 1957, scholarship funds have been received from large business and publishing companies. Prior to that time, contributions were small and made individually. Today NEF provides financial support through scholarship grants for advanced study in nursing. As of 1974, over half a million dollars in scholarship funds were shared by 564 nurses.

Criteria for receiving an award include licensure as a registered nurse, membership in the American Nurses' Association, references, academic achievement and potential contribution to nursing. For more detailed information, write Nurses' Educational Funds, Inc., 10 Columbus Circle, New York, N.Y. 10019. A complete list of donors and recipients is published in *Nursing Outlook*.

American Nurses' Foundation Grant Program

The purpose of the American Nurses' Foundation (ANF) is the promotion of nursing research through financial support of research and by dissemination of the research findings. American Nurses' Foundation publications include: *International Directory of Nurses With Doctorates; ANF Newsletter; Nursing Research Report; Content and Dynamics of Home Visits of Public Health Nurses* Part I and II; *Role of the Nurse in the Outpatient Department;* and *How to Search the Literature.* Abstracts of studies are entered in *Nursing Research* magazine.

Applicants for ANF grants must indicate the role of the nurse or nurses in the project proposed, and submit details of the research methodology and statistical design. Nurses who wish to be considered should submit the research design and a letter to the ANF Director, 2420 Pershing Road, Kansas City, Missouri 64108.

Fellowships through ICN and ANA

The International Council of Nurses awards a $6,000 fellowship annually. From state nurses association nominees, the American Nurses' Association selects a candidate to receive the fellowship, which is sponsored by the Minnesota Mining and Manufacturing Company, for postbasic nursing studies. Two male nurses received the 1975 fellowships; this was the first time two awards were given in one year. Applications may be obtained by writing the Department of Nursing Education, ANA headquarters.

In late spring of 1975, the first ten fellows were selected for the ANA Registered Nurse Fellowship Program for Ethnic/Racial Minority Groups. This program is scheduled for a six-year period. Each fellow selected is expected to complete a doctorate degree in mental health and/or related areas from an accredited institution. The fellow must work in the areas of mental health or social and behavioral science in ethnic/racial minority communities. Applicants include nurses from Afro-American, Asian American, Native American and Spanish-surnamed ethnic minority groups. The ANA fellowship program has been funded for a total of $955,407 by the National Institute of Mental Health, Department of Health, Education, and Welfare. Each nurse-fellow is eligible for an annual award of up to $7,500 for a period of three years.

Sigma Theta Tau Honor Society

Sigma Theta Tau promotes nursing research through research grants. Nursing's honor society has been awarding grants for research since 1965. Over $61,000 has been distributed to fifty-two individual projects. Grant proposals should be submitted to Sigma Theta Tau, 1100 West Michigan Street, Indianapolis, IN 46202.

The National Student Nurses' Association

The National Student Nurses' Association (NSNA) awarded scholarships in 1974 to candidates evaluated on the basis of demonstrated academic excellence, community involvement, and financial need. These were sponsored through the Breakthrough to Nursing minority group recruitment project. Each recipient receives a $2,000 award sponsored jointly by the Brown Shoe Company and NSNA. Black, Spanish, and American-Indian minority groups are invited to submit an application for consideration.

In 1974, the Brown Shoe Scholarship Program awarded ten scholarships to students enrolled in basic nursing programs. Schools of nursing were asked to nominate one student on the basis of contribution to the nursing profession, local and national health related activities, academic achievement, and economic need.

STATE AND FEDERAL AID

Financial aid for students who demonstrate need may be obtained through state and federally funded financial assistance programs such as the Basic Educational Opportunity Grant, Supplemental Educational Opportunity Grant, Veterans Scholarships, National Direct Student Loan Program (NDSL), College Work-Study Program (CWS), and the Nursing Student Loan Program.

Basic Educational Opportunity Grant Program

The Basic Educational Opportunity Grant Program (BEOG) is a federal program for beginning college students who demonstrate a need for financial assistance. The federal government grants up to $1,400 to full-time students who qualify. Only high school seniors and persons entering college for the first time are considered eligible.

Supplemental Educational Opportunity Grant Program

Students from low-income families may apply for grants under the SEOG program. Awards ranging from $200 to $1,500 in an academic year may be given. The award may be cumulative for a maximum of eight semesters or its equivalence and is limited to $4,000 for four years. Half-time students are eligible.

Nursing Student Scholarship and Loan Programs

Students who are enrolled in nursing programs and exhibit exceptional financial need may qualify for a grant of up to $1,500 a year. Loans up to $2,500 are available under the Nursing Student Loan Program. Three percent a year interest is paid by the federal government. Repayment of the loan must begin no later than nine months after ceasing to be a full-time student and must be paid in full within ten years. Part or all of the loan may be cancelled if the student becomes employed in areas where a nurse shortage exists.

General Education Assistance

Under the Guaranteed Loan Program of the Higher Education Act of 1965, students attending colleges, universities, and schools of nursing may borrow money each academic year through private loans, which will be guaranteed by state or federal agencies. Loans may be obtained from local banks and are paid back in installments over a five to ten year period. There are also work-study loans which provide the student with a job fifteen hours a week while carrying a full-time academic load, or forty hours a week on holidays or during the summer. The job pays as much or more than the minimum wage and is usually associated with the college or university. Information about work-study loans or the guaranteed student loan program can be obtained from the Bureau of Higher Education, U.S. Office of Education Financial Aid Programs, U.S. Office of Health Education, and Welfare, Washington, D.C. 20202.

FINANCIAL AID FOR PRACTICAL NURSES

Practical nursing students may receive scholarships awarded by the National Licensed Practical Nurses Educational Foundation. Scholarships are awarded twice annually. Announcements of recipients are made on June 1 and December 1. The deadline for applications for the June 1 scholarship is April 15. Deadline for applications for the December 1 scholarships is October 15. Applicants for scholarships must show financial need, academic competence, and satisfactory character references.

Acceptance for enrollment into an approved school of practical nursing must be confirmed by the director of the program to which the applicant has applied. Applications are carefully studied and evaluated by the Awards

Committee. The Awards Committee consists of the executive director of the NLPNEF, Inc., two practical nurse educators, two LPNs appointed by the Board of Trustees, the ex-officio president of the National Licensed Practical Nurses Educational Foundation, Inc. A copy of *Rules for Awarding Scholarships* and application forms may be obtained from NAPNES.

SOURCES OF FINANCIAL ASSISTANCE FOR NURSING EDUCATION AND/OR INFORMATION

LOCAL

High school guidance counselor
Service clubs, fraternal organizations, labor unions
Church (or religious denomination at national level)
Veterans Administration
Nursing organizations

STATE

State Department of Education (maintains list of scholarships and loans)
State nursing associations

FEDERAL

Basic Educational Opportunity Grant Award
    Basic Grants, P.O. Box 84, Washington, DC
Division of Nursing, Bureau of Health Manpower, Health Resources Administration
    9000 Rockville Pike, Bethesda, MD 20014
Office of Guaranteed Student Loans, U.S. Office of Education
    Washington, DC 20202
Bureau of Indian Affairs, Department of the Interior
    P.O. Box 1788, Albuquerque, NM 87103

NATIONAL ORGANIZATIONS

National League for Nursing
    10 Columbus Circle, New York, NY 10019
Hattie M. Strong Foundation
    1625 Eye Street, N.W. #409, Washington, DC 20006
National Licensed Practical Nurses Educational Foundation, Inc.
    250 W. 57th St., New York, NY 10019
United Student Aid Funds, Inc.
    200 E. 42nd St., New York, NY 10022
National Scholarship Service and Fund for Negro Students
    1776 Broadway, New York, NY 10019
United Scholarship Service, Inc.
    P.O. Box 18285, Capitol Hill Station, Denver, CO 80218

FOR BROAD INFORMATION:

Scholarships, Fellowships, Educational Grants and Loans for Registered Nurses,
    Pub. No. 41-408, NLN, 10 Columbus Circle, New York, NY 10019
Scholarships and Loans for Beginning Education in Nursing, Pub. No. 41-410, NLN,
    10 Columbus Circle, New York, NY 10019

Practical/vocational nursing students may participate in the following financial aid programs:

1. National Direct Student Loan.

2. Educational Opportunity Grants.

3. Local Institutional Scholarships.

4. State Scholarships.

5. Basic Educational Opportunity Grants.

SUMMARY

The Nurse Training Act authorizes millions of dollars for nursing through teaching facilities construction grants, financial distress, traineeships, nurse practitioner programs, student loans and scholarships, and capitation grants for basic nursing education programs. Additional federal money is available for general education through the provisions of the Higher Education Act of 1965, and the Basic Educational Opportunity Grant Program. There are local, state, and national organizations which provide financial assistance. Financial assistance may be provided through loans, scholarships, grants, fellowships, and traineeships. Monies are available for high school graduates wishing to enter a basic nursing program; graduate nurses wishing to obtain further nursing education; and nurses who wish to carry out studies and nursing-related research. The first source which should be consulted for information concerning financial assistance is the director of the program the student plans to enter, or the director of the program in which the student is currently enrolled. Additional information can be obtained from the NLN.

SUGGESTED ACTIVITIES

- Interview the Director of Financial Aid in your institution and report to the class on financial aid available for nursing students.

- Trace the history of federal aid for nursing education beginning with the appropriation of the government monies for the Cadet Nurse Corps during World War II.

- Read at least three articles on nursing scholarships, grants, or loans and write a summary for class recitation.

REVIEW

A.   Multiple Choice. Select the best answer.

1.   The names of contributors and recipients of the Nurses' Educational Funds, Inc. award are published in
     a. Nursing Outlook   c. Journal of Practical Nursing.
     b. American Journal of Nursing.   d. The American Nurse.

2.   A financial award for advanced studies in nursing is sponsored by
     a. Altrusa International.   c. The 3 M Company.
     b. The Brown Shoe Company.   d. Church Women United.

3.   The promotion of nursing research through financial support and dissemination of the research findings is the purpose of the
     a. International Council of Nurses.
     b. National Licensed Practical Nurses Educational Foundation, Inc.
     c. Nurses' Educational Funds, Inc.
     d. American Nurses' Foundation Grant Program.

4.   Legislation authorizing millions of dollars for nursing is called the
     a. Federal Scholarship Grant.
     b. Nurse Training Act.
     c. Nurse Practice Act.
     d. Nursing Student Assistance Program.

B.   Match the following items in Column II to the correct statement in Column I.

Column I	Column II
1. Federal program which provides financial aid to students enrolled in nursing programs who have exceptional financial need.	a. Basic Educational Opportunity Grant
2. Federal program for beginning college students who have need for financial assistance.	b. National Licensed Practical Nurses Educational Foundation, Inc.
3. Federal program for financial aid for students from low-income families.	c. Nurses' Educational Funds, Inc.
4. Provides scholarships for practical nurses.	d. Nursing Student Scholarship and Loan Program
5. Provides scholarship grants for advanced study in nursing.	e. Supplementary Opportunity Grants Program

C.   Briefly answer the following questions.

   1. Name the two nursing leaders honored by memorial funds through the Nurses' Educational Funds, Inc.

   2. List three ethnic minority groups eligible for a fellowship from the American Nurses' Association Fellowship Program funded by the National Institute of Mental Health.

   3. What are the four categories used as a basis for the Brown Shoe Scholarship for basic nursing students?

   4. Name three programs offering financial assistance to practical nursing students.

chapter 23
PROFESSIONAL
LITERATURE

STUDENT OBJECTIVES

- Identify sources of professional literature.
- Explain the general content of various nursing periodicals.
- Identify resources in locating specific articles in nursing periodicals.

Most often, the student nurse is oriented to periodical literature through a course bibliography. An instructor researches the literature and lists specific articles which are relevant to the lesson plan. However, the student must learn to utilize reference material. As a graduate, the ability to locate specific information is an absolute necessity. A professional person never stops learning. Education does not stop on graduation day. Excellence in practice requires a continuous quest for further knowledge. Self-discipline is an asset in developing a self-study enrichment program by regularly reading professional literature.

Periodical literature refers to publications which are published at regular intervals. *Professional literature* refers to articles in professional magazines or journals. Such articles usually contain new concepts, approaches, professional positions on current issues, reports of studies, and so forth. This literature, collectively, is the growing body of knowledge; a professional person has the responsibility to keep abreast of new concepts and trends.

There are many nursing periodicals published at the national and international level. In this chapter, the content of a selection of periodicals will be briefly summarized. This does not infer lack of circulation or quality of other nursing periodicals not mentioned; it would be impossible to include descriptions of all the professional journals in one chapter.

THE AMERICAN JOURNAL OF NURSING

As the official publication of the American Nurses' Association, the *American Journal of Nursing* is a widely read, monthly, professional nursing periodical. Articles represent a variety of pertinent subjects which are of interest to all members of the nursing profession. Students can supplement and enhance course content by reading relevant articles from past and current issues. Special features of the AJN are the Test Yourself page, a column on money management principles for nurses, and a programmed instruction unit which is an invaluable self-learning aid.

Reprints of articles may be ordered in unlimited quantities in accord with a current price schedule. The minimum order, however, is twenty-five reprints of any one article. Order reprints from the Educational Services Division of the American Journal of Nursing Company, 10 Columbus Circle, New York, N.Y. 10019.

THE AMERICAN JOURNAL OF MATERNAL-CHILD NURSING

The American Journal of Nursing Company publishes *MCN,* which is designed for nurses interested in all aspects of maternal-child health. *MCN*'s goal is to assist the practicing nurse in giving high quality care to individuals and families during phases of childbearing and childrearing. Published six times a year, *MCN* is a valuable reference on this specialty in nursing.

NURSING OUTLOOK

Nursing Outlook, the official magazine of the National League for Nursing, is published monthly. Articles correlate well with nursing curricula at all levels.

Subscriptions are available through the National League for Nursing, 10 Columbus Circle, New York, N.Y. 10019. A substantial subscription discount is given to individual members of the NLN. Reprints of articles may be ordered through the American Journal of Nursing Company.

NURSING RESEARCH

Nursing Research, a cosponsored publication of the American Nurses' Association and the National League for Nursing, is issued bimonthly by the American Journal of Nursing Company. Nursing research and findings constitute the majority of articles. Reprints of articles are available through the American Journal of Nursing Company.

In 1970, when it became apparent that current issues and trends could be disseminated in a more concise and economical manner, the American Journal of Nursing Company decided to publish the *Contemporary Nursing Series.* The soft-covered book consists of reprints of selected articles from the *AJN, Nursing Outlook* and *Nursing Research.*

OCCUPATIONAL HEALTH NURSING

The *Occupational Health Nursing* journal is the official publication of the American Association of Industrial Nurses, Inc. It contains information pertinent to occupational health nursing which meets the needs of the industrial nurse practitioner. The journal may be ordered from Charles B. Slack, Inc., 6900 Grove Road, Thorofare, New Jersey 08086.

JOURNAL OF ALLIED HEALTH

The American Society of Allied Health Professions publication is the *Journal of Allied Health.* The main purpose of this journal is to provide recent data on research and developments in allied health education and practice. All of the major allied health occupations are represented; reference to historical backgrounds is also included. The Journal is issued quarterly and may be ordered from Charles B. Slack, Inc., 6900 Grove Road, Thorofare, New Jersey 08086.

THE JOURNAL OF PSYCHIATRIC NURSING
AND MENTAL HEALTH SERVICES

This publication is designed for nursing personnel involved in all aspects of psychiatric nursing. Articles are presented that will assist nurses in understanding the emotional patterns and mental capacities of their patients. The Journal is published six times per year and may be ordered from Charles B. Slack, Inc., 6900 Grove Road, Thorofare, New Jersey 08086.

THE JOURNAL OF OBSTETRIC, GYNECOLOGIC
AND NEONATAL NURSING

The *JOGN* is the official journal of the Nurses' Association of the American College of Obstetricians and Gynecologists. The purpose of this publication is to disseminate information relevant to maternal-child health nursing. Included are research articles which provide an avenue for the exchange of innovative concepts, new techniques and theories. Members of the Nurses' Association of the American College of Obstetricians and Gynecologists receive the journal as part of their annual membership dues. Nonmembers may order from Harper and Row Publishers, Inc., 2350 Virginia Ave., Hagerstown, Maryland 21740.

GERONTOLOGICAL NURSING

Gerontological Nursing is aimed at helping nurses meet the needs of the aged members of society. All nursing personnel are involved in caring for the elderly, which form a great part of the population. Care of the aged has increased at a result of political and social awareness of their needs. It is imperative that knowledge of community resources and the needs of the elderly patient be available to all. Current governmental policies concerning the provision of health care and nursing care for the elderly are explored in this publication. The publisher is Charles B. Slack, Inc., 6900 Grove Road, Thorofare, New Jersey 08086.

NURSING '76*

This journal provides practical information relevant to the personal and professional needs of nurses. Articles deal with the nurse-patient relationship and clincial nursing. The text is presented in a concise, easy to understand format, and is well illustrated. Created specifically for nurses and guided by eminently qualified nursing editors, each monthly issue highlights specific detailed instructions for a new clinical procedure. Problem-solving techniques are emphasized. Subscribers may obtain, at no cost, answers to personal questions from article authors. The journal is published monthly by Intermed Communications, Inc., 414 Benjamin Fox Pavilion, Jenkintown, PA 19046.

NURSING CLINICS OF NORTH AMERICA

Nursing Clinics is published quarterly by W. B. Saunders, West Washington Square, Philadelphia, PA 19105. Each issue of the publication focuses on one or two specific topics. There is a guest editor for each issue and nursing experts in the field are asked to submit articles. The topics deal with all aspects of nursing, including clinical practice, administration and education. The issues are all indexed and are hard-covered.

*The title is updated annually.

THE JOURNAL OF CONTINUING EDUCATION IN NURSING

Continuing education is a steadily growing concern for all nurses. Many nurses in the mid-seventies were faced with the task of developing adult education programs deserving of continuing education unit credits. The *Journal of Continuing Education in Nursing* provides information pertaining to federal involvement and Congressional action. Model programs and self-study plans provide invaluable professional assistance. This journal is published six times per year and may be ordered from Charles B. Slack, Inc., 6900 Grove Road, Thorofare, New Jersey 08086.

NURSING UPDATE

Nursing Update is a ready reference source and comes in a three-hole punched form, ready for insertion in a sturdy binder which is supplied at no cost with every five new subscriptions. This publication assists the nurse to keep abreast of the expanding nursing profession. Articles are based upon practical situations and include nursing techniques, patient-instruction guidelines, equipment updating, charts, and checklists. Special features include review quizzes, article summaries, and annual cumulative indexes. In-service education programs and nursing schools utilizing the core curriculum include *Nursing Update* as an invaluable supplement to instructional materials. The periodical is published monthly and may be ordered from Nursing Update, P.O. Box 1245, Darien, CT 06820.

THE JOURNAL OF NURSING EDUCATION

This journal is specifically designed for nursing educators seeking new ideas in education. Two issues per year are focused on items of a general theme; two issues are centered on a specific area of interest for nursing educators at various levels. Basic nursing education, continuing education, research in nursing education, degree program teaching, and learning concepts are features. This quarterly publication may be ordered from Journal of Nursing Education Subscriptions, P.O. Box 582, Hightstown, N.J. 08520.

IN-SERVICE TRAINING AND EDUCATION

Nursing educators and in-service directors, concerned with the on-the-job training and the educational development of new nursing graduates, will find this journal useful. Articles are geared toward content and teaching methods as well as solutions to problems encountered in in-service education. Stress is placed on clinical application of new concepts. Issues are published quarterly by Health Care Publications, Inc., P.O. Box 696, 125 Elm Street, New Canaan, Connecticut 06840.

THE JOURNAL OF NURSING ADMINISTRATION

Aimed to meet the managerial needs of nursing service administrators and educators, articles in this periodical are written to cover staffing and personnel needs. Bound volumes are available for each year of publication. These volumes are an excellent reference source for nursing administrators who wish to keep abreast of current trends in health care delivery. This journal is published monthly except April, August, and December by Contemporary Publishing, Inc., 12 Lakeside Park, Wakefield, MA 01880.

NURSING DIGEST

Articles cover all clinical areas and are presented to keep nurses intellectually stimulated and up-to-date on professional issues. Issues include relevant articles from the areas of fine arts, highlights from history, politics, medical science, education, behavior, and human affairs, in economical, time-saving, digest form. Special features include a Professional Opportunities section with listings of available positions. *Nursing Digest* is published bi-monthly by Nursing Digest, Inc., 607 North Avenue, Wakefield, Massachusetts 01880.

THE JOURNAL OF PRACTICAL NURSING

As the official publication of the National Association for Practical Nurse Education and Service, Inc., this journal has been meeting the growing needs of the licensed practical nurse since 1951. Features include job listings, articles on clinical nursing skills, and current legislative action affecting economic security and health care. Readers may submit articles based on a personal professional experience. Each issue has been approved by NAPNES for one contact hour of continuing education which may earn a reader 1.2 Continuing Education Units annually by completing the Self-Evaluation question and answer column. Subscriptions are available from NAPNES, Inc., 122 East 42nd St., Suite 800, New York, N.Y. 10017.

NURSING CARE

This national magazine is the official publication of the National Federation of Licensed Practical Nurses. It reflects the diversified role of the licensed practical nurse whose principal concern is the care of the patient. The monthly issues are a valuable learning tool for students enrolled in practical nursing programs. *Nursing Care* carries updated information on nursing techniques in all clinical specialties. Physicians, professional nurses, and practical nurses write informative articles at a reading level easy to understand. Special features include a book review, new products column, a listing of educational opportunities, and available scholarships and a pharmacology quiz. The journal may be ordered from Nursing Care, 75 East 55th Street, New York, N.Y. 10022.

GUIDES TO PERIODICAL LITERATURE

The nursing student and the graduate nurse must know how to locate articles on a specific topic. There are several resources which are invaluable tools for the nurse who needs specific information about nursing or nursing-related topics.

Yale University received a grant from the United States Public Health Service which funded the development of *Nursing Studies Index.* The index serves as a guide to nursing literature published in English, from 1900 through 1959. The design makes the index appropriate for use by all nurses and individuals seeking information on any aspect of nursing. This index is published in four volumes.

The American Journal of Nursing Company publishes the *International Nursing Index.* The first volume was published in 1966 and it is regularly updated. Topics are listed in alphabetical order, with all the relevant articles listed beneath the general topic. Another valuable tool to locating periodical literature is the *Cumulative Index to Nursing Literature,* first published in 1956.

Nurses doing research on a single topic should use one of these three indices to locate relevant articles. However, if the study involves several topics, the nurse might like to obtain a bibliography which includes all articles published on each of the topics. The *computerized bibliographic literature search* is available at most larger libraries. The nurse should make her request known to the reference librarian. For a small charge, the library will obtain a comprehensive bibliography via a computerized network of library resources.

The Interagency Council on Library Resources for Nursing is an interdisciplinary group of representatives from ANA, AMA, NAPNES, NSNA, the Medical Library Association, the Special Library Association, the American Library Association, and Mugar Library in Boston. The council meets several times

Abbreviation	Full Title
AORN J	Association of Operating Room Nurses Journal
Am J NURS	American Journal of Nursing
IN-SERV TRAIN EDUC	In-Service Training and Education
INT NURS REV	International Nursing Review
J CONTIN EDUC NURS.	The Journal of Continuing Education in Nursing
J NURS ADMIN	Journal of Nursing Administration
J NURS EDUC	The Journal of Nursing Education
J PRACT NURS.	Journal of Practical Nursing
J PSYCHIATR NURS	Journal of Psychiatric Nursing and Mental Health Services
MATERNAL-CHILD NURS J.	Maternal-Child Nursing Journal
NURS CARE	Nursing Care
NURS CLIN NORTH AM	The Nursing Clinics of North America
NURS DIGEST	Nursing Digest
NURS FORUM	Nursing Forum
NURS OUTLOOK	Nursing Outlook
NURS PAP.	Nursing Papers
NURS RES	Nursing Research
NURS '76	Nursing '76
NURS TIMES	Nursing Times
NURS UPDATE.	Nursing Update
OCCUP HEALTH NURS.	Occupational Health Nursing

Fig. 23-1 Abbreviations of nursing publications as they appear in indices of nursing periodicals

a year to discuss and plan nursing library resources. The council also acts as an advisory committee.

THE NURSE'S BOOK SOCIETY

The only book club designed exclusively for members of the nursing profession is The Nurse's Book Society. The editors select a wide variety of book titles, from which a member is free to select those which are most interesting or applicable. Books are selected to represent all clinical areas of medicine and surgery. The Book Club *News* is sent to each subscriber fifteen times a year and it describes the current selections. Book selections purchased for professional purposes are tax deductible. For information write The Nurse's Book Society, Riverside, New Jersey 08075.

American Journal of Nursing Company 10 Columbus Circle New York, NY 10019	*The American Journal of Nursing* *Nursing Research* *Contemporary Nursing Series*
National League for Nursing 10 Columbus Circle New York, NY 10019	*Nursing Outlook* *Pamphlets*
Charles B. Slack, Inc. 6900 Grove Road Thorofare, NJ 08086	*The Journal of Cont Educ in Nurs* *Occupational Health Nursing* *Journal of Allied Health* *The Journal of Psychiatric Nursing and* *Mental Health Services* *Gerontological Nursing*
Harper and Row, Publishers, Inc. 2350 Virginia Avenue Hagerstown, MD 21740	*The Journal of Obstetric, Gynecological and Neonatal Nursing*
Intermed Communications, Inc. 414 Benjamin Fox Pavilion Jenkintown, PA 19046	*Nursing '76*
Nursing Update P.O. Box 1245 Darien, CT 06820	*Nursing Update*
Journal of Nursing Education Subscriptions P.O. Box 582 Hightstown, NJ 08520	*The Journal of Nursing Education*
Health Care Publications, Inc. P.O. Box 696 125 Elm Street New Canaan, CT 06840	*In-Service Training and Education*
Contemporary Publishing, Inc. 12 Lakeside Park Wakefield, MA 01880	*The Journal of Nursing Administration* *Nursing Digest*

.Fig. 23-2 Publishers of nursing periodicals

SUMMARY

The publications mentioned are a mere sampling of the nursing journals available to nurses. There are excellent periodicals published by the state nurses associations. Although some are concerned primarily with local issues, they do publish articles of interest to the entire nursing profession. These publications are generally included in the membership fees and are sent to members only.

Subscriptions to professional journals are tax deductible as a professional expense. Some journals are offered at special group rates. By ordering personal copies of the journal most suited to personal and professional needs, the nurse is assured of prompt delivery and ready access to vital reference materials. The rapid rate of changes occurring in the health occupations necessitates reading on a regular basis if the nurse is to incorporate new ideas and concepts into her everyday practices.

SUGGESTED ACTIVITIES

- Make a large wall or bulletin board collage using covers of nursing journals.

- Submit an original case study, or an article based on a personal nursing experience, to a journal that publishes student material.

- Write a letter to the editor of a nursing journal and include suggestions for articles or columns which would be beneficial to students enrolled in basic nursing education programs.

REVIEW

A.   Multiple Choice. Select the best answer.

1. The only journal which invites readers to submit personal questions to authors is
   a. Nursing '76.   c. American Journal of Nursing.
   b. Nursing Digest.   d. Nursing Outlook.

2. Continuing education credit for the self-evaluation section of the Journal of Practical Nursing has been approved by
   a. American Nurses' Association.
   b. National League for Nursing.
   c. National Association for Practical Nurse Education and Service, Inc.
   d. National Federation of Licensed Practical Nurses.

3. A pharmacology quiz designed to assist the student practical nurse and graduates of practical nurse programs is included in
   a. Nursing Research.   c. American Journal of Nursing.
   b. pharmacology textbooks.   d. Nursing Care.

4. Money spent on nursing texts and periodicals is a legitimate professional expense which is
   a. worthwhile.   c. usually reimbursed.
   b. tax deductible.   d. a good investment.

5. Nurse educators are finding it beneficial to supplement the textbook with
   a. clinical practice.   c. films.
   b. periodical literature.   d. harder tests.

B. Match the periodicals in Column II with the correct description in Column I.

Column I

1. "Test Yourself" is a special feature of this journal.

2. A compilation of selected articles from three professional nursing magazines in soft cover.

3. A journal designed for health care workers who have interests in the geriatric patient.

4. The official publication of the National League for Nursing.

5. The official publication of the Nurses' Association of the American College of Obstetricians and Gynecologists.

6. Contains information on legislative status of continuing education proposals.

Column II

a. Journal of Obstetric, Gynecologic and Neonatal Nursing

b. American Journal of Nursing

c. Nursing Outlook

d. Gerontological Nursing

e. Journal of Continuing Education in Nursing

f. Contemporary Nursing Series

g. Journal of Nursing Education

C. Briefly answer the following questions.

1. List four magazines published by the American Journal of Nursing Co.

2. List four nursing organizations that publish a magazine on the national level.

chapter 24
CONTINUING
EDUCATION

STUDENT OBJECTIVES

- Explain the purpose of continuing education.
- List sources which sponsor continuing education programs for nurses.
- Explain the rationale for mandatory continuing education.

Nurses are becoming increasingly aware of their need for continuing education and its effect upon their careers as licensed practitioners. Continuing education provides the nurse with the opportunity for intellectual growth and aids in maintaining standards of nursing practice. It also promotes increased competency in the performance of nursing skills. Continuing education programs are designed to meet the learning needs of nurses and the changing health care needs of the consumers. Nurses are actively involved in planning continuing education programs or working with the sponsors of programs in order to ensure quality, relevance, and approval for credit by state nurses associations.

OFFERINGS IN CONTINUING EDUCATION

Academic credit may be received for certain college courses, but in general the continuing education courses, seminars, workshops, and in-service programs do not provide academic credits. The acquisition of an academic degree is not the goal in continuing education. The primary objective is to maintain competency in nursing practice.

Clinical Nursing	Foundations of Nursing	Specialties	Nursing Service/ Administration
Mental Health Concepts	Death & Dying	Trauma Nurse Specialist Program	Leadership Skills
Drug Addiction	Intravenous Therapy	Independent Nursing Practice	Professional Roles
Alcoholism	Pharmacology	Emergency Care	Record Keeping
Hypertension–The Silent Disease	Nursing Assessment	Respiratory Care	Interpersonal Relations
Anaphylaxis	Team Nursing	Amputee Rehabilitation	Team Leadership
Child Abuse	Refresher Course	Peritoneal Dialysis	Charge Nurse Duties
Cancer	Principles of Asepsis	Kidney Dialysis Machines	Innovative Teaching
Restorative Nursing	The Unconscious Patient	Intensive Coronary Care	Behavioral Objectives
Arrhythmia			Clinical Supervision
Coronary Bypass			Clinical Evaluation
Ostomies			Nursing Management
Pulmonary Surgery			

Fig. 24-1 Sample topics for continuing education programs

Sponsoring Agencies

Continuing education programs are currently being offered by health organizations, governmental agencies, colleges, and universities. Examples of sponsoring agencies include the American Heart Association, American Cancer Society, state and local departments of health, rehabilitation institutes, American Association of Critical Care Nurses, Lung Association, American Nurses' Association, state nurses associations, and the National League for Nursing.

Employing Agencies

The employing agency has a responsibility for providing opportunities for the individual nurse to participate in continued learning programs. In most instances, in-service education departments in hospitals attempt to meet the ultimate goal of improved patient care and service. Smaller institutions do not generally have the resources to hire a qualified educational staff but may compensate for the deficiency by permitting nursing personnel to attend approved conferences and workshops.

Educational Institutions

Educational institutions such as secondary public schools, community colleges, and universities are committed to the concept of adult education. They make an effort to meet the learning needs of all members of the community by providing learning experiences which enable the individual to develop expertise in a given skill.

MEASUREMENTS AND RECORDS

Individual participation in noncredit continuing education programs is measured by units based upon ten contact hours per one *continuing education unit* (CEU). This standard of measurement applies to institutional and organizational learning experiences. A certificate is generally granted upon completion of a given program that has been approved for credit. CEU credit is not awarded for activities such as employing agency orientation training programs, reading and discussion groups, work experience, or other informal educational experiences difficult to measure. In-service programs can be considered one type of continuing education, but the two terms are not synonymous. A required number of contact hours can be attained through staff development programs, institutes, seminars, workshops, radio and television conferences, independent study, and published articles. Continuing education units and traditional academic course credits are not interchangeable.

Origin of the Continuing Education Unit

The CEU method of measuring noncredit continuing education is not used solely by the nursing profession. Representatives of thirty-four national organizations and agencies met in Washington, D.C. in July, 1968, to organize the National Task Force on the Continuing Education Unit. This Task Force is currently responsible for the development and evaluation of programs and

Contact Hours	CEU Values	Contact Hours	CEU Values	Contact Hours	CEU Values
5	0.5	10	1.0	60	6.0
6	0.6	20	2.0	70	7.0
7	0.7	30	3.0	80	8.0
8	0.8	40	4.0	90	9.0
9	0.9	50	5.0	100	10.0

Fig. 24-2 Conversion table for contact hours and continuing education units

projects involving the CEU. The American Nurses' Association was represented at the organizational meetings of the task force and endorsed the CEU as a method of measurement of noncredit continuing education in nursing. The National League for Nursing has also stated that the CEU should be utilized as the standard unit of measurement for noncredit programs.

Recording Mechanisms

Sponsoring agencies follow the task force's criteria in recording information on permanent records. Basic information is recorded by all sponsoring agencies and includes:

- Name of the participant
- Social security number
- Title of course
- Workshop or activity
- Dates of attendance
- Format of course
- Number of CEUs awarded.

Recording must be done in a systematic manner in order for the data to be universally understood and transferable. This accumulation of information

Name of participant	Social Security No.
Address of participant	License Number
City, State, County	State(s) in which licensed
Title of Course, Workshop, or Activity	
Dates of Attendance	
Contact Hours	CEUs Awarded

Fig. 24-3 Sample of permanent record of continuing education

may be important at local, state, and national levels. Currently, employing agencies may use the CEU record when determining an individual's eligibility for promotion and salary increases. On the other hand, the employee has a written record to support claim to increased competency based on the participation in learning activities.

It is the responsibility of the individual nurse to record attendance at all programs for which credit is given. When the accrued credits total twenty contact hours, the information should be submitted for recording on the permanent record. There generally is a small charge by the state nurses association for the recording service; therefore, it is impractical to submit for recording each credit as it is earned.

LEGISLATIVE ACTION

Approximately one hundred million dollars are paid annually in malpractice suits. In Washington, D.C. the Federal Commission on Medical Malpractice, comprised of twenty-one members, has studied the problem. One of the recommendations made by the commission is that health practitioners be required to engage in continuing education in their fields if they wish to maintain licensure. It is felt that malpractice could be reduced with continuing education. The legal aspects of continuing education for license renewal are being studied by legislatures throughout the country.

Mandatory Continuing Education

Compulsory continuing education is a relatively new concept for the nursing profession, but it really is not a new idea to other professions. Teachers, for example, have been required to maintain their teaching certificates and provide basis for salary increments, by continuing and updating their education. Mandatory education will be a controversial topic for nurses until educational opportunities become more readily accessible to them. The State of California legislatures were the first to pass a bill requiring continuing education for relicensure to practice nursing. Advocates for mandatory continuing education justify their position by stating that it is a necessity for upgrading nursing practice and must be mandatory in order to assure the consumer of quality nursing services.

Mandatory continuing education does not affect a nurse's initial license to practice nursing. It is concerned with license renewal only. Many nurses are under a misconception that once a license is granted, they are totally educated as a practicing nurse and no longer need formal organized learning activities.

Voluntary Continuing Education

Nurses who are forced to attend compulsory continuing education programs for a certain number of credit points may not necessarily become better nurse practitioners. This is the familiar argument of nurses who have maintained a competent level of practice for years through in-service education, on-the-job learning, and reading of relevant professional literature. Some persons have benefited from self-directed learning activities.

Voluntary participation occurs only if the individual nurse is motivated by a sense of moral obligation or desires knowledge for scholastic reasons. The percentage of professional nurses who belong to the American Nurses' Association and practical nurses who belong to their professional organizations is very low. This would indicate that in a voluntary system, total involvement and commitment will not be achieved. Many practicing nurses are not motivated to learn new concepts; they do not feel a need to improve their nursing skills. In order for continuing education to effectively promote quality patient care, it must reach all practitioners. Continued education will not reach all practitioners unless it is mandated.

PROFESSIONAL GROUP INVOLVEMENT

Continuing education needs are continually being studied to ensure the establishment of programs which are meaningful and available to everyone. Program planning for the future is currently under way. Present programs and courses of action are continually evaluated so as to be educationally sound. Persons attending meetings, workshops, or courses should check to see if the program has been approved by the Continuing Education Recognition Program (CERP). Interstate transfer of recognition of continuing education programs is being planned by state nurses associations.

National League for Nursing

The National League for Nursing has enlisted health education leaders to promote interdisciplinary education and to coordinate continuing education programs on a regional basis, in order to extend continuing education opportunities and aviod duplication of programs. A statement on NLN's role in continuing education in nursing was issued in February, 1974, along with *Guidelines for the Development of Continuing Education Programs in Nursing.*

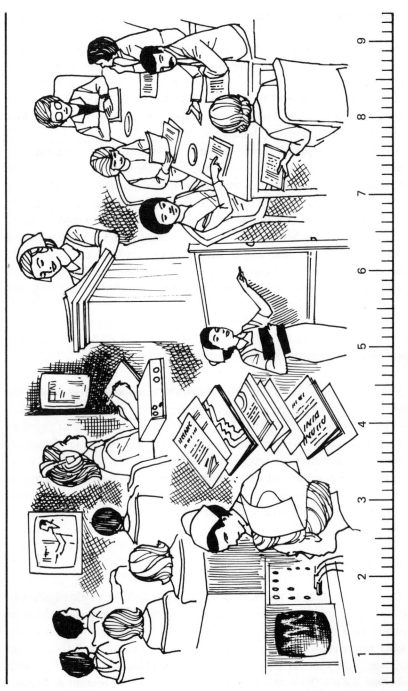

Fig. 24-4 Measuring continuing education

American Nurses' Association

The American Nurses' Association has issued guidelines to state nurses associations for the establishment of systems of recognition for participation in continuing education programs. Some state nursing associations now keep files for members by recording CEUs earned through approved programs. The state nurses associations have also developed criteria and standards for evaluating continuing education programs. Those which meet the criteria are approved and can offer CEUs to participants. The ANA has issued a paper, *Standards for Continuing Education in Nursing,* prepared by the ANA Council on Continuing Education and approved by the ANA Commission on Nursing Education. Goals and objectives are stated and financial resources available for administering programs are outlined.

National Federation of Licensed Practical Nurses, Inc.

The NFLPN has made an official statement regarding continuing education, which declares that "continuing education includes organized educational experiences which should be planned so as to meet the needs of licensed practical nurses in the satisfactory fulfillment of their role as health workers." NFLPN recognizes improved patient care as the primary goal of continuing education for all nurses.

IMPLICATIONS FOR THE INDIVIDUAL NURSE

It is imperative that the selection of continuing education activities be meaningful to the participant's present position in nursing. Nurses may use the ANA's *Interim Statement on Continuing Education in Nursing* as a guide in determining the quality of continuing education programs. The American Nurses's Association Commission on Nursing Education developed guidelines for the state nurses associations to use in the evaluation and approval of continuing education programs. Information is readily obtainable from the state or ANA offices.

Nurses traditionally are concerned with technical skills and procedures. They are not always motivated to fully understand the principles and theoretical concepts underlying the activity. Quality patient care is based on educationally sound nursing practices. Self-assessment of personal and professional goals is essential in planning to meet any educational needs. Resources available to attain the established goals must be studied. Planning should provide for continuity of learning experiences whenever any educational endeavor is undertaken.

Haphazard undertakings often fail to lead to a fruitful reward for time, effort, and money spent. For the working nurse, time is an important factor to consider.

The concept of continuing education is here to stay and should be accepted as an opportunity to develop basic nursing abilities into a competent practice which does not suffer from obsolescence. Learning is a continuous process from birth to death, but it must be properly directed if it is going to assure the development of a capable and effective professional nurse.

SUMMARY

Meeting continuing education needs is an individual responsibility. It is the obligation of the nurse, who is responsible to the patient, to maintain current and relevant knowledge and skills in her field. It is important for each nurse to realize that the attainment of a certificate or degree is not an end in itself. Rather, it is to be viewed as a beginning foundation upon which to build. Every nurse must continue her education if she is to continue to provide safe, quality nursing care. Additional education is also necessary for a nurse to become more highly skilled and competent. Although many may feel that meeting the continuing education requirement is a heavy burden, it should be viewed as an opportunity to improve nursing practice and to develop a sense of self-confidence, security, and professional pride.

SUGGESTED ACTIVITIES

- Debate whether continuing education should be mandatory or voluntary.

- Interview a district or state nurses association representative to discuss current continuing education recognition programs in the school locality.

- Attend a workshop as a class activity and evaluate it as a continuing education experience. Select a program that will correlate with the basic curriculum.

REVIEW

A.   Multiple Choice. Select the best answer.

   1.   The initials CERP stand for
       a. Certified Educational Research Programs.
       b. Continuing Education Recognition Programs.
       c. Certificate in Educational Research Planning.
       d. Continuing Education for Registered Pharmacists.

2. The first state to pass legislation requiring continuing education for nursing relicensure was
   a. New York.
   c. Illinois.
   b. Florida.
   d. California.

3. The ultimate responsibility for meeting continuing education rests with the
   a. hospital's in-service staff.
   c. professional ogranizations.
   b. schools of nursing.
   d. individual.

4. Ten contact hours of participation in approved noncredit continuing education yields
   a. ten continuing education units.
   b. five continuing education units.
   c. one continuing education unit.
   d. two continuing education units.

5. Mandatory continuing education would affect
   a. license renewal.
   c. initial licensing and renewal.
   b. initial licensing.
   d. none of these.

B. Match the items in Column II to the correct statement in Column I.

Column I	Column II
1. Learning activities undertaken by motivated persons seeking to improve skills and increase knowledge.	a. Continuing education
	b. Continuing Education Unit
2. Learning activities planned by the employing agency for the purpose of continued learning.	c. In-Service education
	d. Mandatory continuing education
3. The standard of uniform measurement of an organized continuing education experience.	e. Voluntary continuing education
4. Compulsory education requirement concerned with license renewal.	
5. Credit or noncredit learning activities not directed toward the attainment of an academic certificate or degree.	

C.   Briefly answer the following questions.

1.   What is the primary objective of continuing education?

2.   Name three types of organizations currently offering continuing education programs for nurses.

3.   List three sponsoring agencies of continuing education.

4.   What is the employing agency's responsibility in continuing education?

5.   State the benefits received from continuing education for each of the following:

The Nurse

The Patient

The Employing Agency

6.   Explain the rationale of advocates of mandatory continuing education.

7.   What agency is responsible for the development and evaluation of programs and projects involving the continuing education unit?

GLOSSARY

Acupuncture: Insertion of needles into the body to relieve pain or cure disease.

Advanced placement: Student is given credit for required courses through examination rather than by taking and passing the course.

Articulation: A common or shared bond, interest, or body of knowledge which permits easy flow; in education, the development of programs which facilitate exit and entry at a higher level.

Assault: A threat or attempt to physically hurt another person.

Bargaining agent: Organization certified by a government agency to represent a group of employees for the purpose of collective bargaining.

Bargaining unit: A group of employees recognized as appropriate, who have the right to bargain collectively with the employer.

Battery: The act of hurting or beating another person.

Bedlam: A state of uproar and confusion; originally referred to hospital in the Reformation period which accepted the mentally ill.

Bloodletting: The removal of blood from the body as a means of treating disease.

Breach of contract: When one of the parties in a contract fails to fulfill all the terms of the agreement.

Breech: A type of delivery when the buttocks are the presenting anatomy at birth.

Caduceus: Emblem of the medical profession representing Aesculapius' staff entwined with serpents of wisdom.

Caesarean section: A surgical procedure done to remove a baby from the womb of the mother.

Career ladder: The articulation of educational programs which permits advancement without loss of credit or repetition.

Certification: The process of granting recognition to an individual who has met the established qualifications or criteria of an agency or organization.

Challenging examination: A tool which is used to assess levels of knowledge in order to grant credit for courses not taken.

Collective bargaining: A bilateral determination of conditions of employment by employer and employee which results in a legal contract.

Computer technology: The use of machines to process data.

Continuing education unit: The measurement of participation in continuing education programs whereby ten hours of participation are equivalent to one continuing education unit.

Contract: A legally binding agreement between two or more parties.

Core curriculum: A curriculum design which enables a student to leave a career program at various levels, with a career attained, and the option to continue to another higher level or career.

Cybernetics: Science involving comparative study of automatic control systems.

Defamation: Verbal or written remarks which harm an individual's reputation.

Eclampsia: A pathological condition during pregnancy related to hypertension and the excretion of protein in the urine.

EEG: Electroencephalograph; an instrument which records brain waves.

EKG: Electrocardiograph; an instrument used to record heart rhythmicity.

Endorsement: The acceptance, by a state, of a license issued by another state.

Enrichment studies: A program designed to assist a student who has not met all of the admission requirements of a professional school.

Euthanasia: Killing a person as an act of mercy.

External degree: A degree conferred when all requirements have been met by the applicant, and credit is given for knowledge and skills regardless of when or how achieved.

False imprisonment: Unwarranted restriction of the freedom of an individual.

Fellowship: Appointment of a person to a position which grants an allowance (monetary).

Gerontology: The study of aging.

Grant: A gift of money which may be given under certain conditions; usually to fund a specific project.

Holistic: The emphasis is on the interrelatedness of parts and wholes.

Hospice: An innlike abode which provides food and shelter for travelers.

Hospital costs: Those expenses incurred by hospitals in the treatment of patients.

Informed consent: When a person agrees to participate after he is told what his participation involves, including dangers.

Invasion of privacy: The disturbance or revelation of those things an individual holds as confidential.

Liable: Obligated or accountable by law.

Libel: Written form of defamation.

License: Permission to practice granted after all requirements have been met by an individual.

Ligature: A thread or filament which is tied to occlude blood vessels.

Loan: Money lent for the borrower's temporary use, which must be paid back.

Malpractice: Any professional act which causes damage, injury or loss to the patient or client.

Midwife: Woman experienced in assisting another women during labor and delivery.

Milieu: Environment.

Negligence: Failure to do something that an equally qualified person would have done in a similar circumstance.

Obstetrics: The study of human reproduction.

Oncological: Related to cancer.

Open curriculum: An educational system which allows the student to enter and leave the system and one which utilizes all past education and experience.

Palliative: To minimize the severity of symptoms rather than a cure for disease.

Paramedical specialists: Persons who supplement the work of highly trained medical professionals.

Patient day: Twenty-four hour period during which various hospital services are rendered and upon which costs are determined.

Pediatrics: The study of problems and diseases of young children.

Percussion: Tapping in order to distinguish resonance.

Primary Care: Refers to health care to individuals and families which emphasizes maintenance of health, provided by one qualified health care professional.

Reciprocity: Synonymous term for endorsement.

Registration: Listing of a license with the state, usually for a fee.

Responsibility: The state of being held to blame or accountable.

Resume: A summary of an individual's education, career experiences and qualifications.

Right: The power or privilege to which one is justly entitled.

Rooming-in: An arrangement in a hospital obstetrical unit which allows the mother and newborn to share a room.

Sanatoria: Early Greek establishments which provided therapy, diet and exercise programs.

Scholarship: A gift of money usually associated with recognition of academic excellence.

Slander: The verbal form of defamation.

Sorcery: The use of black magic, witchcraft and the calling upon evil spirits to exert supernatural power over human beings and physical conditions.

Stipend: A monetary allowance paid on a regular basis.

Technology: Application of scientific principles in a practical manner.

Terminal education: Courses of study planned so that the student completes the necessary requirements of predetermined career goals. Work preparation is achieved without further formal education necessary.

Tort: A legally wrongful act.

Traineeship: Monies given to cover the specific training or education of individuals.

Trephination: Surgery performed with a trephine, a circular sawlike edged instrument used to cut out round pieces of the skull.

University without walls: A baccalaureate nursing program which allows a registered nurse to take courses at a college other than the one which will confer the degree.

Upward mobility: The opportunity to have increased status and earning power through higher education.

Wet Nurse: Female who breastfeeds infants belonging to other mothers.

Xenodochia: Shelters, originated by the Hebrews, which provided medical and nursing care for travelers.

ABBREVIATIONS OF ORGANIZATIONS AND PROGRAMS

AHA	American Hospital Association
AMA	American Medical Association
ANA	American Nurses' Association
ANF	American Nurses' Foundation Grant Program
ASHA	American Speech and Hearing Association
BEOG	Basic Educational Opportunity Grant Program
CAI	Computer-Assisted Instruction
CPEP	College Proficiency Examination Program
CERP	Continuing Education Recognition Program
CEU	Continuing Education Unit
CMI	Computer-Managed Instruction
CWS	College Work-Study Program
DHEW	Department of Health, Education and Welfare
HMO	Health Maintenance Organization
HSA	Health Systems Agencies
ICN	International Council of Nurses
JCAH	Joint Commission of Accreditation of Hospitals
LEGS	Learning Experience Guides
MLT	Medical Laboratory Technician Program
NAPNES	National Association for Practical Nurse Education and Service, Inc.
NDSL	National Direct Student Loan Program
NEF	Nurses' Educational Funds, Inc.
NFLPN	National Federation of Licensed Practical Nurses
NLN	National League for Nursing

NLNE	National League of Nursing Education
NLPNEF	National Licensed Practical Nurses Educational Foundation
NLRA	National Labor Relations Act
NSNA	National Student Nurses' Association
PSRO	Professional Standards Review Organization
SEOG	Supplemental Educational Opportunity Grant Program
UWW	University Without Walls Program
VA	Veterans Administration
VISTA	Volunteers in Service to America
WHO	World Health Organization
YWCA	Young Women's Christian Association

BIBLIOGRAPHY

SECTION 1 INFLUENCES OF THE PAST

Chapter 1 Primeval Medicine and Nursing

Ackerknecht, Erwin H. *A Short History of Medicine.* New York: The Ronald Press Co., 1968.

Bettmann, Otto L. *A Pictorial History of Medicine.* Springfield, IL: Charles C. Thomas,Publisher, 1962.

Casteglioni, Arturo. *A History of Medicine.* New York: Alfred A. Knopf, 1941.

Clendening, Logan. *Source Book of Medical History.* New York: Dover Publications, 1960.

Dietz, Lena Dixon, and Lehozky, Aurelia R. *History and Modern Nursing.* 2d ed. Philadelphia: F.A. Davis Co., 1968.

Depierri, Kate P. "One Way of Unearthing the Past." *American Journal of Nursing* 68:521, March 1968.

Dolan, Josephine A. *History of Nursing.* 12th ed. Philadelphia: W.B. Saunders Co., 1969.

Germino, V.H. et al. "Acupuncture." *Physician's Associate* 2:50-56, April 1972.

Gordon, B.L. *Medicine Throughout Antiquity.* Philadelphia: F.A. Davis Co., 1949.

Green, John R. *Medical History for Students.* Springfield, IL: Charles C. Thomas,Publisher, 1968.

Griffin, Gerald Joseph, and King, Joanne. *History and Trends of Professional Nursing.* 7th ed. St. Louis: The C.V. Mosby Co., 1973.

Haggard, Howard W. *Devils, Drugs and Doctors.* New York: Blue Ribbon Books, 1929.

Inglis, Brian. *A History of Medicine.* Ohio: The World Publishing Co., 1965.

Jamieson, Elizabeth M.; Sewall, Mary F.; and Suhrie, Eleanor B. *Trends in Nursing History.* 6th ed. Philadelphia: W.B. Saunders Co., 1966.

Kelly, Cordelia W. *Dimensions of Professional Nursing.* 2d ed. New York: Macmillan Co., Inc., 1968.

Levin, Simon S. *Adam's Rib: Essays on Biblical Medicine.* Los Altos, CA: Geron-X, 1970.

Major, Ralph H. *A History of Medicine.* vol. 1. Springfield, IL: Charles C. Thomas, Publisher, 1954.

McCleary, Elliott H. "Windows on Medicine's Past." *Today's Health* 47:70, October 1969.

Rush, Phillip D. "A Walk Through Medicine's Past." *Today's Health* 45:47, January 1967.

Sigerist, Henry E. *A History of Medicine.* vol. 1. New York: Oxford University Press, 1951.

Singer, Charles, and Underwood, E. Ashworth. *A Short History of Medicine.* 2d ed. New York: Oxford University Press, 1962.

Chapter 2 The Influence of Christianity

Castiglioni, Arturo. *A History of Medicine.* New York: Alfred A. Knopf, 1941.

Dietz, Lena Dixon, and Lehozky, Aurelia F. *History and Modern Nursing.* 2d ed. Philadelphia: F.A. Davis Co., 1967.

Green, John R. *Medical History for Students.* Springfield, IL: Charles C. Thomas, Publisher, 1968.

Griffin, Gerald Joseph, and Griffin, Joanne King. *History and Trends of Professional Nursing.* 7th ed. St. Louis: C.V. Mosby Co., 1973.

Kelly, Cordelia W. *Dimensions of Professional Nursing.* 2d ed. New York: Macmillan Co., 1968.

Major, Ralph H. *A History of Medicine.* vol. 1. Springfield, IL: Charles C. Thomas, Publisher, 1954.

Nelson, S. "The Influence of Christianity on the Care of the Sick Up to the End of the Middle Ages." *South African Nursing Journal* 40:18, August 1973.

Singer, Charles, and Underwood, E. Ashworth. *A Short History of Medicine.* 2d ed. New York: Oxford University Press, 1962.

Walker, Kenneth. *The Story of Medicine.* New York: Oxford University Press, 1955.

Chapter 3 Medieval Health Care

Ackerknecht, Erwin H. *A Short History of Medicine.* New York: The Ronald Press Company, 1968.

Bettmann, Otto L. *A Pictorial History of Medicine.* Springfield, IL: Charles C. Thomas Publisher, 1962.

Castiglioni, Arturo. *A History of Medicine.* New York: Alfred A. Knopf, 1941.

Dietz, Lena Dixon, and Lehozky, Aurelia R. *History and Modern Nursing.* 2d ed. Philadelphia: F.A. Davis Co., 1967.

Green, John R. *Medical History for Students.* Springfield, IL: Charles C. Thomas Publisher, 1968.

Griffin, Gerald Joseph, and Griffin, Joanne King. *History and Trends of Professional Nursing.* 7th ed. St. Louis: C.V. Mosby Co., 1973.

Kelly, Cordelia W. *Dimensions of Professional Nursing.* 2d ed. New York: Macmillan Co., 1968.

Major, Ralph H. *A History of Medicine.* vol. 1. Springfield, IL: Charles C. Thomas Publisher, 1954.

Singer, Charles, and Underwood, E. Ashworth. *A Short History of Medicine.* 2d ed. New York: Oxford University Press, 1962.

Walker, Kenneth. *The Story of Medicine.* New York: Oxford University Press, 1955.

Chapter 4 The Dark Ages and New Ideas

Ackerknecht, Erwin H. *A Short History of Medicine.* New York: Ronald Press Co., 1968.

Bettmann, Otto L. *A Pictorial History of Medicine.* Springfield, IL: Charles C. Thomas,Publisher, 1962.

Castiglioni, Arturo. *A History of Medicine.* New York: Alfred A. Knopf, 1941.

Dickens, Charles. *Martin Chuzzlewit.* 1844. New York: E.P. Dutton and Co.

Dietz, Lena Dixon, and Lehozky, Aurelia R. *History and Modern Nursing.* 2d ed. Philadelphia: F.A. Davis Co., 1967.

Green, John R. *Medical History for Students.* Springfield, IL: Charles C. Thomas, Publisher 1968.

Griffin, Gerald Joseph, and Griffin, Joanne King. *History and Trends of Professional Nursing.* 7th ed. St. Louis: C.V. Mosby Co., 1973.

Inglis, Brian. *A History of Medicine.* New York: The World Publishing Co., 1965.

Kelly, Cordelia W. *Dimensions of Professional Nursing.* 2d ed. New York: Macmillan Co., 1968.

Major, Ralph H. *A History of Medicine.* vol. 1. Springfield, IL: Charles C. Thomas, Publisher, 1954.

Moore, Mary Lou. "Bright Spot in the 18th Century." *American Journal of Nursing* 69:1705, August 1969.

Singer, Charles, and Underwood, E. Ashworth. *A Short History of Medicine.* 2d ed. New York: Oxford University Press, 1962.

Walker, Kenneth. *The Story of Medicine.* New York: Oxford University Press, 1955.

SECTION 2 THE BIRTH OF ORGANIZED NURSING

Chapter 5 The Nightingale Concept

Abel-Smith, Brian. *A History of the Nursing Profession.* London: Heinemann Educational Books Ltd., 1966.

Banworth, Calista. "A Living Memorial to Florence Nightingale." *American Journal of Nursing* 40:491–497, May 1940.

Bettmann, Otto L. *A Pictorial History of Medicine.* Springfield, IL: Charles C. Thomas, Publisher, 1962.

Bishop, William J. "Florence Nightingale's Message for Today." *Nursing Outlook* 8:246–247, 1960.

Bullough, Vern L., and Bullough, Bonnie. *The Emergence of Modern Nursing.* 2d ed. New York: The Macmillan Co., 1969.

Cooper, Lenna F. "Florence Nightingale's Contribution to Dietetics." *Journal of the American Dietetic Association* 30:121-127, 1954.

Dietz, Lena Dixon, and Lehozky, Aurelia R. *History and Modern Nursing.* Philadelphia: F.A. Davis Co., 1967.

Dodge, Bertha S. *The Story of Nursing.* Boston: Little, Brown and Co., 1965.

Dolan, Josephine A. *History of Nursing.* 12th ed. Philadelphia: W.B. Saunders Co., 1969.

Griffin, Gerald Joseph, and Griffin, Joanne King. *History and Trends of Professional Nursing.* 7th ed. St. Louis: C.V. Mosby Co., 1973.

Isler, C. "Florence Nightingale, Rebel with a Cause." *RN* 33:35, May 1970.

Jamieson, Elizabeth M.; Sewall, Mary F.; and Suthrie, Eleanor B. *Trends in Nursing History.* Philadelphia: W.B. Saunders Co., 1966.

Kelly, Cordelia W. *Dimensions of Professional Nursing.* 2d ed. New York: Macmillan, Co., 1968.

Nightingale, Florence. "Florence Nightingale at Harley Street." *Midwife and Health Visitor* 7:26, January 1971.

Nightingale, Florence, ed. "To the Probationer Nurses in the Nightingale Fund School at St. Thomas' Hospital." *International Nursing Review* 18, no. 171:3-5.

Roberts, Mary. "Florence Nightingale as a Nurse Educator." *American Journal of Nursing* 37:775, July 1937.

Roxburgh, R. "Miss Nightingale and Miss Clough: Letters from the Crimea." *Victorian Studies* 13:71, September 1969.

Roy, B. "Follow the Lady with the Lamp." *The Nursing Journal of India* 60:259, August 1969.

Seymer, Lucy R. "Mary Crossland of the Nightingale Training School." *American Journal of Nursing* 61:86, 1961.

Shaw, B.L. "Florence Nightingale, Kaiserswerth Revisited." *RN* 33:53, May 1970.

Spalding, Eugenia Kennedy, and Notter, Lucille E. *Professional Nursing.* 7th ed. Philadelphia: J.B. Lippincott Co., 1968.

Walker, Kenneth. *The Story of Medicine.* New York: Oxford University Press, 1955.

Widmer, Carolyn L. "Grandfather and Florence Nightingale." *American Journal of Nursing* 55:569-571, 1955.

_____. "Florence Nightingale. The Early Years." *RN* 33:39, May 1970.

_____. "Florence Nightingale. The Call to War." *RN* 33:42, May 1970.

_____. "Florence Nightingale. The Great Experiment." *RN* 33:46, May 1970.

_____. "Florence Nightingale. The Final Years." *RN* 33:50, May 1970.

_____. *Florence Nightingale.* (081H) Oradell, NJ: Medical Economics Co., 1975.

Chapter 6 The Vanguards of Nursing in America

Achiwa, Goro. "Linda Richards in Japan." *American Journal of Nursing* 68:1716, August 1968.

Becker, Betty Glore, and Hassler, Sister Ruth Ann. *Vocational and Personal Adjustments in Practical Nursing.* 2d ed. St. Louis: C.V. Mosby Co., 1974.

Bullough, Vern L., and Bullough, Bonnie. *The Emergence of Modern Nursing* 2d ed. New York: Macmillan Co., 1969.

Christy, Teresa E. "Portrait of a Leader: Annie Warburton Goodrich." *Nursing Outlook* 18:46, August 1970.

"Civil War Nurses, North and South." *RN* 34:46–47, April 1971.

Cook, Sir Edward. *A Short Life of Florence Nightingale.* Edited by Rosalind Nash. New York: Macmillan Co., 1927.

Dietz, Lena Dixon, and Lehozky, Aurelia R. *History and Modern Nursing.* 2d ed. Philadelphia: F.A. Davis Co., 1967.

Dock, Lavinia, and Stewart, Isabel. *A Short History of Nursing.* New York: G.P. Putnam's Sons, 1931.

Dodge, Bertha S. *The Story of Nursing.* Boston: Little, Brown and Co., 1965.

Dolan, Josephine A. *History of Nursing.* 12th ed. Philadelphia: W.B. Saunders Co., 1968.

"Early Days in the First American Training School for Nurses." *American Journal of Nursing* 73:1574, September 1973.

Griffin, Gerald Joseph, and Griffin, Joanne King. *History and Trends of Professional Nursing.* 7th ed. St. Louis: C.V. Mosby Co., 1973.

Jamieson, Elizabeth M., and Sewall, Mary F. *Trends in Nursing History.* 4th ed. Philadelphia: W.B. Saunders Co., 1954.

Jensen, Deborah M. *History and Trends of Professional Nursing.* St. Louis: C.V. Mosby Co., 1959.

Kleinert, M.N. "Linda Richards and the New England Hospital." *Journal of American Medical Women Association* 23:828, September 1968.

Seymer, Lucy. *Florence Nightingale.* New York: Macmillan Co., 1950.

Smith, Cecil Woodham. *Florence Nightingale.* New York: McGraw-Hill Book Co., 1951.

Chapter 7 The Evolution of Nursing Education

Brown, Esther Lucile. *Nursing for the Future.* New York: Russell Sage Foundation, 1967.

Cherescavich, Gertrude. "Florence, Where Are You?" *The Nursing Clinics of North America* vol. 6, no. 2. Philadelphia: W.B. Saunders Co., June 1971.

Christy, Teresa E. *Cornerstone for Nursing Education.* New York: Teachers College Press, 1969.

Copp, L.A. "Critical Concerns and Commitments of a New Department of Nursing. . .University of Manchester." *International Journal of Nursing Studies* 11:203–210, December 1974.

Dietz, Lena Dixon, and Lehozky, Aurelia R. *History and Modern Nursing.* Philadelphia: F.A. Davis Co., 1967.

Frank, Sister Charles Marie, and Heidgerken, Loretta E. *Perspectives in Nursing Education.* Washington, D.C.: Catholic University of America Press, 1963.

Griffin, Gerald Joseph, and Griffin, Joanne King. *History and Trends of Professional Nursing.* 7th ed. St. Louis: C.V. Mosby Co., 1973.

Johnston, Dorothy F. *History and Trends of Practical Nursing.* St. Louis: C.V. Mosby Co., 1966.

Mitchell, N.J. et al. "Clothing Design for Operating Room Personnel." *Lancet* 2:1133–1136, 9 November 1974.

Smith, Dorothy M. "Is It Too Late?" *Nursing Clinics of North America* vol. 6, no. 2. Philadelphia: W.B. Saunders Co., June 1971.

Chapter 8 The Historical Development of Specialization

Adams, G.F., and McIllwraith, P.L. *Geriatric Nursing.* New York: Oxford University Press, 1963.

Bean, Margaret. "The Nurse-Midwife Today." *American Journal of Nursing* May 1971.

Burgess, Ann C., and Lazare, Aaron. *Psychiatric Nursing in the Hospital and the Community.* Englewood Cliffs, NJ: Prentice-Hall, 1973.

Clausen, Joy, et al. *Maternity Nursing Today.* New York: McGraw-Hill Co., 1973.

Davies, Winifred Talog. *Orthopedics for Nurses.* 4th ed. Revised by Elizabeth Stone. Baltimore: Williams and Wilkins Co., 1971.

Douglas, Ann M. "Psychiatric Nursing in the Curriculum: Purpose and Process." *Curriculum and Instruction.* Washington, D.C.: The Catholic University of America Press, 1970.

Friesner, Arlyne, and Raff, Beverly. *Obstetric Nursing.* New York: Medical Examination Publishing Co., 1974.

Hamilton, Persis Mary. *Basic Maternity Nursing.* 3d ed. St. Louis: C.V. Mosby Co., 1975.

Hirschberg, Gerald G.; Lewis, Leon; and Thomas, Dorothy. *Rehabilitation.* Philadelphia: J.B. Lippincott Co., 1964.

Ingalls, A. Joy, and Salerno, M. Constance. *Maternal and Child Health Nursing.* St. Louis: C.V. Mosby Co., 1975.

Jamieson, Elizabeth M., and Sewall, Mary F. *Trends in Nursing History.* 4th ed. Philadelphia: W.B. Saunders Co., 1954.

Newton, Kathleen, and Anderson, Helen C. *Geriatric Nursing.* St. Louis: C.V. Mosby Co., 1966.

Obrig, Alice. "A Nurse-Midwife in Practice." *American Journal of Nursing* May 1971.

Powell, Mary. *Orthopedic Nursing.* 6th ed. Baltimore: Williams and Wilkins Co., 1968.

Smith, Dorothy W. "Medical-Surgical Nursing in the Curriculum: Purpose and Process." *Curriculum and Instruction.* Washington, D.C.: The Catholic University of America Press, 1970.

Stevens, Marion Keith. *Geriatric Nursing for Practical Nurses.* Philadelphia: W.B. Saunders Co., 1966.

SECTION 3 EDUCATION FOR NURSES

Chapter 9 The RN: Diploma Schools and Associate Degree Programs

Brown, Esther Lucile. *Nursing for the Future.* New York: Russell Sage Foundation, 1967.

Evans, Patricia A. "University Without Walls Nursing Program." *Associate Degree Education for Nursing Current Issues, 1974.* New York: National League for Nursing, 1974.

Frank, Sister Charles Marie, and Heidgerken, Loretta E. *Perspectives in Nursing Education.* Washington, D.C.: The Catholic University of America Press, 1968.

Graduates of Diploma Schools of Nursing. no. G-115. Kansas City, MO: American Nurses' Association.

"Hospital Schools as Vital as Ever." *Hospitals* 49:69-71, January 1975.

Lenburg, Carrie B. "Innovations in Nursing Education – The Regents External Degree Program in Nursing." *Associate Degree Education for Nursing Current Issues, 1974.* New York: NLN, 1974.

Meleis, A.I. et al. "Operation Concern: a Study of Senior Nursing Students in Three Nursing Programs." *Nursing Research* 23:461-468, November/December 1974.

Montag, Mildred L. *Community College Education for Nursing.* New York: McGraw-Hill Book Co., Blakiston Division, 1959.

Rasmussen, Sandra, ed. *Technical Nursing/Dimensions and Dynamics.* Philadelphia: F.A. Davis Co., 1972.

Rauffenbart, Suzanne. "National Legislation – Implications for Diploma Programs." *The Changing Role of the Hospital and Implications for Nursing Education.* New York: NLN, 1974.

Sheahan, Sister Dorothy. "Degree, Yes – Education, No." *Nursing Outlook* 22:26, January 1974.

Wozniak, Dolores. "External Degrees in Nursing." *American Journal of Nursing* pp. 1014-1018, June 1973.

Zeitz, Ann N.; Howard, Lelia D.; Christy, Elva M.; and Tax, Hariette Simington. *Associate Degree Nursing.* St. Louis: C.V. Mosby Co., 1969.

Chapter 10 The RN: Baccalaureate, Master, and Doctoral Programs

A Statement of Concern About Degree Programs for Nursing Students That Have No Major in Nursing. New York: NLN, 1971.

Baccalaureate and Masters Degree Programs in Nursing Accredited by NLN-1973-74. Pub. no. 15-1310R. New York: NLN, 1973.

Baccalaureate Education for Graduates of Diploma and Associate Degree Programs. Pub. no. 15-1150. New York: NLN, 1964.

Baccalaureate Programs Accredited for Public Health Nursing Preparation-1973-74. Pub. no. 15-1313. New York: NLN, 1973.

Brown, Esther Lucile. *Nursing for the Future.* New York: Russell Sage Foundation, 1967.

Characteristics of Baccalaureate Education in Nursing. Pub. no. 15-1319. New York: NLN, 1968.

Characteristics of Graduate Education in Nursing. Pub. no. 15-1318. New York: NLN, 1968.

College Education: Key to a Professional Career in Nursing-1973-74. Pub. no. 15-1311. New York: NLN, 1973.

Criteria for the Appraisal of Baccalaureate and Higher Degree Programs in Nursing. Pub. no. 15-1251. New York: NLN, 1972.

Davis, Fred, ed. *The Nursing Profession. Five Sociological Essays.* New York: John Wiley and Sons, 1967.

Directory of Career Mobility Opportunities in Nursing Education. Pub. no. 19-1485. New York: NLN Division of Research, 1973.

Doctoral Programs in Nursing/Nurse Scientist Graduate Training Grants Program-1973. Pub. no. 15-1448. New York: NLN, 1973.

Extending the Boundaries of Nursing Education – The Preparation and Roles of the Clinical Specialist. Pub. no. 15-1367. New York: NLN, 1969.

Extending the Boundaries of Nursing Education – The Preparation and Roles of the Functional Specialist. Pub. no. 15-1397. New York: NLN, 1970.

Extending the Boundaries of Nursing Education – The Preparation and Role of the Nurse Scientist. Pub. no. 15-1342. New York: NLN, 1968.

Facts About Nursing. New York: American Nurses' Association, 1973.

Frank, Sister Charles Marie, and Heidgerken, Loretta E. *Perspectives in Nursing Education.* Washington, D.C.: Catholic University of America Press, 1968.

From Diploma School to College: Two Case Studies on Changing Patterns Within Institutions for Nursing Education. New York: The National Commission for the Study of Nursing and Nursing Education, 1972.

Liebow, Phoebe Recht. "Learning the UWW Way." *American Journal of Nursing* pp. 694-695, April 1974.

Millard, R.M. et al. *Developing Nursing Programs in Institutions of Higher Education.* no. 14-1533. New York: NLN Divison of Nursing, 1974.

Ozimek Dorothy. *The Baccalaureate Graduate in Nursing: What Does Society Expect?* no. 15-1520. New York: NLN, 1974.

_____ . *Accreditation of Baccalaureate and Masters Degree Programs in Nursing.* no. 15-1519. New York: NLN, 1974.

Schools of Nursing/R.N.-1973. no. 41-1484. New York: NLN, 1973.

Some Statistics on Baccalaureate and Higher Degree Programs in Nursing — 1974-1975. no. 19-1609. New York: NLN, 1976.

State-Approved Schools of Nursing — RN. Pub. no. 19-1479. New York: NLN, 1973.

Chapter 11   The LPN: Vocational Education

Brown, Esther Lucile. *Nursing for the Future.* New York: Russell Sage Foundation, 1967.

Chayer, Mary Ella. *Nursing in Modern Society.* New York: G.P. Putnam's Sons, 1947.

Dietz, Lena Dixon, and Lehozky, Aurelia. *History and Modern Nursing.* Philadelphia: F.A. Davis Co., 1967.

Clinical Teaching. New York: National Association for Practical Nurse Education and Service, 1953.

Frank, Sister Charles Marie, and Heidgerken, Loretta E. *Perspectives in Nursing Education.* Washington, D.C.: The Catholic University of America Press, 1968.

Kerr, Elizabeth E. et al. *An Analysis of Selected Educational Programs in Practical Nursing.* Iowa City: The University of Iowa Press, April 1970.

Knopf, Lucille; Tate, Barbara L.; and Patrylow, Sarah. *Five Years After Graduation. Practical Nurses' Nurse Career-Pattern Study.* no. 19-1399. New York: NLN, 1970.

Lee, Jane A.; Herzog, Ruth R.; and Morrison, John K. Jr. *Licensed Practical Nurses in Occupational Health.* DHEW Pub. no. (N 10SH) 74-102. OH: National Institute for Occupational Safety and Health, 1974.

Parkhurst, R. "The New Nurse." *Nursing Care* 7:18-21, November 1974.

"Practical Nurse Education." *Nursing Outlook* pp. 366-369, July 1955.

Practical Nurse Testing Services. New York: The Psychological Corporation, 1970.

Practical Nursing Curriculum. Suggestions for Developing a Program of Instruction Based Upon the Analysis of the Practical Nurse Occupation, pp. 1-9 and 15. Washington, D.C.: United States Government Printing Office, 1950.

State-Approved Schools of Nursing – L.P.N./L.V.N. 1974. Pub. no. 19-1517. New York: NLN.

Tate, Barbara L., and Knopf, Lucille. *Nurse Career-Pattern Study.* part 1. Practical Nursing Programs. New York: NLN, 1968.

Tomlinson, Robert M.; Langdon, Lois M.; Huck, John F.; and Hindhede, Lois A. *Background, Characteristics and Success of Practical Nursing Applicants. Students and Graduates.* Urbana, IL: University of Illinois Press, September 1971.

"What are we Doing about the Practical Nurse?" *ANA in Review 1*, no. 3:1, Autumn 1954.

Chapter 12 Technical vs. Professional Nursing

Alfano, Genrose J. "Healing or Caretaking – Which Will it Be?" *The Nursing Clinics of North America.* vol. 6, no. 2. Philadelphia: W.B. Saunders Co., June 1971.

Allen, Virginia O. "Associate Degree Graduates: Generalists or Specialists?" *Journal of Nursing Education* 13:4-7, April 1974.

_____ . *Community College Nursing Education.* New York: John Wiley and Sons, 1971.

Ashkenas, Thais Levberg. *Aids and Deterrents to the Performance of Associate Degree Graduates in Nursing.* New York: National League for Nursing, 1973.

Bowar, Susan. "Enabling Professional Practice Through Leadership Skills." *The Nursing Clinics of North America.* vol. 6, no. 2. Philadelphia: W.B. Saunders Co., June 1971.

Caladarci, Arthur P. "What About the Word Profession?" *American Journal of Nursing* pp. 468-470, March 1974.

Dietz, Lena Dixon, and Lehozky, Aurelia. *History and Modern Nursing.* Philadelphia: F.A. Davis Co., 1967.

Loomis, M.E. "Collegiate Nursing Education: An Ambivalent Professionalism." *Journal of Nursing Education* 13:39-48, November 1974.

Matheney, Ruth V. "Technical Nursing Practice." *Associate Degree Education for Nursing Current Issues, 1974.* New York: NLN, 1974.

Miller, Michael H. "Work Roles for the Associate Degree Graduate." *American Journal of Nursing* pp. 468-470, March 1974.

Montag, Mildred L. *Community College Education for Nursing.* New York: McGraw-Hill Book Co., 1959.

Peplau, Hildegard E. "A.N.A. and the Professional Nurse." *Associate Degree Education for Nursing Current Issues, 1974.* New York: NLN, 1974.

Rasmussen, Sandra, ed. *Technical Nursing/Dimensions and Dynamics.* Philadelphia: F.A. Davis Co., 1972.

SECTION 4 HEALTH CARE AND THE CONSUMER

Chapter 13 Contemporary Health Care

Amenta, Madalon M. "Free Clinics Change the Scene." *American Journal of Nursing* 74:284-288, February 1974.

Bricker, P.W. et al. *The Changing Role of the Hospital and Implications for Nursing Education.* no. 16-1551. New York: NLN Department of Diploma Programs, 1974.

Brown, Elta. "Nursing: A Health Care Specialty." *The Nursing Clinics of North America.* vol. 6, no. 2. Philadelphia: W.B. Saunders Co., June 1971.

Brown, Esther Lucile. *Nursing for the Future.* New York: Russell Sage Foundation, 1967.

Christensen, V.A. "Nursing in a Changing World." *Journal of Psychiatric Nursing* 12:39-43, November/December 1974.

Claflin, M. et al. *Community Health Services in the Health Care Delivery System.* no. 21-1524. New York: NLN, 1974.

Clark, Carolyn Chambers. *Nursing Concepts and Processes.* Albany, NY: Delmar Publishers, 1977.

"Community Services and Residential Institutions for Children." *Children Today* 3:15-17, November/December 1974.

Cornell, S.A. et al. "Computerized Schedules and Care Plans." *Nursing Outlook* 21:781-784, December 1973.

Daugherty, M.C. "A Cultural Approach to the Nurse's Role in Health-Care Planning." *Nursing Forum* 11, no. 3: 311-322, 1972.

Evang, K. "Human Rights – Health for Everyone." *World Health* 3:11, November 1973.

Evans, M. "The Future Role of Nurses in the Delivery of Health Care in Urban Areas." *The Australian Nurses' Journal* 3:38-40, December 1973.

Farmer, R. "Community Care – A Model System." *International Journal of Nursing Studies* 11:21-32, June 1974.

Flomenhoft, K. et al. "Family Therapy Training: a Statewide Program for Mental Health Centers. . ." *Community Psychiatry* 25:789-791, December 1974.

Frank, D. "The Process of Implementing the Nurse's Role in a Neighborhood Center." *Journal of Psychiatric Nursing* 12:33-38, March/April 1974.

Fredericks, M.A. et al. "Demographic Findings and Health Care: A Model for Student Nurses." *Hospital Progress* 54:72, May 1973.·

Freeman, R. "Nurse Practitioners in the Community Health Agency." *Journal of Nursing Administration* 4:21-24, November/December 1974.

French, Ruth M. *The Dynamics of Health Care.* 2d ed. New York: McGraw-Hill Book Co., 1974.

Gentry, J.T. "A More Rational Approach to Health Care Delivery." *Nursing Digest* 2:25-35, March 1974.

Gilchrist, J.M. et al. "The Nature of Nursing in the Health Care Structure." *Nursing Papers* 5:3-13, December 1973.

HMO Sourcebook, 1973 Edition. Prepared under the supervision of Gerald Seifert, J.D., Rockville, MD: Health Law Center, Aspen Systems Corporation.

Hammerman, J. "Health Services: Their Success and Failure in Reaching Older Adults." *American Journal of Public Health* 64:253-256, March 1974.

Health Care Needs — Basis for Change. Pub. no. 20-1332. New York: National League for Nursing.

"Interdependence: Changing Practice Styles for Improved Health Care." (editorial) *P.A. Journal* 3:3-4, Fall 1973.

Janzen, Sharon Ann. "Psychiatric Day Care in a Rural Area." *American Journal of Nursing* pp. 2216-2217, December 1974.

Jeppson, D.H. "Projected Changes in the Health Care Delivery System. The Effects on LP/VNs." *Journal of Practical Nursing* 23:20, July 1973.

Johnson, E.F. "Modern Implementation of Denmark's Tradition of Health Care Delivery." *Health Services Reports* 88:624-630, August/September 1973.

Jones, A. et al. "Nursing Center for Family Health Services . . . Freeport, Long Island, New York." *Nursing Digest* 2:38-41, Summer 1974.

Lewis, Mary Ann. "Child-Initiated Care." *American Journal of Nursing* 74: 652-655, April 1974.

Leininger, M. "Health Care Delivery Systems for tomorrow — possibilities and guidelines." *Washington State Journal of Nursing* 45:10-16, Winter 1973.

Mancioux, M. "A New Concept — Family Care." *International Nursing Review* 20:85, May/June 1973.

McKay, H. "Membership Patterns and Attitudes of Hospital Nurses." *Nursing Times* 70:1547-1549, 3 October 1974.

Mauksch, I. "Nursing Practice in a Changing World." *Minnesota Nursing Accent* 46:55-58, December 1974.

Mechaber, J. et al. "Analysis of the Triage System in a Neighborhood Health Center . . . Rochester Neighborhood Health Center." *Journal of Nursing Administration* 4:29-32, November/December 1974.

Morrow, J.F. et al. *Developing Strategies to Effect Change.* no. 52-1537. New York: NLN Division of Community Planning, 1974.

Mosey, A.C. "Meeting Health Needs." *Nursing Digest* 2:93-96, May 1974.

Murray, Ruth. *Nursing Concepts for Health Promotion.* Englewood Cliffs, NJ: Prentice-Hall, 1975.

Novak, B. "Home Nursing Care Program on an Indian Reservation." *Public Health Reports* 89:545-550,November/December 1974.

Pluckhan, M.L. "A Problem Affecting the Delivery of Health Care." *Nursing Forum* 11, no. 3:300-310, 1972.

"Professional Nursing in Health Care Delivery Systems: Position Statement of the Board of Directors, Texas Nurses' Association August 1974." *Texas Nursing* 48:5, September 1974.

Schlotfeldt, R.M. "New Modes of Health Care." *Washington State Journal of Nursing* 45:3, Fall 1973.

_____. "Planning for Progress." *Nursing Outlook* 21:766-769, December 1973.

Schuler, S. et al. "The Theme is Change . . . V.A. Hospital, Providence, Rhode Island." *Journal of Psychiatric Nursing* 12:15-22, July/August 1974.

Scott, J.M. "The Changing Health Care Environment: Its Implications for Nursing." *American Journal of Public Health* 64:364-369, April 1974.

Shannon, Gary W., and Dever, G.E. Alan. *Health Care Delivery: Spatial Perspectives.* New York: McGraw-Hill Book Co., 1974.

Todd, M.C. "U.S. Health Care and You." *Journal of Practical Nursing* 24:14, July 1974.

Trail, Ira D. "The Legal Implications of Community Nursing Care." *The Nursing Clinics of North America* vol. 9, no. 3. Philadelphia: W.B. Saunders Co., September 1974.

Velie, L. "The Shocking Truth About our Childrens' Health Care." *Readers Digest* 104:170, May 1974.

Wagner, Doris. "Nursing in an HMO." *American Journal of Nursing* pp. 236-238, February 1974.

"WHO Studying New Health Care Systems." *RANF Review* 5:7, July 1974.

Williams, A.F. et al. "Interrelationship of Preventive Actions in Health and Other Areas." *Health Services Reports* 87:969-976, December 1972.

Wilson, V.E. et al. "Health Care Policy Issues in the 1970's." *Health Services Reports* 87:879-885, December 1972.

Chapter 14 The Health Care Consumer

"AHA 'Bill of Rights' for Patients." *OR Reporter* 8:15, February 1973.

Annas, George J. et al. "The Patient Rights Advocate." *Journal of Nursing Administration* 4:25-31, May/June 1974.

Annas, George J. *The Rights of Hospital Patients.* American Civil Liberties Handbook. New York: Avon Books, 1975.

Bloom, B.S. et al. "The Rising Cost of CCUs." *RN* 37:4, December 1974.

Carnegie, M. Elizabeth. "The Patient's Bill of Rights." *Jamaican Nurse* 13:31, December 1973/January 1974.

_____. "The Patient's Bill of Rights and the Nurse." *The Nursing Clinics of North America* vol. 9, no. 3. Philadelphia: W.B. Saunders Co., December 1974.

Curran, W.J. "The Patient's Bill of Rights Becomes Law. . .Minnesota Law." *Nursing Digest* 2:29-31, September 1974.

"Disclosing Clinical Risks to Patients." *Regan Reports on Nursing Law* 15:1, December 1974.

Eddy, Lyndall, and Westbrook, Linde. "Multi-disciplinary Retrospective Patient Care Audit." *American Journal of Nursing* 75:961-963, June 1975.

Englehardt, S. "How to Avoid Needless Surgery." *Readers Digest* 105: 162-165, December 1974.

Ennis, Bruce, and Siegel, Loren. *The Rights of Mental Patients.* American Civil Liberties Handbook. New York: Avon Books, 1975.

Gaylin, W. "The Patient's Bill of Rights." *Nursing Digest* 1:89-91, November 1973.

Hanna, Karolyn K. "Nursing Audit at a Community Hospital." *Nursing Outlook* 24:33-37, January 1976.

"How to Pay Less for Prescription Drugs." *Consumer Report* 40:48-53, January 1975.

Long, Edna S. "How to Survive Hospitalization." *American Journal of Nursing* 74:486-488, March 1974.

Mahoney, M. "Patients Are People, Too!" *Family Health* 6:24, August 1974.

Maisel, A.Q. "How to Hold Down Rising Hospital Costs." *Readers Digest* 105:147-150, November 1974.

Novak, Benjamin J., and Cohn, Ronald E. "From the Patient's Point of View." *Nursing Care* pp. 28-29, June 1975.

PSRO. Program Information and Resources. Chicago: AMA, Division of Medical Practice, 1975.

Quinn, N.K., and Somers, A.R. "The Patient's Bill of Rights. A Significant Aspect of the Consumer Revolution." *Nursing Outlook* 22:240-244, April 1974.

Ramphal, Marjorie. "Peer Review." *American Journal of Nursing* 74:63-67, January 1974.

Rozovsky, L.E. "A Canadian Patient's Bill of Rights." *Dimensions in Health Service* 51:8-10, December 1974.

Ryan, John L. "The Single Room: A Right for Every Patient's Privacy." *Nursing Digest* pp. 46–47, September/October 1975.

Symposium on Current Legal and Professional Problems. "The Patient's Bill of Rights and the Nurse." *The Nursing Clinics of North America.* vol. 9. Philadelphia: W.B. Saunders Co., September 1974.

"The Patient's Bill of Rights." *Jamaican Nurse.* 13:31, December 1973/ January 1974.

"The Patient's Bill of Rights is a 12 Point Lesson Plan." *In-Service Training Education* 2:28, October 1973.

Chapter 15 New Roles and New Responsibilities for Nurses

Andrus, L.H. et al. "Assistants to Primary Physicians in California." *Western Journal of Medicine* 122:80–86, January 1975.

Aradine, C.R. "Development of a Family Health Service. Experiences of a Clinical Nurse Specialist." *Journal of Nursing Administration* 4:45–51, January/February 1974.

Barkin, R.M. "Directions for Statutory Change: The Physician Extender." *American Journal of Public Health* 64:1132–1137, December 1974.

Bates, B. "Doctor and Nurse: Changing Roles and Relations." *Nursing Digest* 2:70–75, October 1974.

Beletz, Elaine E. "Is Nursing's Public Image up to Date?" *Nursing Outlook* NLN 22, no. 7:432–435, July 1974.

Birenbaum, A. "The Pediatric Nurse Practitioner and Preventive Community Mental Health." *Journal of Psychiatric Nursing* 12:14–19, September/ October 1974.

Brown, Esther Lucile. *Nursing for the Future.* New York: Russell Sage Foundation, 1967.

_____ . *Nursing Reconsidered: A Study of Change.* part 1. Philadelphia: J.B. Lippincott Co., 1970.

Browning, Mary H., and Lewis, Edith P. *The Expanded Role of the Nurse.* no. C-10. Kansas City, MO: ANA.

Building for the Future. no. NP-47. Kansas City, MO: ANA.

Burd, M. "Changing Responsibilities." *World of Irish Nursing* 3:218–220, December 1974.

Charles, G. et al. "Physicians' Assistants and Clinical Algorithms in Health Care Delivery." *Annals of Internal-Medicine* 81:733–739, December 1974.

Christensen, V.A. "Nursing in a Changing World." *Journal of Psychiatric Nursing* 12:39–43, November/December 1974.

Creighton, Helen et al. "What will Nursing be Like in the '80's?" part 1. *The Maryland Nurse* 3:1-4, June 1972.

Creighton, Helen, and Squaires, G. Marjorie. "School Nurses: Legal Aspects of Their Work." *The Nursing Clinics of North America.* vol. 9, no. 3. Philadelphia: W.B. Saunders Co., September 1974.

DeAngelis, Catherine, and Curran, William J. "The Legal Implications of the Extended Roles of Professional Nurses." *The Nursing Clinics of North America.* vol. 9, no. 3. Philadelphia: W.B. Saunders Co., September 1974.

"Define Nurse Roles." *Pelican News* 30:8, Winter 1974.

Distributive Nursing Practice: Development and Fusion of the Roles. New York: National Council of School Nurses, 1972 (pamphlet).

"Divided We Fall." (editorial) *Nursing Outlook* 22:159, March 1974.

DuGas, Beverly Witter. "Nursing's Expanded Role in Canada." *The Nursing Clinics of North America.* vol. 9, no. 3. Philadelphia: W.B. Saunders Co., September 1974.

Episodic Nursing Practice: Refinement and Expansion of the Roles. New York: National Council of School Nurses, 1972 (pamphlet).

Ford, Loretta C. "Interdisciplinary Education for Nurses in the Expanded Role: The Way of the Future." *Building for the Future* no. NP-47. Kansas City, MO: ANA, 1975.

_____ . "Nurse Practitioners: What the Future Holds." *American Nurse* 6:4, November 1974.

_____ . "One Nurse's View of Pediatric Nurse Practitioners." *Pediatrics* 54:534-537, November 1974.

Frank, D. "The Process of Implementing the Nurse's Role in a Neighborhood Center." *Journal of Psychiatric Nursing* 12:33-38, March/April 1974.

Freeman, R. "Nurse Practitioners in the Community Health Agency." *Journal of Nursing Administration* 4:21-24, November/December 1974.

Functions and Qualifications for an Occupational Health Nurse in a One-Nurse Service. no. CH-1. Kansas City, MO: ANA.

Galloway, B.T. "The Nurse as a Professional Manager." *Hospitals* 48:89, November 1974.

Gilchrist, J.M. "The Roles and Functions of Nursing." *Nursing Papers* 5: 25-30, December 1973.

Gortner, S.R. "Scientific Accountability in Nursing." *Nursing Outlook* 22: 764-768, December 1974.

Guidelines for Short-Term Continuing Education Programs Preparing the Geriatric Nurse Practitioner no. GE-3. Kansas City, MO: ANA.

Guidelines for Short-Term Continuing Education Programs for the Nurse Clinician in Intensive Neonatal Care and the Nurse Clinician in Intensive Maternal-Fetal Care. no. MCH-4. Kansas City, MO: ANA.

Hanton, E. Michael. *The New Nurse.* Bangor, ME: L.H. Thompson, 1973.

Haupt, Roberta Lyn. "Pediatric Nurse Practitioner." *The Nursing Clinics of North America.* vol. 9, no. 3 Philadelphia: W.B. Saunders Co., September 1974.

Henrion, R.P. "Family Nurse Therapist: A Model of Communication." *Journal of Psychiatric Nursing* 12:10-13, November/December 1974.

Hinsvark, Inez G. "Implications for Action in the Expanded Role of the Nurse." *The Nursing Clinics of North America.* vol. 9, no. 3. Philadelphia: W.B. Saunders Co., September 1974.

Houtz, D.T. et al. *Crisis in Nursing – Changing Roles.* National League for Nursing pub. no. 20-1503. New York: Council of Hospital Related Institutional Services, 1973.

Januska, Charlotte et al. "Development of a Family Nurse Practitioner Curriculum." *American Journal of Nursing* 22:103, February 1974.

Jones, A. et al. "Nursing Center for Family Health Services. . .Freeport, Long Island, New York." *Nursing Digest* 2:38-41, Summer 1974.

Judge, D. "The New Nurse: a Sense of Duty and Destiny." *Modern Health Care* 2:21-27, October 1974.

Kohnke, Mary F.; Zimmern, Ann; and Greenidge, Jocelyn. *The Independent Nurse Practitioner.* New York: Trainex Corp., 1974.

Lambertsen, Eleanor C. "Let's Get the Nurse's Role into Focus." *Nursing Digest* 2:92-96, Summer 1974.

_____ . "The Changing Role of Nursing and its Regulation." *The Nursing Clinics of North America.* Philadelphia: W.B. Saunders Co., September 1974.

Linton, C.B. et al. "The Role of the Nurse in Patient Teaching as Previewed by Physicians in Madison and Jackson Counties." *Alabama Nurse* 3:16-17, December 1974.

McAtee, P.A. et al. "Nurse Practitioners for Children — Past and Future." *Pediatrics* 54:578-582, November 1974.

McKay, H. "Membership Patterns and Attitudes of Hospital Nurses." *Nursing Times* 70:1547-1549, 3 October 1974.

McLaren, P.M. et al. "The Community Nurse Goes to Jail." *Nursing Outlook* 22:35-39, January 1974.

McNelly, P. "Extending the Nursing Role in a Patient Care Setting." *Journal of Continuing Education in Nursing* 2:36-42, July/August 1971.

Maglacas, A.M. "Effective Nursing Practice in the Health Care Services." *Newsette* 9:21-25, April/June 1969.

Mauksch, I. "Nursing Practice in a Changing World." *Minnesota Nursing Accent* 46:55-58, December 1974.

Mechaber, J. et al. "Analysis of the Triage System in a Neighborhood Health Center. . .Rochester Neighborhood Health Center." *Journal of Nursing Administration* 4:29-32, November/December 1974.

Nuckolls, K.B. "Who Decides What the Nurse Can Do?" *Nursing Outlook* 22:626-631, October 1974.

Nurse Clinician and Physicians' Assistant: The Relationship Between Two Emerging Practitioner Concepts. New York: National Council of School Nurses, 1972 (pamphlet).

"Nurse in Private Practice – a New Role." *Nursing News* (Connecticut) 47:1, November 1974.

"Nurses and Physicians' Assistants Vis-a-Vis." *New Jersey State Nurses Association News* 4:20-22, September/October 1974.

Nursing at the Crossroads. no. R-11. Kansas City, MO: ANA.

Olsen, Lois. "The Expanded Role of the Nurse in Maternity Practice." *The Nursing Clinics of North America.* vol. 9, no. 3. Philadelphia: W.B. Saunders, September 1974.

"PA's Step Out on Their Own." *Medical World News* 16:23-25, 13 January 1975.

Preparing Registered Nurses for Expanded Roles. DHEW pub. no. (NIH) 74-31. Kansas City, MO: ANA, 1973.

Recommendations on Educational Preparation and Definition of the Expanded Role and Functions of the School Nurse Practitioner. no. CH-3. Kansas City, MO: ANA.

Rodgers, J.A. "The Clinical Specialist as a Change Agent." *Journal of Psychiatric Nursing* 12:5-9. November/December 1974.

Schweer, S.F. et al. "The Extended Role of Professional Nursing – Patient Education." *International Nursing Review* 20:174, November/December 1973.

Scope of Practice for the Pediatric Nurse Practitioner. Reprinted from *The American Nurse.* no. AN-1. Kansas City, MO: ANA, July 1974.

Smith, Stuart L., and English, John. "Nurse-Therapists in a General Hospital's Psychiatric Unit." *Nursing Digest* pp. 58-60, September/October 1975.

Stevens, B.J. "A Second Look at 'New Position Descriptions'." *Journal of Nursing Administration* 3:21-23, November/December 1973.

Sweet, B.R. "Patients' Reactions to Male Midwives." *Nursing Times* 70:1619-1620, 17 October 1974.

"The Nurse Practitioner Question." *American Journal of Nursing* 74:2188-2191, December 1974.

The Nurse in Research: ANA Guidelines on Ethical Values. no. D-31. Kansas City, MO: ANA.

The Nurse Practitioner: Preparation and Practice. no. R-16. Kansas City, MO: ANA.

The Role of the Nurse in Drug Abuse Treatment. no. NP-45. Kansas City, MO: ANA.

Trail, Ira D. "The Legal Implications of Community Nursing Care." *The Nursing Clinics of North America.* vol. 9, no. 3. Philadelphia: W.B. Saunders Co., September 1974.

Chapter 16 The Health Care Team

Allied Health Education. Directory Missouri/Illinois. St. Louis: Health Delivery Systems, 1974.

Andrus, L.H. et al. "Managing the Health Care Team." *PA Journal* 3:5-22, Fall 1973.

Bakke, Kathy. "Primary Nursing: Perceptions of a Staff Nurse." *American Journal of Nursing* 74:1434.

Campbell, Emily, and Johnson, Betty. "It's Time to be Realistic About the Work Load." *American Journal of Nursing* 66, no. 6:1282, June 1966.

Clark, Carolyn Chambers. *Nursing Concepts and Processes.* Albany, NY: Delmar Publishers, 1977.

Cooper, Signe Skott. *Contemporary Nursing Practice.* part 1. New York: McGraw-Hill Book Co., 1970.

Douglass, Laura Mae. *Review of Team Nursing.* St. Louis: C.V. Mosby Co., 1973.

DuVal, M.K. "Together We Stand." *Journal of Allied Health* 2:45-50, Spring 1973.

Golden, A.S. et al. "Non-physician Family Health Teams." *Nursing Digest* 11:49-54, September 1974.

Griffin, N.M. "Health Manpower: Trends and Issues." *Journal of School Health* 44:310-313, June 1974.

Mase, D.J. "Allied Health – Today and Tomorrow." *Journal of Allied Health* 2:56-66, Spring 1973.

McAnulty, Elizabeth. "Can a Team Leader Become Involved." *American Journal of Nursing* 65, no. 7:128-132, July 1965.

Nolan, Mary. "Team Nursing in the OR." *American Journal of Nursing* 74, no. 2:272-274, February 1974.

Parramore, B., and Yeager, W. "Team Nursing in Public Health." *Nursing Outlook* June 1968.

Pellegrino, Ed. "Allied Health Concept – Fact or Friction?" *Journal of Allied Health* 3:79-84, Spring 1974.

Peterson, Grace G. *Working with Others for Patient Care.* 2d ed. Dubuque, IA: William C. Brown and Co., 1973.

Pittsburgh Mercy Hospital Staff. *A Manual for Team Nursing.* St. Louis: The Catholic Hospital Association, 1968.

Ramphal, Marjorie. "A Rationale for Assignments." *American Journal of Nursing* 67, no. 8:1630, August 1967.

Robinson, Alice M. "Primary Nurse: Specialist in Total Care." *RN* 37:31, 1974.

Saunders, Mary. "Primary Nursing Care in a Hospital Setting." *Developing Strategies to Effect Change.* New York: NLN, 1974.

Sister Regina Elizabeth. "The Team Assignment Plan." *Hospital Progress* 46, no. 2:76-82, February 1965.

Smith, Elizabeth, and Huber, Barbara. *Concepts in Leadership for the Licensed Practical Nurse.* St. Louis: C.V. Mosby Co., 1973.

Stevenson, Neva. "The Better Utilization of Licensed Practical Nurses." *Nursing Outlook* 65, no. 7:34, July 1965.

Swansburg, Russell C. *Team Nursing.* New York: G.P. Putnam's Sons, 1968.

Tappan, Frances M. *Toward Understanding Administrators in the Medical Environment.* New York: Macmillan Publishing Co., 1968.

Todd, M. "Medicine and the Allied Health Professions." *Journal of Allied Health* 3:73-78, Spring 1974.

SECTION 5 THE NURSING COMMUNITY AND THE LAW

Chapter 17 Professional Organizations

"Academy of Nursing Governing Council." *Journal of Nursing Administration* 3:43, July/August 1973.

Beaman, A.L. "From a Mustard Seed." *Journal of Continuing Education in Nursing* 2:43, July/August 1971.

Bowman, R.A. "The Nursing Organization as a Political Pressure Group." *Nursing Forum* 12, no. 1:72-81, 1973.

Bridges, Daisy Caroline. *A History of the International Council of Nurses 1899-1964.* Philadelphia: J.B. Lippincott Co., 1967.

Cahoon, M.C. "A Canadian Council of Nurse Researchers." *Nursing Papers* 6:7-8, Fall 1974.

Christie, L.S. "A Chance for the Nursing Profession?" *Nursing Times* 67: 1375-1376, 4 November 1971.

Collins, J.M. "The Making of an Organization." *Occupational Health Nursing* 20:14-17, November 1972.

"Dynamics of a Local Unit." *Reporter* 7:4, October 1974.

Evans, A. "The Need for a Strong Nurses' Organization." *Australian Nurses Journal* 4:27, August 1974.

Facts About Nursing. no. D–41 5M. Kansas City, MO: ANA, 1974.

Ford, B. "Caring is . . . Speaking out for Nurses and Nursing." *Colorado Nurse* 74:1, November 1974.

Freeman, R.B. "N.L.N. at Twenty: Challenge and Change." *Nursing Outlook* 20:376–384, June 1972.

"Guide for Organizing an Agency Chapter." *Alabama Nurse* 31:9, December 1974.

Hall, C.M. "Who Controls the Nursing Profession?" *Australian Nurses' Journal* 3:29–32, August 1973.

Higgs, Z. et al. "Nursing Leadership Needed for Our Transitional Times." *Journal of New York State Nurses Association* 5:20–24, November 1974.

Illustrious Past, Challenging Future. no. R–4, Kansas City, MO: ANA.

Jarrett, L. "The Modern Student Nurse and her Professional Organization." *International Nursing Review* 18, no. 1:31–39, 1971.

Newcomb, R.F. "Nursing Finds a New National Voice." *RN* 36:60, March 1973.

Nightingale, A. "A Professional Organization." *New Zealand Nursing Journal* 66:9, December 1973.

Russey, F. "A Constituent League in Action." *Nursing Outlook* 19:325–327, May 1971.

Scott, D. et al. "Reflections on Convention." *New Jersey State Nurses Association News* 4:1–10, November/December 1974.

Turnbull, J. "Keep your Powder Dry." *New Zealand Nursing Journal* 68:26, August 1974.

"Unified Effort by R.N.'s is Termed Key to Power." *OR Reporter* 9:1, June 1974.

Walsh, Margaret E. *The Health Profession Education Organization and the Governmental Process.* no. 14–1541. New York: NLN, 1974.

Widmer, C.L. "Sigma Theta Tau: Golden Anniversary." *Nursing Outlook* 20:786–788, December 1972.

Chapter 18 Nursing Practice Acts and Licensure

Agree, B.C. "The Threat of Institutional Licensure." *American Journal of Nursing* 73:1758–1763, October 1973.

"A.N.A. Issues State Board Guidelines." *Washington State Journal of Nursing* 46:7, Spring 1974.

Beswetherick, M.A. "What Does 'RN' after your Name Really Mean?" *Canadian Nurse* 68:27-28, October 1972.

"Citizenship No Longer Requisite for Licensure." *CHART* 71:2, March 1974.

Creighton, Helen. "Institutional Licensure." *Supervisor Nurse* 5:11, March 1974.

Driscoll, V. "Liberating Nursing Practice." *Nursing Outlook* 20:24-28, January 1972.

Dunkley, Pearl H. "The A.N.A. Certification Program." *The Nursing Clinics of North America* vol. 9, no. 3. Philadelphia: W.B. Saunders Co., September 1974.

Egelston, E.M. "Continuing Education: A Requirement for Professional Membership or a Necessity for Relicensure." *The Journal of Continuing Education in Nursing* 5:12-20, May/June 1974.

_____. "Institutional Licensure: What's Up?" *Nursing Care* 7:26-30, January 1974.

Forni, P.R. "Trends in Licensure and Certification." *Journal of Nursing Administration* 3:17-23, September/October 1973.

Guy, J.S. "Institutional Licensure: A Dilemma for Nurses." *The Nursing Clinics of North America* vol. 9. Philadelphia: W.B. Saunders Co., September 1974.

Hall, Virginia C. "Legal Problems Stemming from the Nurse and Medical Practice Acts." *Building for the Future.* no. NP 47 2M. Kansas City, MO: ANA, 1975.

Hershey, N. "Nursing Practice Acts and Professional Delusion." *Journal of Nursing Administration* 4:36-39, July/August 1974.

Hick, F. "Dimensions of Licensing." *Texas Nursing* 48:4-7, June 1974.

"Individual Licensure and Quality Nursing." *Regan Reports on Nursing Law* 14:1, June 1973.

Kelly, L.Y. "Institutional Licensure." *Nursing Outlook* 21:566-572, September 1973.

_____. "Nursing Practice Acts." *American Journal of Nursing* 74:1310-1319, July 1974.

Lipman, M. "Your Rights Before a State Disciplinary Board." *RN* 36:44, December 1973.

Mike, L.H. "What is Institutional Licensure?" *Supervisor Nurse* 4:39, August 1973.

"Nurses Battle Institutional Licensure." (editiorial) *AORN Journal* 18:1089-1090, December 1973.

Petrowski, Dorothy D., ed., and Partheymuller, Margaret T., ed. *Forces Affecting Nursing Practice.* Washington, D.C.: Catholic University of America Press, 1969.

Roemer, R. "Trends in Licensure, Certification, and Accreditation: Implications for Health-Manpower Education in the Future." *Journal of Allied Health* 3:26-33, Winter 1974.

"Says State License Safeguards Nurses." *OR Reporter* 9:13, August 1974.

"Should Institutional Licensure Replace Individual Licensure?" *American Journal of Nursing* 74:444, March 1974.

Stahl, A.G. "State Boards of Nursing: Legal Aspects." *The Nursing Clinics of North America.* vol. 9. Philadelphia: W.B. Saunders, September 1974.

Thomas, L.A. "A Solution to the Licensure Problem." *Hospitals* 48:77-80, 16 July 1974.

"Trouble in Texas: Institutional Licensure for R.N.'s?" *RN* 37:29, April 1974.

Chapter 19   Legal Rights and Responsibilities

Allen, M. "Ethics of Nursing Practice." *Canadian Nurse* 70:22-23, February 1974.

"A.N.A. Code for Nurses." *South Carolina Nursing* 21:46-47, Winter 1973-1974.

Amundson, N.E. "Labor Relations and the Nursing Leader." Regular column appearing in the *Journal of Nursing Administration.*

Armington, Catherine L. "Legal Implications in Emergency Services." *The Nursing Clinics of North America.* vol. 9, no. 3. Philadelphia: W.B. Saunders Co., September 1974.

Berger, Al. "Legal Corner: What Would You Do . . ." *Pennsylvania Nurse* 27:7, March 1972.

Bergman, R. "Ethics – Concepts and Practice." *International Nursing Review* 20:140, September/October 1973.

Bramson, Helen Kitchen. "Malpractice: What Can the Nurse Say?" *Nursing Care* pp. 30-31, May 1975.

Cazalas, M.W. "Legalities and Nursing." *Association of Operating Room Nurses Journal* 13:79-86, May 1971.

Cleland, Virginia S. "A Professional Model for Collective Bargaining." *American Nurse* 6:10-12, December 1974.

——————. "To End Sex Discrimination." *The Nursing Clinics of North America.* vol. 9, no. 3. Philadelphia: W.B. Saunders Co., September 1974.

"Code of Ethics for the Licensed Practical/Vocational Nurse." *Journal of Practical Nursing* 21:33, June 1971.

Creighton, Helen. "Ten Commandments in Nursing." *Nursing '73* 3:7-8, January 1973.

Creighton, Helen. *Changing Legal Attitudes: The Effect of the Law on Nursing.* no. 20-1512. New York: NLN Council of Hospitals and Related Institutional Nursing Services, 1974.

_____. "Malpractice and the Nurse." *IMPRINT* 20:154, October 1973.

_____. "The Malpractice Problem." *The Nursing Clinics of North America.* vol. 9, no. 3. Philadelphia: W.B. Saunders Co., September 1974.

_____. "Your Legal Risks in Emergency Nursing Care." *Nursing '73* 3:23-25, April 1973.

_____. *Law Every Nurse Should Know.* 3d ed. Philadelphia: W.B. Saunders Co., 1975.

Creighton, Helen, and Squaires, G. Marjorie. "School Nurses: Legal Aspects of Their Work." *The Nursing Clinics of North America.* vol. 9, no. 3. Philadelphia: W.B. Saunders, September 1974.

Denison, J.M. "Which Brothers Do We Keep? The Ethics and Politics of Caring." *Canadian Nurse* 68:19-20, May 1972.

Driscoll, J. "Nursing Accountability." *Point of View* 11:14, April 1974.

Economically Speaking, Are You Talking to Yourself? no. EC-87, Kansas City, MO: ANA.

Ede, L. et al. "The 'Good Samaritan Law' and the Nurses' Immunity for Emergency Care." *Occupational Health Nursing* 20:10-15, September 1972.

"Expanding Horizons in Medical Ethics." (editorial) *Supervisor Nurse* 5:7, April 1974.

Fagin, C.M. "Nurses' Rights." *American Journal of Nursing* 75:82-85.

Feld, Lipman G. "The Nurse's Liability for Faulty Injections." *Nursing Care.* 25 April 1974.

Fletcher, J. "Ethics and Euthanasia." *American Journal of Nursing* 73:670-675, April 1973.

Geach, B. "Gifts and Their Significance." *American Journal of Nursing* 1:266-270, February 1971.

Guidelines for the Individual Nurse Contract. no. EC-126. Kansas City, MO: ANA.

Hamilton, H.D. "Legal Aspects: You and the L.P.N." *RN* 34:50, January 1971.

"ICN Code for Nurses: Ethical Concepts Applied to Nursing." *The Philippine Journal of Nursing* 42:239, October/December 1973.

Is There a Difference? no. EC-131. Kansas City, MO: ANA.

Jacox, A. "Collective Bargaining in Academe: Background and Perspective." *Nursing Outlook* 21:700, November 1973.

"Keeping Patients Alive: Who Decides?" *U.S. News* 72:44-49, 22 May 1972.

Kramer, Henry T. "What About Pensions?" *The Nursing Clinics of North America* vol. 9, no. 3. Philadelphia: W.B. Saunders Co., September 1974.

Lancour, Jane. "Legal Aspects of Critical Care Nursing." *The Nursing Clinics of North America.* vol. 9, no. 3. Philadelphia: W.B. Saunders Co., September 1974.

Leininger, M.M. "Conflict and Conflict Resolutions: Theories and Processes Relevant to the Health Professions." *American Nurse* 6:17-22, December 1974.

Lipman, M. "Joint Statements/Your Legal Safeguard." *RN* 34:40, April 1971.

_____. "When Should a Nurse Blow the Whistle?" *RN* 34:50, October 1971.

McNabb, B.W. "The Nurse — and the Medical Record." *Supervisor Nurse* 2:17, November 1971.

"Mediator Predicts No Rash of Strikes." *Association of Operating Room Nurses Journal* 20:1046, December 1974.

Menor, N. "Professionalism in Nursing." *Newsette* 11:24-27, January/March 1971.

"New International Code of Ethical Concepts Issued by ICN." 1973 *Mississippi RN* 36:3-4, March 1974.

"New Legal Aid." *Queen's Nursing Journal* 16:183, November 1973.

"Nurse Sues over Bargaining Right and Wins." *American Journal of Nursing* 74:32, January 1974.

"Nurses' Notes as Vital Legal Evidence." *Regan Report on Nursing Law* 12:1, June 1971.

"Nurses' Pledge." *Ghana Nurse* 6:1, December 1970.

"Nursing Service Problem: Standing Orders." *Regan Report on Nursing Law* 14:4, February 1974.

"Nursing Service Problem: Restraining Patients." *Regan Report on Nursing Law* 14:4, November 1973.

Passos, J.Y. "Accountability: Myth or Mandate?" *Journal of Nursing Administration* 3:16-22, May/June 1973.

"Patient Care After Shock Therapy: Nursing Liability." *Regan Report on Nursing Law* 13:2, September 1972.

"Recuperating Patients: Duty to Observe and Aid." *Regan Report on Nursing Law* 14:2, February 1974.

Reinders, Agnes A. "Nursing and Some Large Moral Issues." *The Nursing Clinics of North America* vol. 9, no. 3. Philadelphia: W.B. Saunders Co., September 1974.

"Restraining Patients: Duty to Observe Results." *Nursing Digest* 2:95-96, February 1974.

Rose, V. "Careless Talk Can Cause Misery." *Nursing Mirror* 136:14, 5 January 1973.

Rozovsky, L.E. "The Doctor, the Nurse and the Law." *Canadian Hospital* 40: 32-33, January 1971.

Rubsanon, David S. "Doctor and the Law." *Medical World News* 15, no. 21:33, 24 May 1974.

Schlotfeldt, R.M. "Nurses, Physicians and Physicians' Assistants: An Anecdote." *CHART* 71:5, February 1974.

Schutt, B.G. "Collective Action for Professional Security." *American Journal of Nursing* 73:1946, November 1973.

Simer, P. "What do you Expect from your Employer?" *Point of View* 11: 3-4, 15 November 1974.

Stanton, Marjorie. "Political Action and Nursing." *The Nursing Clinics of North America.* vol. 9, no. 3. Philadelphia: W.B. Saunders Co., September 1974.

"Terminal Patients and 'no code' Orders." *Regan Report on Nursing Law* 14:1, November 1973.

"The Code for Nurses." *Florida Nurse* 21:4, December 1973.

The Health Law Center, and Streiff, Charles J. ed. *Nursing and the Law.* 2d ed. Rockville, MD: Aspen Systems Corp., 1975.

"These Are Your Professional Rights . . ." *Reporter* 7:3, December 1974.

Trail, Ira D. "The Legal Implications of Community Nursing Care." *The Nursing Clinics of North America.* vol. 9, no. 3. Philadelphia: W.B. Saunders Co., September 1974.

"Vice is Being Afraid of Virtue." *Occupational Health* (London) 23:108-109, April 1971.

"Visitor's Safety: Nurses Share Responsibility." *Regan Report on Nursing Law* 13:2, January 1973.

Weber, L.J. "Ethics and Euthanasia – Another View." *American Journal of Nursing* 73:1228-1231, July 1973.

"What Are Your Ethical Standards?" *Nursing '74* 4:29-33, March 1974.

What Every Nurse Should Know About Signed Written Agreements. no. EC-130. Kansas City, MO: ANA.

"When Patients Leave Against Advice: Restraints." *Regan Report on Nursing Law* 14:2, March 1974.

Wieman, B. "A Key for Nurses to Avoid Legal Entanglement." *Hospital Forum* (California) 14:11, October 1971.

Wittner, D. "Life or Death." *Today's Health* 52:48-53, March 1974.

Young, Fannie Belle. "Rural Nursing Practice and Questions of Legality." *The Nursing Clinics of North America.* vol. 9, no. 3. Philadelphia: W.B. Saunders Co., September 1974.

Zimmerman, Ann. "Models for a Multi-Purpose Organization. The Industrial Model." *American Nurse* 6:7-9, December 1974.

SECTION 6 OPPORTUNITIES TO GROW

Chapter 20 Employing Agencies and Job Opportunities

Aynes, Edith A. *From Nightingale to Eagle: An Army Nurse's History.* Englewood Cliffs, NJ: Prentice-Hall, 1973.

Beisel, J.J. "Recognition of Professional Preparation: the Key to Job Evaluation in Health Care Facilities." *Nursing Digest* 2:54-58, January 1974.

Employment Outlook for Registered Nurses, Licensed Practical Nurses, Hospital Attendants. no. 1700-9, Washington, D.C.: U.S. Department of Health, Education and Welfare Publication, 1972-1973.

"Equal Opportunities for Men and Women." *Midwives Chronicle* 86:348-349, November 1973.

"Fourth Annual Guide to Finding the Right Position." *RN* 36:G1, December 1973.

Frost, M. "Job Satisfaction." *Nursing Mirror* 137:9, 2 November 1973.

Hanger, T.I. "The Employment Process." *Supervisor Nurse* 5:40, August 1974.

_____. "Your Next Job Interview: How to Use it to Your Best Advantage." *Nursing '74* 4:45-48, September 1974.

Hanley, M. et al. "Summary report of the task force on the working environment of nurses." *Virginia Nurse Quarterly* 41:11, Summer 1973.

Hurka, S.J. "Organizational environment and work satisfaction." *Dimensions in Health Service* 51:41-43, January 1974.

Kavalier, F. "Are Agencies for You?" *Nursing Times* 69:1102-1103, 23 August 1973.

Lee, Jane A.; Herzog, Ruth R.; and Morrison, John H. Jr. *Licensed Practical Nurses in Occupational Health.* Cincinnati: U.S. Department of Health, Education, and Welfare Public Health Service, 1974.

Luneski, I.D. ed. "Temporary Nursing: Is It for You?" *RN* 36:46-50, September 1973.

"New Position Descriptions in Nursing." *Journal of Nursing Administration* 3:17-20, November/December 1973.

Nichols, G.A. "Important, Satisfying, and Dissatisfying Aspects of Nurses' Jobs." *Supervisor Nurse* 5:10-15, January 1974.

"Recommended Minimum Employment Standards for Registered Nurses."
Colorado Nurse 74:2-4, January 1974.

Reid, M.F. "How to Get the Job You Want." *Nursing Times* 70:970-971,
20 June 1974.

Reres, M. "Employment Opportunities – Assessing Growth Potential." part 1.
American Journal of Nursing 74:670-676, April 1974.

Samuel, B.A. "Working Conditions of Nurses in Some Hospitals in U.P." *Nursing Journal of India* 65:23-24, January 1974.

Stevens, B.J. "A Second Look at 'new' position descriptions." *Journal of
Nursing Administration* 3:21-23, November/December 1973.

Thomson, W. "On Being Interviewed." *Nursing Times* 68:520-521, 27 April
1972.

Walsh, W.J. "Preparing a Resume." part 2. *American Journal of Nursing*
74:677-679, April 1974.

Chapter 21   New Dimensions in Nursing Education

A Guide for Establishing Statewide Master Planning Committees. New York:
National Commission for the Study of Nursing and Nursing Education, 1972.

*A Model for an Upward Mobility Nursing Education Program at the Junior
College Level.* Project Proposal submitted by Modesto Junior College,
2 March 1971.

Allen, Virginia O. *Community College Nursing Education.* New York: John
Wiley and Sons, 1971.

Allyn, Nathaniel C. "College Credit by Examination." *Nursing Outlook* 17,
no. 4:44-46, April 1969.

Beckes, I. et al. *Financial Management for Schools of Nursing.* no. 16-1549,
New York: NLN Department of Diploma Programs, 1974.

Bourosma, Franklin. "Innovative Teaching Techniques." *Associate Degree
Education for Nursing Current Issues, 1974.* no. 23-1539. New York:
NLN.

Brickner, P.W. et al. *The Changing Role of the Hospital and Implications for
Nursing Education.* no. 16-1551. New York: NLN Department of Diploma
Programs, 1974.

Brown, Esther Lucile. *Nursing for the Future.* New York: Russell Sage Foundation, 1967.

Bruton, M.R. "The Process of Curriculum Revision." *Nursing Outlook* 22:
310-314, May 1974.

Burnett, C.N. "A Closer Look at Core." *Journal of Allied Health* 2:107-112,
Summer 1973.

Burnside, Helen. "Practical Nurses Become Associate Degree Graduates." *Nursing Outlook* 17, no. 4:47, April 1969.

Drage, Martha O. "Core Courses and a Career Ladder." *American Journal of Nursing* 71:1356-1358, July 1971.

Evans, Patricia A. "University Without Walls Nursing Program." *Associate Degree Education for Nursing Current Issues, 1974.* New York: NLN, 1974.

Faunce, R.C. and Bossing, N.L. *Developing the Core Curriculum.* Englewood Cliffs, NJ: Prentice-Hall, 1951.

Formi, P.R. "Implementation of the Open Curriculum in a Midwestern Region." *Journal of Continuing Education in Nursing* 4:5-13, November/December 1973.

Frank, Sister Charles Marie, and Heidgerken, Loretta E. *Perspectives in Nursing Education.* Washington, D.C.: Catholic University of America Press, 1968.

Geissler, E.M. "A New Way of Looking at Old Ideas." *International Nursing Review* 21:169-171, November/December 1974.

Gelber, M. et al. *Associate Degree Education for Nursing Current Issues, 1974.* no. 23-1539. New York: NLN Department of Associate Degree Programs, 1974.

Genn, N. "Where Can Nurses Practice as They're Taught?" *American Journal of Nursing* 74:2212-2215, December 1974.

Graduates of Diploma Schools of Nursing. no. G-115. Kansas City, MO: ANA.

Grant, E. Louise. "The RN Writes her Own Transfer Credit." *Nursing Outlook* 14, no. 5:39-40, May 1966.

Hangartner, Rev. Carl A., S.J. "College Credit Equivalency and Advanced Standing." *Nursing Outlook* 14, no. 5:30-32, May 1966.

Hauer, R.M. et al. "Coming of Age of a Refresher Program . . . Beth Israel Medical Center, New York." *American Journal of Nursing* 75:88-91, January 1975.

"Hospital Schools as Vital as Ever." *Hospitals* 49:69-71, January 1975.

Ketefian, S. "Trends in Curricular Innovations in Nursing Education." *International Nursing Review* 21:139-142, September/October 1974.

Kinsinger, Robert E. "A Core Curriculum for the Health Field." *Nursing Outlook* vol. 15, February 1967.

Kramer, Ruth E. "A Core Curricular Approach in Allied Health Education." *Journal of Practical Nursing* p. 23, October 1973.

Lenburg, Carrie B. "Innovations in Nursing Education – The Regents External Degree Program in Nursing." *Associate Degree Education for Nursing Current Issues, 1974.* New York: NLN, 1974.

Lenburg, Carrie B., ed. *Open Learning and Career Mobility in Nursing.* St. Louis: C.V. Mosby Co., 1975.

Lenburg, Carrie B.; Johnson, Walter L.; and Vahey, Jo Ann T. *Directory of Career Mobility Opportunities in Nursing.* New York: NLN Division of Research, 1973.

"Let's Examine the Challenge Examination for the Registered Nurse Student." *Nursing Outlook* 17, no. 4:48, April 1969.

Lidz, Clara Gray. "Computer-Managed Instruction in Nursing." *Associate Degree Education for Nursing Current Issues, 1974.* no. 23-1539. New York: NLN.

Love, I.D. "Graduation – the end or the Beginning?" *Australian Nurses Journal* 4:38–40, September 1974.

Lyond, William, and Schmidt, Mildred S. "Credit for What you Know." *American Journal of Nursing* pp. 101-104, January 1969.

Major, D.M. "Nursing School Courses for Non-Nurses." *Nursing Outlook* 22:769-772, December 1974.

Mannion, S.E. "Upgrading L.P.N.'s to R.N.'s." *Journal of Practical Nursing* 19, no. 9:31, September 1969.

Meleis, A.I. et al. "Operation Concern: A Study of Senior Nursing Students in Three Nursing Programs." *Nursing Research* 23:461-468, November/December 1974.

Merrill, Lois J. "Articulated Curriculum – Associate Through Master's Degree." *Associate Degree Education for Nursing Current Issues, 1974.* no. 23-1539. New York: NLN.

Montag, Mildred L. *Community College Education for Nursing.* New York: McGraw-Hill Book Co., Blakiston Division, 1959.

Ozimek, Dorothy. *The Baccalaureate Graduate in Nursing: What Does Society Expect?* no. 15-1520. New York: NLN.

Perry, J. Warren. "Career Mobility in Allied Health Education." *Journal of the American Medical Association* 21, no. 1:107-110, 6 October 1969.

Ramphal, Marjorie. "Needed: A Career Ladder in Nursing." *American Journal of Nursing* 68, no. 6:1234-1236, June 1968.

Rasmussen, Sandra, ed. *Technical Nursing Dimensions and Dynamics.* Philadelphia: F.A. Davis Co., 1972.

Rauffenbart, Suzanne. "National Legislation – Implications for Diploma Programs." *The Changing Role of the Hospital and Implications for Nursing Education.* New York: NLN, 1974.

Sheahan, Sister Dorothy. "Degree, Yes – Education, No." *Nursing Outlook* 22:26, January 1974.

Squaires, G. Marjorie. "Planning New Educational Avenues for the Degree Seeking R.N." *Associate Degree Education for Nursing Current Issues, 1974.* no. 23-2539, New York: NLN.

Wozniak, Dolores. "External Degrees in Nursing." *American Journal of Nursing* pp. 1014-1018, June 1973.

Zeitz, Ann N.; Howard, Lelia D.; Christy, Elva M.; and Tax, Hariette Simington. *Associate Degree Nursing.* St. Louis: C.V. Mosby Co., 1969.

Chapter 22 Scholarships, Fellowships, Grants, and Loans

"American Nurses' Foundation." *Washington State Journal of Nursing* 46:15, Fall 1974.

"American Nurses' Foundation Grant Program." *Nursing Research Report* 9:3, October 1974.

"ANF Awards Developmental Grants to Two Nurses." *Nursing Research Report* 8:2, March 1973.

"British Commonwealth Nurses' War Memorial Fund: This Year's Scholars." *Nursing Mirror* 139:40–41, 23 August 1974.

"Foundation Awards Eight Grants for Research." *Nursing Research Report* 9:3, March 1974.

Gortner, S.R. "Research in Nursing . . . The Federal Interest and Grant Program." *American Journal of Nursing* 73:1052–1055, June 1973.

Henderson, J. et al. "How CNF Scholars are Selected." *Canadian Nurse* 69:33–35, May 1973.

"July Grants Include Geriatric, Pediatric Nursing." *Nursing Research Report* 9:4, October 1974.

Kaiser, L.R. "Grantsmanship in Continuing Education." *Journal of Nursing Education* 12:12, January 1973.

"3M Scholarship." *New Zealand Nursing Journal* 66:20, July 1973.

McKeller, S. "Climbing the Career Ladder: Tax dollars can help." *Imprint* 19:17, May 1972.

Montag, M.L. "Nurses' Educational Funds, Inc." *Nursing Outlook* 22:444–447, July 1974.

Nursing Scholarships and Student Loans: Information for Schools. no. (NIH) 73.357. Washington, D.C.: U.S. Department of Health, Education and Welfare Publication, September 1972.

"Raising Funds from Foundations." *Nursing Outlook* 20:108–110, February 1972.

"Scholarships – 1973." *Nursing Journal of India* 63:422, December 1972.

"Scholarships and Bursaries." *New Zealand Nursing Journal* 66:22–23, August 1973.

Scholarships and Loans for Beginning Education in Nursing. no. 41-410. New York: NLN.

"Scholarships Available for AORN Members." *AORN Journal* 19:483–484, February 1974, and 19:617–618, March 1974.

Scholarships, Fellowships, Educational Grants and Loans for Registered Nurses.
no. 41–408. New York: NLN, July 1974.

*Special Project Grants and Contracts Awarded for Improvement in Nurse Train-
ing.* A listing. no. HRA 74-19. Washington, D.C.: U.S. Department of
Health, Education and Welfare Publication.

"The Winston Churchill Memorial Trust: 1975 Churchill Travelling Fellowships." *Nursing Mirror* 139:48, 30 August 1974.

Chapter 23 Professional Literature
No Bibliography – See Chapter Materials

Chapter 24 Continuing Education

Ayers, R.   "In California, Continuing Education Will Be Mandatory." *AORN
Journal* 18:487–493, September 1973.

Chamberlain, J.   "The Crisis in Continuing Education Leadership" *Journal of
Continuing Education in Nursing* 4:9-13, March/April 1973.

Cooper, Signe Skott.   "A Brief History of Continuing Education in Nursing in
the United States." *Journal of Continuing Education in Nursing* 4:5-14,
May/June 1973.

_____ . "Continuing Education Should Be Voluntary." *AORN Journal*
18:471–477, September 1973.

_____ . "This I Believe About Continuing Education in Nursing."
Nursing Outlook 20:579-583, September 1972.

_____ . "Why Continuing Education in Nursing?" *Cardiovascular
Nursing* 8:23-28, November/December 1972.

Cooper, Signe Scott, and Hornback, May Shiga. *Continuing Nursing Education*
New York: McGraw-Hill Book Co., 1973.

Dake, Marcia A.   "CEU-A Means to an End?" *American Journal of Nursing*
74:103-104, January 1974.

Dauria, A.M.   "Evaluating Continuing Education." *Journal of Continuing
Education in Nursing* 4:18-20, July/August 1973.

Del Bueno, D.V.   "A.C.E. Unit Course." *Nursing Outlook* 21:504-505, August
1973.

Gibbs, G.E.   "Will Continuing Education Be Required for License Renewal?"
American Journal of Nursing 71:2175-2179, November 1971.

Gwaltney, B.H.   "Continuing Education in Nursing." *Virginia Nurse Quarterly* 241:7-13, Spring 1973.

Hayter, J.   "Individual Responsibility for Continuing Education." *Journal of
Continuing Education in Nursing* 3:31-38, November/December 1972.

Hornback, May Shiga. "Measuring Continuing Education." *American Journal of Nursing* 73:1576-1577, September 1973.

Klutas, E.M. "The Occupational Health Nurse Views Future Needs in Continuing Education: What Do We Want? Where Do We Get It?" *Occupational Health Nursing* 21:9-15, September 1973.

Kondrath, Andrew S. "Iowa Goes All Out-Continuing Education for Health Care Personnel." *American Vocational Journal* May 1973.

Lembright, K.A. "Structuring for . . . Continuing Education Programs Within the American Heart Association." *Journal of Continuing Education in Nursing* 1:41-45, July 1970.

Lysaught, J.P. "Continuing Education: Necessity and Opportunity." *Journal of Continuing Education in Nursing* 1:5-10, September/October 1970.

McGriff, Erline P. "A Case for Mandatory Continuing Education in Nursing." *Nursing Outlook* 20:712-713, November 1972.

_____. "Continuing Education in Nursing." *The Nursing Clinics of North America* vol. 8. Philadelphia: W.B. Saunders, June 1973.

_____. "Mandatory Continuing Education for Nurses." *AORN Journal* 18:479-485, September 1973.

McGriff, Erline P. and Cooper, Signe S. *Accountability to the Consumer through Continuing Education in Nursing.* no. 14-1507. New York: NLN, 1974.

McNeil, D.R. "Structuring for . . . Continuing Education in Nursing Within the University." *Journal of Continuing Education in Nursing* 1:8-11, July 1970.

Popiel, Elda S. "Continuing Education: Provider and Consumer." *American Journal of Nursing* 71:1586-1587, August 1971.

_____. *Nursing and the Process of Continuing Education.* St. Louis: C.V. Mosby Co., 1973.

Tait, E. "A Standard Method for the Recording of Participating in Continuing Education." *Journal of Continuing Education in Nursing* 3:31-34, September/October 1972.

Thomas, B. et al. "A Survey of Continuing Education Needs." *Journal of Continuing Education in Nursing* 4:26-31, May/June 1973.

Walsh, Margaret E. "The Role of NLN in Continuing Education in Nursing." *Journal of Continuing Education in Nursing* 3:44-48, May/June 1972.

Walton, M.H. "Structuring for . . . Continuing Education Within the Hospital Nursing Service." *Journal of Continuing Education in Nursing* 1:12-17, July 1970.

Weldy, A.A. "Structuring for . . . Continuing Education Within the Professional Association." *Journal of Continuing Education in Nursing* 1:36-40, July 1970.

Wood, Lucile A. "Continuing Education: The Nurse and the Legislative Process." *Journal of Continuing Education in Nursing* 4:19-23.

_____ . "A Reality for LP/VNs: Continuing Education." *Nursing Care* pp. 27-28, March 1974.

_____ . "ANA Sets Standards for Continuing Education." *American Journal of Nursing* 74:31, January 1974.

_____ . "Continuing Education in Nursing: Necessity and Opportunity." New York: National Commission for the Study of Nursing and Nursing Education Office, 1972.

_____ . "Continuing Education Will Be Mandatory for California Nurses." *Modern Hospital* 120:32, March 1973.

_____ . "Excerpts from an Interim Statement on Continuing Education in Nursing." *Virginia Nurse Quarterly.* 40:65-74, Winter 1972.

_____ . "Landmark Statements from the American Hospital Association." *Journal of Continuing Education in Nursing* 1:32-35, July 1970.

_____ . "Report from Florida. . .Recognition for Continuing Education." *Journal of Continuing Education in Nursing* 4:31-37, July/August 1973.

_____ . "Should Continuing Education Be Mandatory?" *American Journal of Nursing* 73:442-443, March 1973.

_____ . "Some Thoughts on Structuring for Continuing Education in Nursing." *Journal of Continuing Education in Nursing* 1:5-7, July 1970.

_____ . "The Comparative Study of Continuing Professional Education." *Journal of Continuing Education in Nursing* 3:4-11, May/June 1972.

_____ . "The Role of the Practitioner in Continuing Education. The Qualities of an Educational Climate." *Journal of Continuing Education in Nursing* 1:16-20, November/December 1970.

AUDIO-VISUAL MATERIALS TO SUPPLEMENT SECTIONAL TOPICS

SECTION 1 INFLUENCES OF THE PAST (Chapters 1–4)

SECTION 2 THE BIRTH OF ORGANIZED NURSING (Chapters 5–8)

Film Strips: *A History of American Nursing.* For 35 mm filmstrip projectors
  AS–05 Silent, with mimeographed narration $12 Sale
  AS–06 with 33 1/3 RPM 12" record and mimeographed narration $17 Sale

Slides: *A History of American Nursing* 128 (2" x 2") slides from filmstrip.
  AT–01 slides — $36 Sale
  AT–02 slides with record — $42 Sale
  AT–03 record — $6 Sale

Film: *The Ruth Sleeper Story.* 16 mm sound. 34 minutes
  3627 Black and White   Rental $15

             Order from: The American Journal of Nursing Company
                           Film Library
                           c/o Association-Sterling Films
                           600 Grand Avenue
                           Ridgefield, NJ   07657

SECTION 3 EDUCATION FOR NURSES (Chapters 9–12)

Films: *Idea With a Future: The Associate Degree Nursing Program*
  3580   Color   26 minutes   Rental $15

Vertical Mobility: A Nursing Disease?
3661   Black and White   30 minutes   Rental $25

> Order from: The American Journal of Nursing Company
> Film Library
> c/o Association-Sterling Films
> 600 Grand Avenue
> Ridgefield, NJ   07657

SECTION 4 HEALTH CARE AND THE CONSUMER (Chapters 13-16)

Films:

3552   *Almost a Miracle.*   Color.   26 minutes.   Rental $15

3560   *Challenge to Serve.*   Color.   20 minutes.   Rental $20

3660   *Should RNs Initiate Change in Nursing Practice in Poverty Areas?*
Black and White.   30 minutes.   Rental $25

3659   *Should Nursing Functions be Revised to Include the Expanded
Role of the RN?*   Black and White.   30 minutes.   Rental $25.

3640   *This is Nursing.*   Color.   25 minutes.   Rental $20.

3654   *Consumer Views of Nursing.*   Black and White.   30 minutes.
Rental $25

3658   *Should Nurses Control Nursing Practice in Every Agency?*   Black
and White.   30 minutes.   Rental $25

3600   *Nurses: Crisis in Medicine.*   Black and White. 53 minutes.   Rental
$20.

3601   *Nurses: Crisis in Medicine.*   Color.   53 minutes.   Rental $25.

S 06   *Ethical – Legal Aspects of Nursing Practice.*   Rental $25 day.

S 05   *Rights of Patients.*   Guest participant Martha T. Mitchell.   Rental
$25 day.

> Order from: The American Journal of Nursing Company
> Film Library
> c/o Association–Sterling Films
> 600 Grand Avenue
> Ridgefield, NJ   07657

A Healthy Choice.   Narrated by E.G. Marshall.

> Order from: Blue Cross Association
> 840 North Lake Shore Drive
> Chicago, IL   60657

Audiocassettes:

AC MO1   *The Changing Health Care System* (Film no. MO1)

AC MO2   *Federal Involvement in Health Care* (Film no. MO3)

AC MO3   *Community Health Service*

    Price: Audiocassette — $9.50 ea Sale

        Film: 16 mm. sound

            30 minute class

            Black and White

            Rental — $20.00 for 1 day use

            Sale — $195.00 ea

AS-09   *Six Steps to Team Nursing*

    With 33 1/3 RPM, 16" Record $19 Sale

AS-10   *Team Relationships in Nursing Care.*

    With 33 1/3 RPM, 16" Record $19 Sale

        Order from: American Journal of Nursing Company

            Educational Services Division

            10 Columbus Circle

            New York, NY   10019

    The Nurse Practitioner — An Interview with

    Dr. Ingeborg Mauksch

    Set of two audiocassettes $10.55

        Order from: Nursing and Health A-V Productions

            Box 17113

            Cincinnati, OH   45217

Overhead Transparencies:

The Meaning of Nursing

The Function and Role of the Nurse

    Six transparencies   Sale $15

        Order from: The Robert J. Brady Company

            Subs of Prentice Hall

            Rtes 197 and 450

            Bowie, MD   20715

SECTION 5 THE NURSING COMMUNITY AND THE LAW
(Chapters 17-19)

Films: 3564 *Just the Facts, Nurse.*   15 minutes.

        Black and White.   Rental $15.

Films/videotapes

S 01 *Nurse Practice Acts*
S 02 *Scope of Practice and Standards of Care*
S 03 *Malpractice*
S 04 *Nursing Torts*
S 05 *Rights of Patients*
S 06 *Ethical-Legal Aspects of Nursing Practice*
S 07 *The Nurse and the Employer*

Seven units dealing with the nurse and the law. Each unit is available on 16 mm film or on videotape. Films and videotapes are for sale. Films may be rented. Prices subject to change without notice.

Each unit 30 minutes. Color. Rental film $25 for one day.

Videotape Sales:
1/2" EIAJ Standard
3/4" A-Matic Videocassette
Sale – $150.00 each

Order film from: The American Journal of Nursing Company
                   Film Library
                   c/o Association-Sterling Films
                   600 Grand Avenue
                   Ridgefield, NJ   07657

Audiovisual Sales:
                   The American Journal of Nursing Company
                   Educational Sales Division
                   10 Columbus Circle
                   New York, NY   10019

Audiocassettes:

AC S01 *Nurse Practice Acts* and *Scope of Practice and Standards of Care.*
AC S02 *Malpractice* and *Nursing Torts.*
AC S03 *Rights of Patients* and *Ethical-Legal Aspects of Nursing Practice.*
AC S04 *The Nurse and the Employer.*

Each for sale $9.50

Order from: The American Journal of Nursing Company
              Educational Services Division
              10 Columbus Circle
              New York, NY   10019

Other sources which offer educational aids are:

The Nursing Team and the Law

no. 22-0501 C   Filmstrip Program. Cassette. Training Guide. Evaluation Test. Price $55.00

no. 22-0501 R   Filmstrip Program. L.P. Record. Training Guide. Evaluation Test. Price $50.00

no. 22-05013   Package of 50 Evaluation Tests. Price $3.00

no. 22-05017   Extra Training Guides. Price $0.25

no. 22-0001   Package of 50 Answer Cards. Price $3.50

Order from: Career Aids, Inc.
5024 Lankershim Blvd.
North Hollywood, CA   91601

Nursing Law. Current Problems and Solutions. Lectures by William A. Regan.

Cassette tapes:

Group A (part 1) Recorded Live, November 1972

Group B (part 2) Recorded Live, April 1973

Price $32.00/set

Order from: Hospital Research and Educational Trust of New Jersey
1101 State Road/Research Park
Princeton, NJ   08540

Audiocassettes: LA-01   *Nurse's Responsibilities to Patients.* 7 minutes.

LA-02   *Nurse's Responsibilities to Agencies, Institutions and Physicians.* 36 minutes

LA-03   *Nurse's Responsibilities for the Negligent Conduct of Others.* 40 minutes

LA-04   *Legal Implications of Nurse's Records.* 26 minutes

Order from: Medical Electronic Educational Services, Inc.
29423 West Six Mile Road
Livonia, MI   48152

Programmed Course: *Nurses' Liability for Malpractice.* Eli P. Bernzweig. 1969.

Order from: McGraw-Hill
Blakiston Division
1221 Ave. of the Americas
New York, NY   10020

SECTION 6 OPPORTUNITIES TO GROW (Chapters 20-24)

Filmstrips:

AS-04   *At Your Request* – (ANA Professional Credential and Personnel Service). 52 frames. Silent, with mimeographed narration. $14 Sale.

Films:

3580   *Idea with a Future: The Associate Degree Nursing Program.* Color 26 minutes. Rental $15.

3661   *Vertical Mobility: A Nursing Disease?* Black and White. 30 minutes. Rental $25 (also audiocassette)

3686   *A Day in the Life . . .* Color. 17 minutes. Rental $20.

M 07   *Dilemmas of Nursing Education.* Narrated by Eleanor Lambertson, RN, EdD. and Inez G. Hensvark, RN., EdD. Rental $20 for one day use.

M 08   *Projections for the Future in Nursing.* Rental $20 per day

S 07   *The Nurse and the Employer.* 30 minute Class. Rental $25 for one day use only. (Also audiocassette)

Order from: The American Journal of Nursing Company
Film Library
Association-Sterling Films
600 Grand Avenue
Ridgefield, NJ   07657

Audiocassettes:

AC MO4   *Vertical Mobility: A Nursing Disease?*
AC SO4   *The Nurse and the Employer*

Audiocassettes $9.50
1/2" EIAJ Standard $125.00
3/4" U-Matic Videocassette $125.00

Booklet:

R-17   *Employment Opportunities.* 16 page supplement from April, 1974 American Journal of Nursing. Single copy – $.75. 25 copies or more – $.65

Order from: The American Journal of Nursing Company
Educational Services Division
10 Columbus Circle
New York, NY   10019

ACKNOWLEDGMENTS

The author wishes to thank the many individuals and agencies who generously and graciously participated in the development of this text.

Each person who consented to appear in a photograph.

The instructors and students who participated in the surveys and studies conducted to (1) test the content validity and correlation of scores on the end review material, (2) evaluate materials designed for use in a core course and (3) determine significant areas of content to be included in the text.

Contributions by Delmar Staff

Director of Publications – Alan N. Knofla
Divisional Editor – Angela R. Emmi
Project Editor – Pamela Culbert
Editorial Assistants – Ruth Saur and Hazel Kozakiewicz
Director of Manufacturing and Production – Fred Sharer
Illustrators – John Orozco, George Dowse, Tony Canabush, Tanya Harrell
Production Specialists – Margaret Mutka, Sharon Lynch, Lee St. Onge, Jean LeMorta, Betty Michelfelder, Patti Manuli, Debbie Monty

Technical Advisor

Aline L. Stolarik, ADN Instructor, College of Lake County

A very special thanks to Marilyn Kasner, Librarian and Research Associate, New York State Nurses Association.

Contributions to Classroom Testing

Portions of the manuscript were evaluated by students and instructors of the following institutions.

Belleville Area College

Black Hawk College

Carl Sandburg College

College of Lake County

Illinois Central College

Illinois Valley Community College

Kaskaskia College

Kennedy – King College

Kishwaukee College

Lewis and Clark Community College

Morton College

Oakton Community College

Parkland College

Rend Lake College

Sauk Valley College

Spoon River College

Thornton Community College

Triton College

Contributions of Content and Illustration

Ruth T. Begay, for figure 13-10.

Toni Bullock for original artwork, figure 1-7.

Josephine A. Dolan and W.B. Saunders Co., figure 1-8.

Dorothy Gehl Lescher, figure 7-9.

Marion G. Howell, figure 19-4.

Anne K. Roe and Mary C. Sherwood, figure 21-3.

Singer and Underwood, *A Short History of Medicine,* The Clarendon Press, Oxford, England, figure 4-7.

ACTION/Peace Corps, figure 20-8.

Albany Medical College, Albany, New York, figures 15-4, 15-5, 15-8, 15-10.

American Hospital Association, Chicago, figure 14-2.

American National Red Cross, Washington, D.C., figures 6-10, 6-11.

American Nurses' Association, figures 6-3, 6-4, 6-6, 6-9, 6-10, 8-1, 8-3, 8-5, 8-8, 12-2, 15-9, 17-1, 17-2.

Berkeley-Charleston-Dorchester Technical Education Center, N. Charleston, S.C. figure 16-4.

Bellevue Hospital, New York, figures 7-3, 7-4, 7-5, 7-6.

Catholic Hospital Association, St. Louis, figure 7-1.

Charles C. Thomas, Publisher, Springfield, Illinois, figures 1-13, 1-15.

Collins-World Publishers, Lakewood, Ohio, figure 2-1.

Cornell University Press, Ithaca, New York, figure 2-5.

Coustable and Co., Ltd., London and McGraw-Hill, New York, figure 5-12.

Deaconess Hospital, Evansville, Indiana, figure 21-2.

Department of Health, Education and Welfare, Public Health Service, Bethesda, Maryland, figures 16-11, 20-3.

District Management Team of St. Thomas' Health District, London, figure 5-10.

Fresno City College, Fresno, California, figure 16-3.

Indian Health Service, figure 13-9.

J. Sargeant Reynolds Community College, Richmond, Virigina, figure 12-3.

Joint Commission on Accreditation of Hospitals, figure 14-4.

Macob County Community College, Center Campus, Mt. Clemens, Michigan, figure 13-4.

Maginnis and Associates, Chicago, figure 19-8.

Mansell Collection, London, figure 1-2.

Mayo Clinic, Rochester, Minnesota, figures 4-15, 4-18.

Memorial Hospital, figure 16-7.

Mercy San Juan Hospital, Carmichael, California, figures 14-5, 14-6.

Michigan Nurses' Association, figure 19-1.

Milwaukee Area Technical College, figure 16-17.

National Aeronautics and Space Administration, figure 20-7.

National Association for Practical Nurse Education and Service, New York, figure 17-4.

National Federation of Licensed Practical Nurses, New York, figure 17-5.

National League for Nursing, New York, figure 21-1.

Navy Department, Bureau of Medicine and Surgery, Nursing Division, figure 20-4.

New York State Nurses' Association, figures 18-1, 18-2, 19-2.

North Central Technical College, Mansfield, Ohio, figure 13-2.

Paramount General Hospital, figure 16-20.

Parke, Davis and Company, Detroit, figures 1-1, 1-3, 1-4, 1-5, 1-6, 1-9, 1-11, 1-14, 1-16, 1-17, 3-5, 3-6, 3-7, 4-8, 4-9, 5-5, 8-4.

Pasadena City College, Pasadena, California, figure 9-8.

Pfizer Inc., New York, figure 16-12.

Photographie Giraudon, Paris, figure 2-4.

Physicians' Record Company, Berwyn, Illinois, figure 4-5.

Presbyterian Hospital, School of Nursing, New York, Florence Nightingale Collection, figures 5-3, 5-7.

Project Primex, University of California, UCLA Extension Center, figure 13-11.

Rush — Presbyterian — St. Luke's Medical Center, Chicago, figure 4-14.

Sigma Theta Tau, and the American Journal of Nursing Co., figure 17-6.

St. Anne's Hospital, Chicago, figures 7-7, 7-8, 9-1, 9-2, 9-3, 9-4, 9-5, 9-6.

St. Dominic's Mission Society, Chicago, figure 3-4.

St. Mary's Hospital, Rochester, Minnesota, figures 4-16, 4-17.

St. Therese Hospital, Waukegan, Illinois, figures 16-18, 19-5, 19-6, 19-7, 20-10.

State of Illinois Department of Registration and Education, figure 18-3.

State University of Iowa, Iowa City, figure 10-1.

Trustees of Sir John Soane's Museum, London, figure 4-3.

United States Air Force, figure 20-6.

United States Army, figure 20-5.

Valencia Community College, Orlando, Florida, figure 13-3.

W.B. Saunders, Philadelphia, figures 6-5, 6-7.

Wayne Community College, Goldsboro, North Carolina, figure 10-3.

Winchester House, Libertyville, Illinois, figure 8-6.

INDEX